Nursing: The Art and Science of Person-Centered Care

Nursing: The Art and Science of Person-Centered Care

Editor: Jim Carrey

FOSTER ACADEMICS

www.fosteracademics.com

www.fosteracademics.com

FOSTER ACADEMICS

Cataloging-in-Publication Data

Nursing : the art and science of person-centered care / edited by Jim Carrey.
p. cm.
Includes bibliographical references and index.
ISBN 978-1-64646-618-4
1. Nursing. 2. Nursing care plans. 3. Nursing--Practice. 4. Nursing services. 5. Medical care. I. Carrey, Jim.
RT41 .N873 2023
610.73--dc23

Foster Academics,
118-35 Queens Blvd., Suite 400,
Forest Hills, NY 11375, USA

ISBN 978-1-64646-618-4 (Hardback)

Contents

Preface

The world is advancing at a fast pace like never before. Therefore, the need is to keep up with the latest developments. This book was an idea that came to fruition when the specialists in the area realized the need to coordinate together and document essential themes in the subject. That's when I was requested to be the editor. Editing this book has been an honour as it brings together diverse authors researching on different streams of the field. The book collates essential materials contributed by veterans in the area which can be utilized by students and researchers alike.

Nursing is the branch of medical science which involves delivering person-centered care. It is also focused on the maintenance of the optimal well-being and quality of life for individuals. The principal roles of nursing include health promotion and prevention of illness, caring for disabled and mentally ill persons, and engaging in healthcare teaching. Nursing also involves providing assistance in healthcare research. On the basis of the patient being cared for, nursing can be divided into various specialties such as mental health, pediatrics and gerontology. This book studies and analyses the central concepts of nursing and its utmost significance in modern times. It strives to provide a fair idea about this area of medical science and to help develop a better understanding of the lastest advances within this field. The book is a vital tool for all researching and studying the field of nursing.

Each chapter is a sole-standing publication that reflects each author´s interpretation. Thus, the book displays a multi-facetted picture of our current understanding of application, resources and aspects of the field. I would like to thank the contributors of this book and my family for their endless support.

Editor

1

The Relationship Between the Quality of Work and Organizational Commitment of Prison Nurses

Ayfer KARAASLAN[1] • Manar ASLAN[2]*

ABSTRACT

Background: Nurses working in prisons are exposed to security problems while serving those who may be uninterested in their own healthcare, face high risks of drug and alcohol addiction, and may have aggressive personalities. For this reason, nurses working in prisons may have more problems with work-related quality of life than their non-prison-nurse peers.

Purpose: This descriptive research study was conducted to evaluate the work-related quality of life and organizational commitment of nurses who work at prisons and detention centers.

Methods: According to 2015 data, approximately 513 nurses currently work in prisons in Turkey. The study group consisted of 224 nurses who currently work in prisons or detention centers. The data were collected by sending a created link address to the e-mail addresses of nurses who work in these facilities. A 13-item sociodemographic information form, including a demographics datasheet, a work-related quality of life scale, and an organizational commitment scale, was used to collect data.

Results: The participants reported a moderate level of work-related quality of life and organizational commitment. Moreover, work-related quality of life was shown to affect organizational commitment, with 20% of the total variance in organizational commitment explained by work-related quality of life.

Conclusions/Implications for Practice: This study supports that work-related quality of life affects organizational commitment positively. Therefore, regulating working conditions by taking into consideration employee security will positively affect job satisfaction in terms of both the institution and the employee. Moreover, as nurses do not only work in hospitals, taking this action should also work in different settings. Administrators should ensure the work-related quality of life of the prison nurses by understanding the difficulties of prison nursing.

Key Words:
prison nurse, work-related quality of life, organizational commitment.

Introduction

Prison Nursing

Prison nursing has been likened to psychiatric nursing and healthcare nursing by some nursing professionals. Actually, prison nursing covers all of these features and more. Goals of prison services include keeping prisoners in custody; establishing a regular, disciplined, and safe environment in prison; providing good conditions for prisoners; and meeting prisoner needs, including healthcare. Prison nursing is unique because prison nurses use all of their knowledge and skills daily in patient care. Groups that prison nurses meet in prison are made up of individuals of low socioeconomic status who have difficult and complex health problems at a vulnerable stage in their lives. Prison nurses have knowledge of prisoners' crimes, hopes, and despair. In this regard, nurses are supporters of prisoner health. Without a doubt, the environment and culture in prisons are different from those in places that nurses have experienced previously. Therefore, prison nurses should be supported for their professional development and should be educated and protected in their profession (Norman & Parrish, 1999).

Prison nurses have a great influence on therapeutic interventions that are intended to prevent mental disorders and promote health (Willmott, 1997). Prison nursing is a service that provides patients with education, physical examinations, drug distribution, compliance and continuity of the treatment, first aid, screenings, personnel training, and postoperative care, in addition to emergency medical services (Flanagan & Flanagan, 2001). Upon examining the duties of prison nursing in Turkey, it is observed that prison nurses work synergistically with prison physicians both as occupational health nurses and for prisoners/sentenced persons, with a priority to create a healthy and secure environment. For prisoners/sentenced persons, prison nurses have duties such as solving health problems; providing guidance; collecting and recording information about health status; performing periodic examinations; referring those with the symptoms of disease for further examination and treatment; administering medicines prescribed by the physician; determining and following up

[1]*MSN, RN, Research Assistant, Faculty of Health Sciences, Department of Nursing, Necmettin Erbakan University, Konya, Turkey* • [2]*PhD, RN, Assistant Professor, Faculty of Health Sciences, Department of Nursing, Trakya University, Edirne, Turkey.*

prisoners with emotional problems, chronic diseases, venereal diseases, malnutrition, and bad habits such as alcohol, cigarette, and drug use; preventing accidents; and providing first aid. In addition, prison nurses have duties such as solving the health problems of employees and their families and guiding them, collecting and recording information about their health status, providing hospital referrals, preventing accidents, determining reasons for absenteeism, and training employees in first aid (Turkish Nursing Association, 2015).

Nurses who work in prison settings are exposed to security problems while serving those who have low levels of education, may not be interested in their own healthcare, are likely addicted to drugs or alcohol, may have an aggressive personality, may have chronic diseases, and may experience sudden changes in mental health status (Doyle, 1999; Flanagan & Flanagan, 2001). For this reason, nurses working in prisons and detention centers may have problems with work-related quality of life (WRQoL) and with organizational commitment (OC) and performance (Beh & Rose, 2007; Doyle, 1999; Flanagan & Flanagan, 2001).

Organizational Commitment

OC, a subject that is frequently studied in the field of organizational behavior, has many definitions. Simply defined, OC is the loyalty and emotional relationship between employees and the organization. It may also be defined as an individual's identity that has been formed with the organization and the associated relative power of participation within that organization (Mahanta, 2012)

The rapid change in health services affects quality of service and makes sustaining OC in specialist staff a critical issue (Christmas & Hart, 2007). Nurses' work stress, burnout, the inadequacy of support mechanisms, heavy workloads, and role confusion are all seen as important factors affecting intention to quit (Chang, 2015; Hayes et al., 2012; O'Brien-Pallas, Murphy, Shamian, Li, & Hayes, 2010).

A high rate of turnover affects the effectiveness of other employees, their perceptions of work, and, therefore, quality of work (Chen et al., 2015). Therefore, many studies have indicated that high employee OC reduces intention to quit, which increases organizational continuity (Bianchi, 2015; Chen et al., 2015).

Work-Related Quality of Life

The following considers separately the words that together comprise the acronym WRQoL. Work (W) is defined as the fulfillment of responsibilities within certain boundaries to produce a result. Work life does not mean only the possibilities provided during the working hours. It includes everything to which employees attach importance, both within and outside the workplace. Quality (Q) is the competence of the service or product being given to meet the expectations of service areas. The concept of WRQoL covers working conditions; employee safety; wages; participation in decision making; positive, emotional reactions and attitudes toward employees' work; and organizational and individual level quality of relationships (Aketch, Odera, Chepkuto, & Okaka, 2012; Battu & Chakravarthy, 2014; Jayakumar & Kalaiselvi, 2012). This concept, which centers on people, is also defined as the process of responding to the needs of employees (e.g., health, safety, economic; Chib, 2012; Parsa, Idris, Samah, Wahat, & Parsa, 2014).

WRQoL aims to increase employee satisfaction and ensure continuity by establishing a positive attitude toward the organization, establishing suitable working environments for employees and the organization, increasing employee productivity and organizational effectiveness, strengthening learning in the workplace, and reducing organizational stress by increasing teamwork and communication (Chib, 2012; Jayakumar & Kalaiselvi, 2012; Parsa et al., 2014).

WRQoL is studied in many areas such as sociology, psychology, education, management, healthcare, and nursing (Vagharseyyedin, Vanaki, & Mohammadi, 2010). Nurses are the largest group of employees in healthcare institutions (Mohammadi et al., 2011; Moradi, Maghaminejad, & Azizi-Fini, 2014). In most countries, nurses have many problems such as work overload, fatigue, inadequate communication, burnout, and absenteeism (Battu & Chakravarthy, 2014; Erat, Korkmaz, Çimen, & Yahyaoğlu, 2011; Nayeri, Salehi, & Noghabi, 2011). These factors, which adversely affect professional performance and WRQoL, may result in medical errors and adverse events in healthcare. Therefore, it is very important to promote WRQoL in nurses (Battu & Chakravarthy, 2014).

Relationship Between Work-Related Quality of Life and Organizational Commitment

Examining the importance of human resources in achieving organizational goals highlights how improving WRQoL has become a main objective of the organization today (Birjandi, Birjandi, & Ataei, 2013). Organizations want to employ and keep individuals who are committed to achieving specific goals, that is, compatible, productive, and committed to organizational goals and objectives. For this reason, OC is a subject that has been much researched and discussed (Altuntaş, 2014). The OC of employees is known to be an important resource for promoting organizational performance. In this respect, WRQoL is seen as a fundamental and interesting issue related to the improvement of employee OC (Faghih Parvar, Allameh, & Ansari, 2013; Farjad & Varnous, 2013; Jayakumar & Kalaiselvi, 2012).

The many studies conducted in various countries on the relationship between WRQoL and OC in nurses concluded that WRQoL has a significant effect on OC (Almalki, FitzGerald, & Clark, 2012; Gifford, Zammuto, & Goodman, 2002; Nayak, Sahoo, & Mohanty, 2015). However, the number of studies of this issue targeting prison nurses is limited. Therefore, this study was designed to evaluate the relationship between the WRQoL and OC of nurses currently working in prisons or detention houses in Turkey.

Prisons in Turkey

Prisons and detention houses in Turkey provide services mandated by the Ministry of Justice. These institutions are classified as closed penitentiary institutions (high-security closed, closed women's, closed juvenile, closed youth), open penitentiary institutions (open detached, open women's), and reformatories for minors. Execution and correction procedures are conducted in prisons and detention centers, and educational, psychosocial, and health services are provided to both sentenced persons and prisoners (Turkey General Directorate of Prisons and Detention Houses [TPDH], 2015).

Sentenced persons have the right to benefit from examination and treatment facilities as well as medical devices to protect their physical and mental health and to diagnosis diseases. These individuals are treated in the infirmaries of institutions and, when the former is unavailable, in the prisoner wards of state and university hospitals. As of 2009, the primary healthcare formerly provided to sentenced persons and prisoners by institutional physicians is being provided by the Ministry of Health within the scope of the general healthcare system through family physicians in accordance with a protocol signed in April 2009. In accordance with this protocol, healthcare services are provided by creating positions for family physicians in each institution containing 1,000 and more sentenced persons and prisoners. According to 2014 data, 11 doctors, four dentists, and 513 nurses currently work in penitentiary institutions in Turkey (TPDH, 2015).

Methods

This descriptive and correlational study was conducted to evaluate the relationship between WRQoL and OC in nurses working in prisons and detention centers that were affiliated with the Ministry of Justice in Turkey. The target research population was all of the 513 nurses working in prisons and detention centers in Turkey, according to 2015 data obtained from the Ministry of Justice, General Directorate of Prisons and Detention Centers. The research sample comprised the 224 nurses (44%) who completed and submitted the questionnaire during the data collection period (June 10 to November 20, 2015).

Ethical Approval

Approval from the ethics committee (2015-281) and permission from the administrative authority (57299965-204. 06.03-527/60504) were obtained. The consent of individual participants was obtained on the front of the questionnaire sheet.

Data Collection Technique and Tools

After correspondence with the Ministry of Justice, an electronic link address was established. The Ministry of Justice sent the link address to the e-mail addresses of all the registered prison nurses in Turkey. The recipients could then access the informed consent form at the front of the questionnaires when they clicked on the link address. The participants responded by opening the questionnaire online after indicating their consent to participate on the informed consent form. After a participant completed the questionnaire, it was sent automatically to the researcher's e-mail address along with the informed consent form.

Data were collected using the sociodemographic information and work characteristics form, the WRQoL scale, and the OC scale. The former obtained descriptive characteristic data using 13 questions (e.g., age, gender, marital status, education) that addressed sociodemographic and work-related variables.

Work-related quality of life scale

The Turkish version of the WRQoL scale, originally developed by Van Laar, Edwards, and Easton in 2007 and translated and validated in its Turkish form by Duyan, Aytaç, Akyıldız, and Van Laar (2013), was used to measure the WRQoL of the participants in this study. The WRQoL scale, scored on a 5-point Likert-type scale, includes 24 items in six subdimensions, including general well-being, home–work interface, job and career satisfaction, control at work, working conditions, and stress at work. The Cronbach's alpha internal consistency coefficient for the scale was .91, and the Cronbach's alphas for the subscales ranged between .75 and .88. The Turkish adaptation study made by Duyan et al. reduced the original scale from 24 to 21 items, earning Cronbach's alphas of .89 for the overall scale and between .67 and .76 for the subscales. Items 6 and 17 on the scale were scored inversely (Duyan et al., 2013).

Organizational commitment scale

The OC scale, created by Meyer and Allen (1991) and tested for validity and reliability by Wasti (2000), was used to measure the OC levels of the participants in this study. The OC scale, scored using a 7-point Likert-type scale, includes 18 items with three subdimensions, including affective commitment (AC), continuance commitment, and normative commitment (NC). The Cronbach's alpha internal consistency coefficient for the subscales ranged between .73 and .86. The Turkish adaptation study conducted by Wasti found that Cronbach's alphas for the subscales ranged between .60 and .80. Items 3, 4, 6, and 7 in the scale were scored inversely, as they expressed negative attitudes (Wasti, 2000). High overall scores for the scale indicate a high level of OC. Permission to use this scale was obtained via e-mail from the researchers who performed the validity and reliability studies on the Turkish version.

SPSS Version 21 (IBM, Armonk, NY, USA) was used for data analysis. Number, percentage, mean, *t* test, one-way analysis of variance, Mann–Whitney *U*, Kruskal–Wallis test, and correlation analysis were used in statistical analysis.

Research Questions

Providing nursing services in prison settings is difficult for employees because of environmental factors including established regimens, security and prison cultures, stressful conditions, and the necessity of multidisciplinary teamwork (Flanagan & Flanagan, 2002; Norman, 1999; Willmott, 1997). Therefore, WRQoL and OC are issues that should be considered in prison nursing. Thus, the following research questions were formed:

1. What are the levels of WRQoL and OC in prison nurses?
2. Do sociodemographic characteristics impact the OC level of these nurses?
3. Do work characteristics impact the OC level of these nurses?
4. Does a significant relationship exist between level of WRQoL and level of OC in prison nurses?

Results

In terms of the sociodemographic characteristics of the participants, 60.7% were male, 58.5% were single, and 62.1% did not have children. Furthermore, 63.8% were less than 27 years old, 68.3% were graduates of a vocational school of health, 80.8% had worked at their current institution for 3 or more years, 67.4% had 0–5 years of professional work experience, and 88.8% worked day shifts. Slightly over half (54.9%) of the participants were responsible for 0–50 convicts on average, 81.7% do not feel that their incomes were adequate in light of their expenditures, 65.6% work in closed prisons, 68.3% expressed that they did not feel secure in their institution, and 56.7% indicated that the institution took security measures for its employees.

The average scores of the participants were 85.76 ± 14.97 for the OC scale and 80.91 ± 14.98 for the WRQoL scale (Table 1). Statistical evaluations were performed to determine whether the scores on the OC scale and its subdimensions were affected significantly by sociodemographic and working characteristic variables. The average AC score was higher in those participants who were less than 27 years old than in those who were 27 years old and older ($Z = -2.771$, $p = .006$; Table 2). Moreover, the average NC score was higher in those with 4 or more years of working experience in their current institution than their > 4-year counterparts ($Z = -2.038$, $p = .042$) and in those with > 6 years of professional nursing work experience than their counterparts with 0–5 years of working experience ($Z = -2.152$, $p = .031$). In addition, the participants who expressed the belief that the institution did not take security measures earned higher average OC scores than those who believed that security measures were taken ($Z = -2.359$, $p = .019$; Table 3).

The average AC and OC scores of those participants who did not perceive their income as adequate were higher ($Z = -2.562$, $p = .003$, and $t = 2.367$, $p = .019$, respectively) than those who did, and the average AC score of the participants who thought that the institution did not take security measures was higher ($Z = -2.441$, $p = .015$) than those who did. Furthermore, the total scale point averages for the NC ($Z = -1.984$, $p = .047$) and OC ($t = -2.994$, $p = .003$) of the participants who did not feel safe were higher (Table 3).

As shown in Table 4, the OC total scale correlated positively with its subdimensions, the WRQoL, and WRQoL subdimensions. A moderately positive relationship was found between the WRQoL and OC ($r = .438$, $p < .05$). The regression analysis indicated that 20% of the total variance of OC was explained by the WRQoL ($R^2 = .2$; Table 5).

TABLE 1.

Average Scores for the OC and WRQoL Scales and Their Subdimensions (N = 224)

Scale and Subdimension	Mean	*SD*	Min	Max
OC Subdimensions	85.76	14.97	47	120
Affective commitment	31.62	7.18	7	42
Normative commitment	29.63	6.92	12	42
Continuance commitment	24.50	7.39	6	42
WRQoL Subdimensions	80.91	14.98	36	105
General well-being	18.97	4.21	8	25
Home–work interface	16.58	5.45	5	25
Job and career satisfaction	16.51	3.31	6	20
Control at work	10.91	3.43	3	15
Working conditions	11.99	2.50	3	15
Stress at work	8.12	2.10	2	10

Note. OC = organizational commitment; WRQoL = work-related quality of life.

Discussion

The sociodemographic data showed a higher number of male than female participants, a higher number of high school graduates than undergraduates, and a higher number of participants less than 27 years old than 27 years old or over. Prison nursing in Turkey is a branch of nursing that is performed mostly by male nurses because of the high number of male convicts and prisoners, by high school graduate nurses, and by nonspecialized nurses (TPDH, 2015). Higher scores on the OC scale are associated with a more positive attitude. The mean score of the OC scale was 85.76 ± 14.97. Considering that the lowest score obtained from the scale was 47 and the highest was 120, it was determined that the OC levels of participants in this study were above average. As there are no similar studies of prison nurses in the literature, the comparison was made with other studies that examined the OC of nurses working in a variety of clinical settings and fields. Duygulu and Korkmaz (2008) and Demirel, Öz, and Yıldırım (2014) used a different OC scale with nurses who were working at hospitals affiliated with the Ministry of Health and its medical faculties. These studies stated that OC levels in the nurses were above average. Çakınberk and Aksel (2009) found a high level of OC using the same scale in their study on midwives and

TABLE 2.

Sociodemographic Characteristics of Nurses According to the OC Scale and Its Subdimensions (N = 224)

			Affective Commitment		Normative Commitment		Continuing Commitment		Total Scale Score	
Characteristic	*n*	%	*M*	*SD*	*M*	*SD*	*M*	*SD*	*M*	*SD*
Age (years)										
< 27	144	64.3	32.65	6.84	29.01	6.88	24.51	7.52	86.17	14.32
≥ 27	80	35.7	29.8	7.45	30.74	6.91	24.49	7.19	85.04	16.13
Z/*t*			−2.771		−1.573		*t* = 0.016		*t* = 0.542	
p			.006		.116		.987		.588	
Gender										
Female	88	39.3	31.28	7.08	29.63	6.73	24.58	7.05	85.49	14.74
Male	136	60.7	31.84	7.26	29.64	7.07	24.46	7.62	85.93	15.17
Z/*t*			−0.561		−0.000		*t* = 0.122		*t* = −0.217	
p			.574		1.000		.903		.829	
Marital status										
Married	93	41.5	30.63	7.53	30.38	6.72	24.29	6.88	85.30	16.07
Single	131	58.5	32.32	6.87	29.11	7.04	24.66	7.75	86.08	14.20
Z/*t*			−1.525		−1.100		*t* = 0.122		*t* = 0.385	
p			.127		.271		.903		.701	
Have children										
Yes	85	38.0	30.99	7.02	30.52	7.00	23.87	6.91	85.38	14.38
No	139	62.1	32.01	7.28	29.09	6.84	24.89	7.66	85.99	14.38
Z/*t*			−1.171		−1.145		*t* = −1.004		*t* = −0.298	
p			.242		.147		.317		.766	
Educational status										
Health vocational high school	153	68.3	32.05	6.54	29.10	6.70	23.95	7.41	85.10	13.59
Undergraduate	71	31.7	30.69	8.38	30.77	7.30	25.70	7.24	87.17	17.61
Z/*t*			−0.695		−1.587		*t* = −1.661		*t* = −0.960	
p			.487		.112		.098		.338	

Note. t = *t* test; *Z* = Mann–Whitney *U* test; OC = organizational commitment.

nurses. Studies that used the same scale on nurses who were working at hospitals affiliated to the Ministry of Health and its medical faculties found OC levels that were above average. A study by Ahmad and Oranye (2010) that compared nurses in Malaysia and England found OC levels of 81.33 ± 15.32 in Malaysian nurses and 68.10 ± 15.19 in English nurses. Although the working environment and attributes of nurses in prisons differ from those of hospitals, this study indicates that their OC is relatively high.

In this study, the average score for WRQoL was 80.91 ± 14.98, an above-average score in light of the scale's score range of 36–105. In the absence of similar studies of prison nurses, the findings of this study were compared with those of prior studies that examined the WRQoL of nurses working in different clinical settings and fields. Almalki et al. (2012) and Nayeri et al. (2011), using the same WRQoL scale as this study, determined that the nurses in their studies had a moderate level of WRQoL. The studies, while obtaining similar research findings, indicate that the WRQoL of nurses is generally moderate.

The AC and OC of those participants who did not perceive their income as adequate were relatively higher than those who did. Different from the findings in the literature, this study determined that perceiving one's wage to be adequate increases OC and reduces intention to quit (Birjandi et al., 2013; Farjad & Varnous, 2013; Gifford et al., 2002). The literature highlights many factors that affect OC, including organizational justice, support resources, and rights (Bayram, 2005). Therefore, the high OC of those in this study who perceived their wages as inadequate may be due to factors other than wage considerations (e.g., job security). In Turkey, nurses working in the public sector have more job security than nurses who work in the private sector. In addition, nurses in public hospitals work regular, 40-hour weeks, whereas nurses in private hospitals typically work between 45 and 60 hours per week. For this reason, nurses prefer to work in the public sector, even if they believe that their salaries are low. Upon considering that most of the participants in this study (80.8%) have been working in their current institution for around 3 years and that 67.4% have

TABLE 3.
Nurses' Work Attributes According to the OC Scale and Its Subdimensions (N = 224)

Characteristic	n	%	Affective Commitment		Normative Commitment		Continuing Commitment		Total Scale Score	
			M	*SD*	*M*	*SD*	*M*	*SD*	*M*	*SD*
Years working in current institution										
< 4	181	80.8	31.96	7.18	29.20	6.66	24.40	7.28	85.55	14.28
≥ 4	43	19.2	30.21	7.08	31.47	7.77	24.95	7.91	86.63	17.76
Z/*t*			−1.500		−2.038		*t* = −0.442		*t* = −0.422	
p			.134		.042		.659		.673	
Years working in the nursing profession										
< 6	151	67.4	31.18	6.75	28.91	6.74	24.57	7.44	85.66	14.16
≥ 6	73	32.6	30.47	7.92	31.12	7.10	24.37	7.32	85.96	16.63
Z/*t*			−1.324		−2.152		*t* = 0.189		*t* = −0.139	
p			.185		.031		.850		.890	
Type of work										
Day shift	199	88.8	31.60	7.24	29.59	6.89	24.57	7.34	85.77	15.08
Night shift	25	11.2	31.76	6.81	29.96	7.33	23.96	7.92	85.68	14.43
Z/*t*			−0.026		−0.282		*t* = 0.390		*t* = 0.028	
p			.979		.778		.670		.733	
Number of prisoners per nurse										
< 51	123	54.9	32.12	6.80	30.26	7.05	23.77	7.35	86.15	14.96
≥ 51	101	45.1	31.01	7.61	28.87	6.73	25.40	7.37	85.28	15.09
Z/*t*			−0.953		−1.708		*t* = −1.642		*t* = 0.435	
p			.341		.088		.102		.664	
Perceive income as adequate										
Yes	41	18.3	28.00	8.73	28.44	8.17	24.37	7.31	80.80	18.57
No	183	81.7	32.43	6.54	29.90	6.61	24.54	7.42	86.87	13.86
Z/*t*			−2.562		−1.080		*t* = −0.133		*t* = −2.367	
p			.003		.280		.895		.019	
Accept institution's security measures as adequate										
Yes	127	56.7	30.57	7.28	28.86	7.56	24.28	7.15	83.72	15.17
No	97	43.3	32.99	6.84	30.65	5.88	24.79	7.72	88.43	14.36
Z/*t*			−2.441		−1.655		*t* = −0.511		*t* = −2.359	
p			.015		.098		.610		.019	
Feel secure										
Yes	71	31.7	29.93	8.18	28.15	7.71	23.35	6.26	81.44	16.01
No	153	68.3	32.41	6.55	30.32	6.44	25.04	7.82	87.76	14.07
Z/*t*			−1.962		−1.984		*t* = −1.595		*t* = −2.994	
p			.050		.047		.112		.003	
Type of prison										
Open	35	15.6	30.14	8.12	27.77	7.48	24.54	6.95	82.46	17.29
Closed	147	65.6	31.99	7.12	29.97	7.02	24.24	7.74	86.20	15.03
High security closed	42	18.8	31.55	6.55	30.02	5.93	25.38	6.52	86.95	12.47
KW/*F*			1.288		2.193		*F* = 0.384		*F* = 1.049	
p			.525		.334		.697		.978	

Note. OC = organizational commitment; *t* = *t* test; *F* = one-way analysis of variance test; *Z* = Mann–Whitney *U* test; KW = Kruskal–Wallis test.

TABLE 4.

Correlation Analysis of the Variables of OC, WRQoL, and Their Subdimensions

Variable	1	2	3	4	5	6	7	8	9	10
1. Organizational commitment (total)	–									
2. Affective commitment	.626**									
3. Normative commitment	.772**	.339**								
4. Continuance commitment	.648**	.029	.294**							
5. Work related quality of life (total)	.438*	.364**	.447**	.127						
6. General well-being	.343**	.263**	.339**	.120	.819**					
7. Control at work	.313**	.231**	.386**	.066	.821**	.534**				
8. Job and career satisfaction	.428**	.401**	.431**	.096	.817**	.576**	.650**			
9. Home–work interface	.346**	.282**	.336**	.141*	.732**	.510**	.517	.563**		
10. Stress at work	.137*	.215**	.126	−.044	.394**	.242**	.271**	.265**	.147*	
11. Working conditions	.348**	.272**	.363**	.122	.807**	.632**	.626**	.625**	.568**	.181**

Note. OC = organizational commitment; WRQoL = work-related quality of life.
$^*p < .05$. $^{**}p < .01$.

worked in their profession for around 5 years, our results may be explained by the largely young and economically concerned profile of our study population.

The AC of participants who felt that the institution did not take sufficient security measures was higher than those who felt their institutions did take sufficient measures. The reason for this difference may be that prison nursing is perceived as a type of occupational nursing. Therefore, prison nurses may prefer to work in prisons than in hospitals, which would positively impact their AC.

The NC and OC were higher among participants who did not feel secure in their institution than among those who did. Many related studies in the literature have identified a positive relationship between job security and OC (Baek & Jung, 2015; Farjad & Varnous, 2013). NC is a concept that involves the sense of responsibility that employees hold toward their organization and the belief that they have liabilities and thus should show loyalty. It is thought that the difference in the findings of this study may be the tendency of employees to be committed to the policies of their institution, which engenders feelings of positive responsibility toward that institution despite feelings of insecurity and results in relatively high NC and OC scores. In addition, nurses are not organized in Turkey, and few have other jobs to go to if they leave work. Thus, many nurses continue to work despite experiencing less-than-ideal working conditions.

Studies on the relationship between WRQoL and OC have been conducted on various categories of professionals, including educators, factory workers, teachers, and healthcare workers (Faghih Parvar et al., 2013; Oshaghi & Aghdam, 2015; Tamini, Yazdany, & Bojd, 2011). However, the number of studies conducted on prison nurses has been limited. Data related to WRQoL and OC in Turkey are particularly rare. It was determined that the OC total scale was correlated positively with its subdimensions, WRQoL, and the subdimensions of the WRQoL (Table 2). According to the results of a study conducted by Gifford et al. (2002) on 276 people at seven different hospitals in the United States, a strong relationship exists between WRQoL and OC. A study conducted on healthcare professionals in India that addressed a study population that was 51.2% nurses concluded that WRQoL had a significant effect on OC (Nayak et al., 2015). In a 2014 study, a positive relationship between WRQoL and OC was found in 59.8% of the nurses at an educational research hospital (Gül, Bol, Selçuk, & Erbaycu, 2014). Erat et al. (2011) examined the effect of WRQoL on motivation in nurses and determined a significant effect on institutional commitment.

Furthermore, this study found a significantly positive relationship between OC and home–work interface and control in the workplace. Similarly, a study conducted at a

TABLE 5.

Regression Analysis of Work-Related Quality of Life and Organizational Commitment

Model	*B*	*SE*	ß	*t*	*p*
Organizational commitment	49.535	5.025	–	9.806	< .001
Work-related quality of life	0.475	0.064	.447	7.369	< .001

Note. $r = .438$, $R^2 = .200$, $F = 55.552$.

1,200-bed hospital in Ankara province (Cihangiroğlu, Uzuntarla, & Özata, 2015) examined the effect of nurse autonomy and participation in decision making on OC and found a significant relationship between participation in decision making and both AC and NC. In addition, Korkmaz and Erdoğan (2014) examined the effect of home–work interface on OC and found that this interface increased OC. Whereas a significantly positive relationship between OC and workplace stress was found in this study, Jamal and Baba (2000) reported in a study of nurses in Canada that work stress was significant and negatively related to OC.

Conclusions

Given the positive relationship between WRQoL and OC, it is recommended that WRQoL be improved to increase OC in nurses. The link between these variables may help managers and leaders reach a more comprehensive understanding regarding how improving WRQoL enhances OC. To increase WRQoL, it may be advisable to adjust or improve working conditions, provide career opportunities for employees, and ensure that an appropriate balance is maintained between home and work. In addition, prisons are places of nursing service, and nurses in prisons should be considered. Thus, the working conditions of nurses and the problems that they encounter in the workplace should be investigated further.

Limitations of the Study

The use of e-mail to collect the data for this study, the low response rate (44%), the lack of prior research into this topic, and the anomalous nature of some of the findings (e.g., the high OC found among participants who felt that their organization lacked adequate security measures, the significantly positive relationship found between OC and workplace stress) all represent limitations of this study and may prevent or limit the generalizability of results.

References

Ahmad, N., & Oranye, N. O. (2010). Empowerment, job satisfaction and organizational commitment: A comparative analysis of nurses working in Malaysia and England. *Journal of Nursing Management, 18*(5), 582–591. https://doi.org/10.1111/j.1365-2834.2010.01093.x

Aketch, J. R., Odera, O., Chepkuto, P., & Okaka, O. (2012). Effects of quality of work life on job performance: Theoretical perspectives and literature review. *Current Research Journal of Social Sciences, 4*(5), 383–388.

Almalki, M. J., FitzGerald, G., & Clark, M. (2012). The relationship between quality of work life and turnover intention of primary health care nurses in Saudi Arabia. *BMC Health Services Research, 12*(314), 1–11. https://doi.org/10.1186/1472-6963-12-314

Altuntaş, Y. S. (2014). Organizational trust, organizational commitment and organizational citizen behaviours. In Ü. Tatar Baykal & E. Ercan Türkmen (Eds.), *Nursing services management* (1st ed., pp. 698–714). Istanbul, Turkey: Akademi Basın Yayıncılık. (Original work published in Turkish)

Baek, Y. M., & Jung, C. S. (2015). Focusing the mediating role of institutional trust: How does interpersonal trust promote organizational commitment? *The Social Science Journal, 52*(4), 481–489. https://doi.org/10.1016/j.soscij.2014.10.005

Battu, N., & Chakravarthy, G. K. (2014). Quality of work life nurses and paramedical staff in hospitals. *International Journal of Business and Administration Research Review, 2*(4), 200–207.

Bayram, L. (2005). A new paradigm in management: Organizational commitment. *Sayıştay Journal, 59,* 125–139. (Original work published in Turkish)

Beh, L., & Rose, R. C. (2007). Linking QWL and job performance: Implications for organizations. *Performance Improvement, 46*(6), 30–35. https://doi.org/10.1002/pfi.139

Bianchi, R. (2015). Occupational and non-occupational strains should be concomitantly considered in research on burnout, organizational commitment, and turnover intention. *International Journal of Nursing Studies, 53,* 403–404.

Birjandi, M., Birjandi, H., & Ataei, M. (2013). The relationship between the quality of work life and organizational commitment of the employees of Darab Cement Company: Case study in Iran. *International Journal of Economics, Business and Finance, 1*(7), 154–164.

Çakınberk, A., & Aksel, İ. (2009). The empirical research of organizational commitment on midwives and nurses in health centers in Malatya. *E-Journal of New World Sciences Academy, 4*(3), 277–298. (Original work published in Turkish)

Chang, C. S. (2015). Moderating effects of nurses' organizational support on the relationship between job satisfaction and organizational commitment. *Western Journal of Nursing Research, 37*(6), 724–745. https://doi.org/10.1177/0193945914530047

Chen, S. Y., Wu, W. C., Chang, C. S., Lin, C. T., Kung, J. Y., Weng, H. C., ... Lee, S. I. (2015). Organizational justice, trust, and identification and their effects on organizational commitment in hospital nursing staff. *BMC Health Services Research, 15,* 363. https://doi.org/10.1186/s12913-015-1016-8

Chib, S. (2012). Quality of work life and organizational performance parameters at workplace. *SEGi Review, 5*(2), 36–47.

Christmas, K., & Hart, K. A. (2007). Workforce shortages are a global issue. *Nursing Economics$, 25*(3), 175–177.

Cihangiroğlu, N., Uzuntarla, Y., & Özata, M. (2015). Analysis of the impact of autonomy and participation on decisions on organizational commitment. *Bartın University Faculty of Economics and Administrative Sciences Journal, 12*(6), 39–52. (Original work published in Turkish)

Demirel, Y., Öz, B. F., & Yıldırım, G. (2014). Assessing the commitment of nurses working in a university hospital to their institutions. *Van Medical Journal, 21*(2), 92–100. (Original work published in Turkish)

Doyle, J. (1999). A qualitative study of factors influencing psychiatric nursing practice in Australian prisons. *Perspective in Psychiatric Care, 35*(1), 29–35. https://doi.org/10.1111/j.1744-6163.1999.tb00565.x

Duyan, E. C., Aytaç, S., Akyıldız, N., & Van Laar, D. (2013). Measuring work related quality of life and affective well-being in Turkey. *Mediterranean Journal of Social Sciences, 4*(1), 105–116. (Original work published in Turkish)

Duygulu, S., & Korkmaz, F. (2008). Nurses' organizational commitment, job satisfaction and reasons for leaving work. *Journal of Cumhuriyet University School of Nursing, 12*(2), 9–20. (Original work published in Turkish)

Erat, Ş., Korkmaz, M., Çimen, V., & Yahyaoğlu, G. (2011). The effect of nurses' work life quality to motivation. *The Journal of Academic, Sport, Health and Medicine, 1*(1), 68–97. (Original work published in Turkish)

Faghih Parvar, M. R., Allameh, S. M., & Ansari, R. (2013). Effect of quality of work life on organizational commitment by SEM (case study: OICO company). *International Journal of Academic Research in Business and Social Sciences, 3*(10), 135–144. https://doi.org/10.6007/IJARBSS/v3-i10/285

Farjad, H. R., & Varnous, S. (2013). Study of relationship of quality of work life (QWL) and organizational commitment. *Interdisciplinary Journal of Contemporary Research in Business, 4*(9), 449–456.

Flanagan, N. A., & Flanagan, T. J. (2001). Correctional nurses' perceptions of their role, training requirements, and prisoner health care needs. *Journal of Correctional Health Care, 8*(1), 67–85. https://doi.org/10.1177/107834580100800105

Flanagan, N. A., & Flanagan, T. J. (2002). An analysis of the relationship between job satisfaction and job stress in correctional nurses. *Research in Nursing and Health, 25*(4), 282–294. https://doi.org/10.1002/nur.10042

Gifford, B. D., Zammuto, R. F., & Goodman, E. A. (2002). The relationship between hospital unit culture and nurses' quality of work life. *Journal of Healthcare Management, 47*(1), 13–25.

Gül, G., Bol, P., Selçuk, N., & Erbaycu, A. E. (2014). The effect of work life quality to level of organizational commitment: An example of education and research hospital. *The Journal of Industrial Relations and Human Resources, 16*(4), 14–30. (Original work published in Turkish)

Hayes, L. J., O'Brien-Pallas, L., Duffield, C., Shamian, J., Buchan, J., Hughes, F., ... North, N. (2012). Nurse turnover: A literature review—An update. *International Journal of Nursing Studies, 49*(7), 887–905. https://doi.org/10.1016/j.ijnurstu.2011.10.001

Jamal, M., & Baba, V. V. (2000). Job stress and burnout among Canadian managers and nurses: An empirical examination. *Canadian Journal of Public Health, 91*(6), 454–458.

Jayakumar, A., & Kalaiselvi, K. (2012). Quality of work life—An overview. *International Journal of Marketing, Financial Services and Management Research, 1*(10), 140–149.

Korkmaz, O., & Erdoğan, E. (2014). Impact of work—Life balance on organizational commitment and employee satisfaction. *Aegean Academic Overview, 14*(4), 541–557. (Original work published in Turkish)

Nayak, T., Sahoo, C. K., & Mohanty, P. K. (2015). Quality of work life plays the mediating role in between workplace empowerment and employee commitment: A study on healthcare employees of an Indian state. *Journal of Health Management, 17*(3), 263–273. https://doi.org/10.1177/0972063415589236

Nayeri, N. D., Salehi, T., & Noghabi, A. A. (2011). Quality of work life and productivity among Iranian nurses. *Contemporary Nurse, 39*(1), 106–118. https://doi.org/10.5172/conu.2011.39.1.106

Mahanta, M. (2012). Personal characteristics and job satisfaction as predictors of organizational commitment: An empirical investigation. *South Asian Journal of Management, 19*(4), 45–58.

Meyer, J. P., & Allen, N. J. (1991). A three-component conceptualization of organizational commitment. *Human Resource Management Review, 1*(1), 61–89. https://doi.org/10.1016/1053-4822(91)90011-Z

Mohammadi, A., Sarhanggi, F., Ebadi, A., Daneshmandi, M., Reiisifar, A., Amiri, F., & Hajamını, Z. (2011). Relationship between psychological problems and quality of work life of intensive care units nurses. *Iranian Journal of Critical Care Nursing (IJCCN), 4*(3), 135–140.

Moradi, T., Maghaminejad, F., & Azizi-Fini, I. (2014). Quality of working life of nurses and its related factors. *Nursing and Midwifery Studies, 3*(2), e19450.

Norman, A. (1999) Prison health care: What is it that makes prison nursing unique? *British Journal of Nursing, 8*(15), 1032–1033. https://doi.org/10.12968/bjon.1999.8.15.6534

Norman, A., & Parrish, A. (1999). Prison health care: Work environment and the nursing role. *British Journal of Nursing, 8*(10), 653–656.

O'Brien-Pallas, L., Murphy, G. T., Shamian, J., Li, X., & Hayes, L. J. (2010). Impact and determinants of nurse turnover: A pan-Canadian study. *Journal of Nursing Management, 18*(8), 1073–1086. https://doi.org/10.1111/j.1365-2834.2010.01167.x

Oshaghi, F. J., & Aghdam, G. F. (2015). Relationship between the quality of work life and organizational commitment and the job satisfaction of Sarcheshmeh Copper industry employees. *SCRO Annual Report Journal, 3*, 1–5.

Parsa, B., Idris, K. B., Samah, B. B. A., Wahat, N. W. B. A., & Parsa, P. (2014). Relationship between quality of work life and career advancement among Iranian academics. *Procedia-Social and Behavioral Sciences, 152*(2014), 108–111. https://doi.org/10.1016/j.sbspro.2014.09.164

Tamini, B. K., Yazdany, B. O., & Bojd, F. B. (2011). Quality of work life as a function of organizational commitment and job burnout of Government and Private Bank Employees in Zahedan city. *The Social Science, 6*(5), 368–374. https://doi.org/10.3923/sscience.2011.368.374

Turkey General Directorate of Prisons and Detention Houses. (2015). *Characteristics of prisons and detention houses.* Retrieved from http://www.cte.adalet.gov.tr (Original work published in Turkish)

Turkish Nursing Association. (2015). *Nursing law/regulations and task, authorities, responsibilities (no. 27515).* Retrieved from http://www.turkhemsirelerdernegi.org.tr (Original work published in Turkish)

Vagharseyyedin, S. A., Vanaki, Z., & Mohammadi, E. (2010) The nature nursing quality of work life: An integrative review of literature. *Western Journal of Nursing Research, 33*(6), 786–804.

Van Laar, D., Edwards, J. A., & Easton, S. (2007). The work-related quality of life scale for healthcare workers. *Journal of Advanced Nursing, 60*(3), 325–333. https://doi.org/10.1111/j.1365-2648.2007.04409.x

Wasti, S. A. (2000). *The reliability and validity of Meyer and Allen's three-component organizational commitment scale.* Paper presented at the Eighth Annual National Conference of Administrative Sciences, Nevşehir, Turkey.

Willmott, Y. (1997). Prison nursing: The tension between custody and care. *British Journal of Nursing, 6*(6), 333–336. https://doi.org/10.12968/bjon.1997.6.6.333

2

Determining Factors That Influence Nurses' Perceptions of Quality Implementations Conducted in Hospitals in Turkey

Emel GÜR[1]* • Dilek EKICI[2]

ABSTRACT

Background: Quality management program implementations in health services are team endeavors that involve all health service personnel. Because they are direct providers of care, nurses are best able to evaluate the influence of quality management program implementations on the health services and quality of care provided by hospitals.

Purpose: The aim of this study was to develop an instrument to determine how nurses perceive the implementation of quality management programs in hospitals. Furthermore, the nurses' perceptions of the influence of these implementations on the quality of patient care and their job satisfaction were examined.

Methods: A descriptive, comparative, cross-sectional online survey was conducted using a convenience sample (N = 388) of practicing nurses working at public and university hospitals where quality management programs were implemented. Nurses' perceptions of the implementations were analyzed using confirmatory factor analysis, whereas the influence of nurses' perceptions of quality management implementations on patient care and job satisfaction was measured using structural equation modeling approaches.

Results: This study revealed that the instrument is valid and reliable for the measurement of participant perceptions of quality management program implementations. Nurses' perceptions were generally negative, and they exhibited negative attitudes toward the implementation of quality management in the institutions where they work. However, the quality management program implementations had little influence on perceptions of the quality of patient care. Participant job satisfaction was lower than average, and the quality management program implementations conducted in the hospitals negatively affected job satisfaction. On the other hand, participants who worked at university hospitals perceived quality management program implementations more affirmatively; patient care quality and job satisfaction were viewed more positively as well.

Conclusions/Implications for Practice: Because nurses do not participate effectively in quality management program implementations, they perceive these efforts as unnecessary and the responsibility of the quality control department. It is very important to ensure that all care-service providers participate to effectively implement quality management programs in hospitals and to encourage the adoption of a culture of patient safety in all institutions.

KEY WORDS:
nurse, quality management, structural equation modeling, patient care, job satisfaction.

Introduction

Organizational structure, technical infrastructure, and labor force insufficiency have been identified as the most important factors affecting medical errors (Ekici, Cerit, Gür, Mert, & Türkmen, 2016; Kohn, Corrigan, & Donaldson, 2000; Pizzi, Goldfarb, & Nash, 2001; World Health Organization [WHO], 2015). Patient safety is a critical factor in providing and maintaining high-quality health services; it comprises the precautions taken by management and healthcare providers to prevent harm to patients. A 5-year study by the WHO (2013) covering five countries concluded that patient safety is the responsibility of individual institutions, and hospitals should make it a priority and handle it comprehensively. Furthermore, generalization and adoption of evidence-based practices, improvement of professional implementation with in-service training, determination of the process for investigating errors, utilizing electronic recording systems, and fostering a culture of patient safety for both managers and employees are very important (WHO, 2013). All healthcare personnel should participate in a culture of patient safety in line with institutional philosophy, report any factors and medical errors that threaten patient and employee safety, and perform diagnosis, treatment, and care without harming the patient (Pizzi et al., 2001; Singla, Kitch, Weissman, & Campbell, 2006).

A culture of patient safety is an important indicator of quality management in health services. Total quality management (TQM) in health services is defined using the target

[1]*MSN, RN, Research Assistant, Department of Nursing, Health Science Faculty, Çankırı Karatekin University, Turkey* • [2]*PhD, RN, Professor, Department of Nursing, Health Science Faculty, Gazi University, Turkey.*

of continuous improvement in patient care, the systematic participation of the healthcare provider team, a determination of the underlying causes of undesired consequences during and after health service provision, and the implementation of corrective and preventive measures. TQM is a program in which the institution integrates continuous improvement and development efforts with management philosophy to generate high-quality services (van Schoten, de Blok, Spreeuwenberg, Groenewegen, & Wagner, 2016).

Various institutions have developed health service standards. Health institutions may apply to standardization programs such as Joint Commission International, European Foundation for Quality Management Excellence Model, and International Organization for Standardization (ISO) to align the quality of their health services with these internationally recognized models. The standards institution measures and assesses service quality and may either approve or disapprove based on established criteria. Similarly, since 2008, quality management program implementations at all health institutions in Turkey must include "Transformation in Health" in their scope. A subsidiary agency of the Ministry of Health assesses and approves the service quality of all health institutions based on Quality System in Health Standards (Health Quality Standards [SCS]). Thus, in Turkey, quality standards related to health services have been in effect for 9 years. As part of this process, the Ministry of Health performs quality audits at hospitals.

The health service standards in Turkey focus on quality management and on the development of quality management systems in hospitals. Related studies in the literature have noted that quality management is related to multiple factors, including organizational behavior and culture, organizational structure, leadership style, teamwork and participation, quality management process, resource management, customer satisfaction, and training and education (Øvretveit, 2000; Talib, Rahman, & Azam, 2011; Wardhani, Utarini, van Dijk, Post, & Groothoff, 2009). When successfully implemented in healthcare institutions, TQM has improved patient and employee satisfaction, the quality and performance of healthcare, and patient safety (Talib et al., 2011).

The WHO suggests that the implementation of quality management at hospitals significantly improves the quality of patient care and safety (WHO, 2015). Because of their responsibility for patient care and clinical experience, nurses have significant roles in ensuring patient safety and care quality (Draper, Felland, Liebhaber, & Melichar, 2008; Stanton, 2004; Stimpfel & Aiken, 2013). Therefore, the perceptions of nurses are important indicators of the quality of patient care (McHugh & Stimpfel, 2012). Various instruments have been developed to measure healthcare service quality (Al-Shdaifat, 2015). However, no study has examined the perception of nurses toward quality implementation in their institutions. The aim of this study was, first, to develop an instrument to determine how nurses perceive the implementation of quality management programs at hospitals and, second, to examine whether the implementations at different institutions varied significantly in terms of nurse perceptions, resulting quality of patient care, and job satisfaction. Thus, the research hypotheses are the following:

H1: Quality management program implementations have a significant and positive effect on the quality of care that patients receive.

H2: Quality management program implementations have a significant and positive effect on the job satisfaction of nurses.

H3: Nurses who work at public hospitals and university hospitals, respectively, hold different perceptions regarding quality implementation.

H4: Nurses who work at public hospitals and university hospitals, respectively, hold different perceptions regarding patient care quality.

H5: Nurses who work at public hospitals and university hospitals, respectively, hold different perceptions regarding job satisfaction.

Methods

Research Design

A descriptive, comparative, cross-sectional design with a self-report survey among a convenience sample of participants was used for this study.

Instruments

The study questionnaire was composed of three parts. The first included nine questions on demographic characteristics, including age, gender, education, tenure, and institution type, as well as the quality certification held by the respondent's institution, information on quality management program implementations, participation in these implementations, and whether an effective error reporting system was used at the institution. The second part was designed to assess the perception of "quality of patient care" using a score ranging from 0 = *dangerously low* to 10 = *very high*. The job satisfaction level of the respondent was measured on a scale of 1–10, with 0 = *not satisfied at all* and 10 = *highly satisfied*. Finally, to assess quality management program implementations in the health sector, related studies in the literature were reviewed to assess the perceptions, attitudes, beliefs, and behaviors of the participants based on an item pool of 28 statements. A focus group study was conducted with six participants to collect ideas and opinions on quality management program implementations. Information from the focus group and study findings were used to compose survey items. Some statements based on the results of the literature review were constituted as follows: "I believe that the quality management program implementations conducted in this institution increase the quality of the care given to patients" (DelliFraine, Langabeer, & Nembhard, 2010; Stanton, 2004); "In the institutions where quality management program implementations are conducted, the personnel consider patient safety as a priority issue"

(Stanton, 2004); and "Quality management program implementations are the duty of the 'Quality Department' only" (Alimo-Metcalfe, Alban-Metcalfe, Bradley, Mariathasan, & Samele, 2008; Draper et al., 2008). Patients consider quality certifications such as ISO, Joint Commission International, and SCS an important factor when selecting institutions at which to receive healthcare services (Øvretveit, 2000). Fourteen of the statements were positive, and 14 were negative. These items were prepared using a 5-point Likert scale (1 = *strongly disagree* to 5 = *strongly agree*).

These statements were sent to six specialists to analyze the content validity of the 28 items and to solicit opinions. The specialists assessed each item using one of the following statements: "not relevant," "somewhat relevant" (item or statement needs revision), "quite relevant" (relevant, but some minor changes are required), and "highly relevant." On the basis of the assessment results, the validity index for the questionnaire was determined as .94. As this value is higher than the minimum acceptable value of .80, the 28 items were accepted as the draft form of the questionnaire (Davis, 1992).

Sample, Setting, and Data Collection

A personalized cover letter was mailed electronically to 932 bedside nurses at public (*n* = 478) and university (*n* = 454) hospitals in Turkey where quality management program implementations had been conducted using e-mail addresses acquired from hospital Web sites. These emails explained the purpose of the study and provided a consent form, with a request for the recipient to participate in the study. Returning the completed consent form was considered agreement to participate. The Participant Information Form and study questionnaire were sent to the participants via a second e-mail. Data were collected from 388 participants (response rate: 42%). Study populations must be at least five times higher than the number of items subject to factor analysis (Child, 2006). Therefore, the sample size was sufficient for analysis in this study, which was conducted from March to December 2017.

Ethical Considerations

An application indicating the objective and scope of the study was submitted to the ethics committee of Gazi University; approval was provided on October 2, 2017 (reference: 77082166-302.08.01).

Data Analysis

Statistical analysis of the data was performed using IBM SPSS Statistics Version 20.00 (IBM, Inc., Armonk, NY, USA) and LISREL Version 8.80 (Scientific Software International, Lincolnville, IL, USA). Age, gender, tenure, presence of a quality department, certificates held by the hospital, participation in quality management program implementations, and perceptions of patient care and job satisfaction of the participants were analyzed using descriptive statistical methods (*M* and *SD*), and the independent *t* test was used to analyze the differences between public and university hospitals.

Exploratory factor analysis (EFA) was used to determine the component structure of developed instrument, and confirmatory factor analysis was performed to show evidence for construct validity. Goodness-of-fit indices (GFIs) were used to determine the sufficiency of the tested structure. Frequently used GFIs in confirmatory factor analysis are as follows: chi-square goodness (χ^2), GFI, comparative fit index (CFI), normed fit index (NFI), nonnormed fit index (NNFI), and root mean square error of approximation (RMSEA). Reliability, which indicates the internal consistency of a structure, was tested using both structural reliability and the Cronbach's alpha coefficient. Finally, after the instrument was developed, structural equation modeling was used to assess the causality between exogenous variables.

Results

Demographic Data

The average age of the participants was 32.97 (*SD* = 7.62) years. More than two thirds (79%, *n* = 307) were female, and 57% (*n* = 220) worked at a public hospital. The average duration of employment at their current hospital was 7.26 (*SD* = 6.89) years.

"Is there any Quality Department in your hospital?" received a "yes" response of 99% (*n* = 385); 372 of the participants (96%) reported that there was no efficient error reporting system at their institution. "What quality certifications does your hospital possess?" was answered with ISO certificate (68%, *n* = 262) and SCS (32%, *n* = 126). Furthermore, 17% of the participants (*n* = 66) stated that they actively participated in quality management program implementations, 29% (*n* = 112) stated that they partially participated, and 54% (*n* = 210) stated that they did not participate. Finally, 31 participants (8%) answered the open-ended question asking about the quality implementations in which they participated. In summary, most of the participants stated that they were involved in TQM issues.

Patient Care

The influence of quality management program implementations on participant perceptions of the quality of patient care was tested using structural equality modeling (Figure 1). According to the results, quality management program implementations conducted in the institutions had a positive and low influence on participant perceptions of the quality of patient care by 2.6% (Table 1). Furthermore, a low-level (.16) correlation was found between the quality management program implementations conducted in the institutions and the perceptions of the quality of patient care (Figure 1). When the created model was assessed using goodness-of-fit criteria (NFI = .94, NNFI = .95, CFI = .96, GFI = .92), acceptable fit was found (Schermelleh-Engel, Moosbrugger, & Müller, 2003). According to the results, quality management program

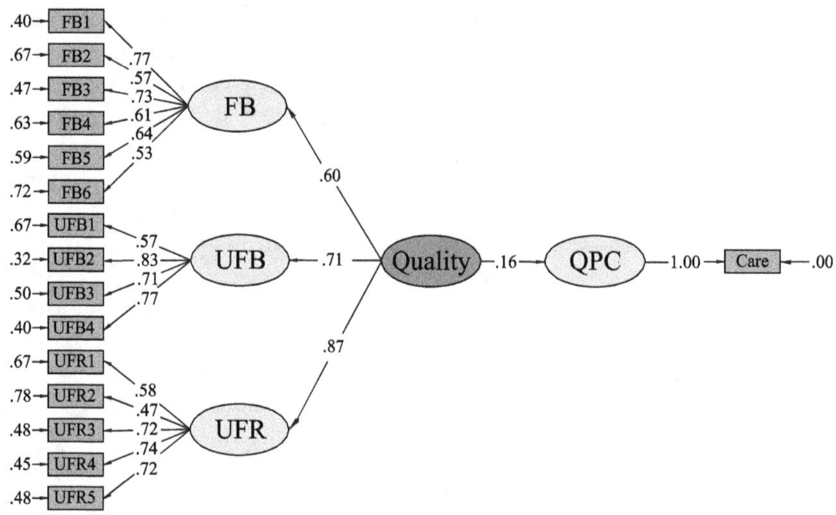

Figure 1. Structural equation modeling of patient care quality. FB = favorable belief; UFB = unfavorable belief; UFR = unfavorable reaction; QPC = quality of patient care. χ^2 = 265.03, *df* = 101, $p < .001$, RMSEA = .065.

implementations influenced the quality of patient care, albeit at a low level (2.6%). This finding partially confirmed H1.

Job Satisfaction

The influence of quality management program implementations on job satisfaction was tested using structural equality modeling (Figure 2). It was determined that quality management program implementations conducted in the hospitals had a negative influence on job satisfaction (−16%; Table 1). Accordingly, the coefficient between quality implementations conducted in the institution and job satisfaction was −.41. When the model was assessed using goodness-of-fit criteria (NFI = .94, NNFI = .96, CFI = .96, GFI = .92), an acceptable fit was found (Schermelleh-Engel et al., 2003). Thus, H2 was rejected.

Differences Between Public and University Hospitals

The independent sample *t* test was performed to assess institution-based differences in perceptions of quality management program implementations. Statistically significant differences were found between favorable beliefs (M = 2.99, SD = 0.81; t = −3.656; $p < .001$), unfavorable beliefs (M = 2.53, SD = .93; t = −3.132; $p < .01$), and total beliefs and attitudes toward quality management program implementations (M = 2.88, SD = 0.65; t = −3.610, $p < .001$). According to the results, participants who worked at public hospitals had less favorable perceptions of quality management program implementations. On the other hand, no statistically significant difference was found for the unfavorable reaction dimension ($p > .05$). Thus, H3 was accepted.

An independent sample *t* test was conducted to assess the difference between patient care quality of the nurses and job satisfaction. A statistically significant difference between patient care quality and job satisfaction was found between the participants at public and university hospitals, respectively ($p < .001$). Perceptions of the participants working at public hospitals were low with respect to both patient care quality (M = 6.02, SD = 2.22; t = −4.843) and job satisfaction (M = 4.25, SD = 2.43; t = −5.527). Accordingly, H4 and H5 were accepted.

Discussion

An item pool composed of 28 items was created using the implementations that were initially conducted. Both positive and negative behaviors, perceptions, beliefs, and attitudes of the nurses were handled in this item pool. The construct validity of the developed items was reviewed using EFA. First, principal component analysis was performed to test the compliance of the size of the working group for factoring, and the Promax rotation method was used for conversion (Costello & Osborne, 2005; Matsunaga, 2011). Structural analysis to determine the factor structures was made using principal axis factoring. Promax was used for rotation, and principal axis factoring was used to set the latent factors underlying the data to zero (Matsunaga, 2011). On the basis of the analysis results, items greater than 1 eigenvalue were gathered under seven components, and their total

TABLE 1.
Structural Correlations and Equations for the Model

	Quality		
Variable	Standard Error	R^2	λ
Quality of patient care	.32	.026	.16
Job satisfaction	.42	.160	−.41

Note. Quality of patient care = λ quality; job satisfaction = λ quality.

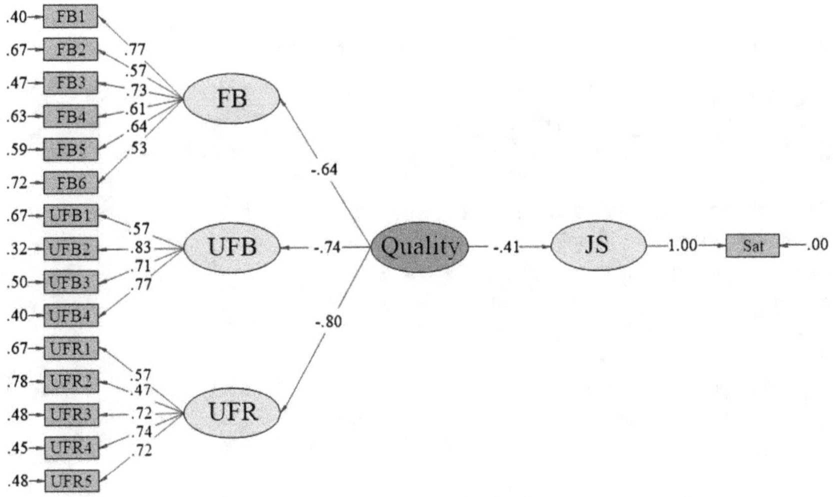

Figure 2. Structural equation modeling of job satisfaction. FB = favorable belief; UFB = unfavorable belief; UFR = unfavorable reaction; JS = job satisfaction. χ^2 = 255.15, *df* = 101, $p < .001$, RMSEA = .063.

contribution to the variance was determined to be 58.856% (Kaiser–Meyer–Olkin = .887, $\chi^2(378) = 3711.907$, $p < .01$). The overlapping and factor load values of the items were assessed during the analysis with respect to whether these meet the acceptance level or not, and 10 items that overlapped and had a low factor load (< .40; DeVellis, 2003) were excluded from the instrument (Items 5, 8, 9, 10, 18, 17, 12, 21, 20, and 23). These items included "I am willing to actively participate in quality implementations in the institution," "Results of quality implementations are shared with all employees," and "I think quality implementations increase employee satisfaction." Second, an EFA of the remaining 18 items was made using principal axis factoring, and the Promax rotation method was used for rotation (Matsunaga, 2011). As a result of these analyses, three more items with a low factor load were excluded from the analysis, including Item 4 (the workload resulting from quality implementations prevents me from providing efficient care to my patients), Item 7 (I think employees meet the standards determined within the scope of quality implementations), and Item 11 (I will be angry if I have to work overtime due to quality implementations). The remaining 15 items, grouped under three components, constitute the survey instrument. GFIs suggested by Schermelleh-Engel et al. were used in the assessment of the theoretical model. In fit-wellness measurements of the proposed theoretical model, χ^2 (with associated degrees of freedom [*df*] and *p* value), relative χ^2 ($\chi^2/df \leq 3.0$), RMSEA ≤ .08, GFI ≥ .90, CFI ≥ .95, and NFI ≥ .95 were used (Schermelleh-Engel et al., 2003). In this research, $\chi^2/df = 2.31$, GFI = .94, NFI = .95, NNFI = .96, CFI = .97, and RMSEA = .058 values indicate that the compliance of the theoretical model in terms of both structure and data was acceptable (Table 2).

Cronbach's alpha reliability and structural reliability were assessed for internal consistency of the data obtained from this instrument. The reliability levels for each dimension were higher than .70, proving the reliability of measurement results (Nunnally & Bernstein, 1994). The Cronbach's alpha value of the instrument was found to be .86. Furthermore, the structural reliability of the three components of the instrument was found to vary between .79 and .81.

Although various methods are available to measure patient care quality in a hospital, nurses are widely accepted as valid and reliable informants for providing opinions related to the quality of patient care (McHugh & Stimpfel, 2012). Furthermore, nurses have opinions about non-documented medical records and about the positive and negative results of implementations. It is suggested that quality management program implementations at hospitals increase the levels of patient care quality and patient safety significantly (WHO, 2015). However, this research found that quality implementations had little influence (2.6%) on participant perceptions of care quality (Figure 1).

Aiken et al. (2012) found that 11%–35% of nurses assessed the level of patient care quality and patient safety at hospitals in 12 countries as poor or fair. Similarly, Cho et al. (2016) found that 65% of Korean nurses perceived the level of patient care quality in South Korea as poor or fair. McHugh and Stimpfel (2012) found that 29% of a sample of nurses in the United States defined the patient care quality in their hospitals as excellent. In this study, the participant perceptions of patient care quality were slightly higher than average (good; $M = 6.47$, $SD = 2.14$). However, 96% of the participants stated that there was no efficient error-reporting system in their institution, whereas 83% stated that they participate in quality improvement implementations either partially or never. Although error reporting systems do not improve the quality of health services, being aware of errors is important to preventing recurrence (WHO, 2008). The American Association of Nurse Executives states that a culture of patient safety should be established by a manager to identify and remedy errors as soon as possible (Vogelsmeier & Scott-Cawiezell, 2007). However, statements of the participants such as "There is no efficient error reporting system in

TABLE 2.
Confirmatory Factor Analysis Results of the Instrument

Factor	*M*	*SD*	Standard Loads	Error Variance	*t*	R^2
Favorable belief						
FB1. I believe that quality implementations conducted in this institution increase the quality of the care given to patients.	3.29	1.15	.77	.40	16.61	.60
FB3. In the institutions where quality implementations are conducted, they support professional development of the personnel.	3.44	1.13	.73	.47	15.31	.53
FB5. The institutions where quality implementations are conducted provide good opportunities for their personnel.	2.79	1.13	.64	.59	12.93	.41
FB4. I think quality implementations increase patient satisfaction.	3.36	1.10	.61	.62	12.29	.38
FB2. Patients place importance on quality certifications such as ISO, JCI, and SCS when selecting institutions at which to receive health services.	2.50	1.15	.57	.67	11.31	.33
FB6. In the institutions where quality implementations are conducted, the personnel consider patient safety as a priority issue.	3.36	1.09	.53	.72	10.28	.28
Unfavorable Belief						
UFB2. Quality implementations increase the work load of the employees therefore I believe it is stressful.	2.54	1.14	.83	.32	18.25	.68
UFB4. I believe quality implementations increase my work load.	2.57	1.09	.77	.40	16.71	.60
UFB3. Frequently conducted quality audits conducted by the quality department bother the employees.	2.43	1.05	.71	.50	14.93	.50
UFB1. Due to intense quality implementations, my willingness to work decreases.	3.07	1.15	.57	.67	11.45	.33
Unfavorable reaction						
UFR4. Each implementation conducted due to quality implementations shall bother me since each implementation shall be based on a standard.	3.14	1.10	.74	.45	15.50	.55
UFR3. I find applied quality implementations are unnecessary.	3.34	1.05	.72	.48	14.99	.52
UFR5. I think quality implementations require a lot of procedures.	2.85	1.18	.72	.48	14.95	.52
UFR1. I am not interested in quality implementations.	3.24	1.18	.58	.67	11.36	.33
UFR2. Quality implementations are the duty of the "Quality Department" only.	2.68	1.10	.47	.78	9.04	.22

Note. χ^2 = 201.22 (df = 87), χ^2/df = 2.31; RMSEA = .058; NFI = .95; NNFI = .96; CFI = .97; GFI = .94. ISO = International Organization for Standards; JCI = Joint Commission International; SCS = Health Quality Standards; FB = favorable belief; UFB = unfavorable belief; UFR = unfavorable reaction.

their institution" and "They participate in quality improvement implementations either partially or never" indicate that their perception about patient care quality as "good" may not be realistic and that the obtained result as the influence on patient care quality is by 2.6% reflects their positive beliefs in quality implementations. On the other hand, unfavorable beliefs and attitudes such as "These implementations are conducted by the Quality Department" and "Quality implementations are not necessary" do not serve to improve the quality of patient care (Table 2). This situation suggests that nurses are not actively included in quality management program implementations and that these programs do not achieve their stated goals.

Nurse satisfaction has been identified in the literature as a factor that increases the quality of patient care (Aiken et al., 2011). However, this study revealed lower-than-average job satisfaction among participants (M = 4.85, SD = 2.54) and that quality management program implementations negatively influenced job satisfaction (−16%). Accordingly, H2, which posits that quality management program implementations have a positive and significant effect on job satisfaction, was rejected. A study conducted in hospitals across 12 countries in Europe and the United States that investigated perceptions of care quality and job satisfaction levels among nurses found job satisfaction levels that were between 11% and 56% (Aiken et al., 2012).

In this research, workload increase after quality management program implementations, decreased willingness to work because of heavy work flows, and the high frequency of quality audits were perceived negatively. In other respects, some of them stated that they found "the applied changes related to quality implementations to be unnecessary," "quality implementations require a lot of procedures," "quality implementations are the duty of the quality department," and "we are not interested in the quality implementations" and other negative reactions. Therefore, the results of this study indicate that quality management program implementations decrease job satisfaction in nurses and that program implementations conducted in Turkish hospitals by top management result in an undesirable situation for employees.

Participants from university hospitals in this study approached quality management program implementations more affirmatively and had more positive views of patient care quality and job satisfaction. In research conducted by Al-Shdaifat (2015), an instrument was developed to assess the perceptions of nurses regarding TQM implementations at private, university, military, and public hospitals in Jordan. As a result, a relationship between the Jordanian hospitals type and implementing TQM was found. It was revealed that nurses who were working at private hospitals had higher levels of perception, which consisted of continuous improvement, teamwork, training, top management commitment, and customer focus, than their peers who were working at other types of hospitals (Al-Shdaifat, 2015). The perceptions, attitudes, and behaviors of hospital managers directly influence the culture of patient safety and quality implementations (van Schoten et al., 2016). Results indicate that differences between hospital types are rooted in the differences in the attitudes and behaviors of top managers in these institutions.

Limitations

The most important limitation of this study is that the research data were collected only from nurses working in Turkey and thus reflect country-specific cultural and proficiency group characteristics. As the study sample was small, the findings may not be generalizable to all healthcare professionals. Furthermore, the findings of the research were limited to the answers of the participants.

The findings of this study indicate that the job satisfaction level of participants was negatively affected (−16%) by the quality management program implementations at their respective hospitals in Turkey. Research findings are limited by the data that were collected. Other factors that may influence the job satisfaction of nurses should be determined and addressed.

Conclusions

According to the findings, the instrument was found to be valid and reliable for measuring participant perceptions of quality implementations. In general, the participants reported negative perceptions of institutional quality management program implementations and little impact (2.6%) on perceptions of care quality. Furthermore, job satisfaction levels of the participants were found to be lower than median (M = 4.85, SD = 2.54; score range: 1–10), with a negative correlation between the quality management program implementations and nurse job satisfaction (−.41).

Implications for Practice

Because nurses do not participate in quality management program implementations, they are likely to perceive these implementations as unnecessary and quality management as the responsibility of the quality department. However, it is very important to make all care-service providers participate to effectively implement quality management programs in hospitals and to adopt a culture of patient safety across an institution. Therefore, TQM implementations should be initially adopted by top management and all managers before being conducted together with all employees.

Acknowledgments

We thank the hospital managers who accepted this study and enabled us to interview their nurses.

Author Contributions

Study conception and design: DE
Data collection: All authors
Data analysis and interpretation: All authors
Drafting of the article: All authors
Critical revision of the article: All authors

References

Aiken, L. H., Cimiotti, J. P., Sloane, D. M., Smith, H. L., Flynn, L., & Neff, D. F. (2011). Effects of nurse staffing and nurse education on patient deaths in hospitals with different nurse work environments. *Medical Care, 49*(12), 1047–1053. https://doi/org/10.1097/MLR.0b013e3182330b6e

Aiken, L. H., Sermeus, W., Van den Heede, K., Sloane, D. M., Busse, R., McKee, M., ... Kutney-Lee, A. (2012). Patient safety, satisfaction, and quality of hospital care: Cross sectional surveys of nurses and patients in 12 countries in Europe and the United States. *BMJ, 344*, e1717. https://doi/org/10.1136/bmj.e1717

Alimo-Metcalfe, B., Alban-Metcalfe, J., Bradley, M., Mariathasan, J., & Samele, C. (2008). The impact of engaging leadership on performance, attitudes to work and wellbeing at work: A longitudinal study. *Journal of Health Organization and Management, 22*(6), 586–598. https://doi/org/10.1108/14777260810916560

Al-Shdaifat, E. A. (2015). Implementation of total quality management in hospitals. *Journal of Taibah University Medical Sciences, 10*(4), 461–466. https://doi/org/10.1016/j.jtumed.2015.05.004

Child, D. (2006). *The essentials of factor analysis* (3rd ed.). London, England: Continuum.

Cho, E., Lee, N. J., Kim, E. Y., Kim, S., Lee, K., Park, K. O., & Sung, Y. H. (2016). Nurse staffing level and overtime associated with patient safety, quality of care, and care left undone in hospitals: A cross-sectional study. *International Journal of Nursing Studies, 60*, 263–271. https://doi/org/10.1016/j.ijnurstu.2016.05.009

Costello, A. B., & Osborne, J. W. (2005). Best practices in exploratory factor analysis: Four recommendations for getting the most from your analysis. *Practical Assessment Research & Evaluation, 10*(7), 1–9.

Davis, L. L. (1992). Instrument review: Getting the most from a panel of experts. *Applied Nursing Research, 5*(4), 194–197. https://doi.org/10.1016/S0897-1897(05)80008-4

DelliFraine, J. L., Langabeer, J. R., II, & Nembhard, I. M. (2010). Assessing the evidence of six sigma and lean in the health care industry. *Quality Management in Health Care, 19*(3), 211–225. https://doi/org/10.1097/QMH.0b013e3181eb140e

DeVellis, R. F. (2003). *Scale development: Theory and applications* (2nd ed.). Thousand Oaks, CA: Sage.

Draper, D. A., Felland, L. E., Liebhaber, A., & Melichar, L. (2008). The role of nurses in hospital quality improvement. *Research Brief, 3*, 1–8.

Ekici, D., Cerit, K., Gür, E., Mert, T., & Türkmen, S. (2016). *Analysis of managerial failures in healthcare.* Ankara, Turkey: Sim. (Original work published in Turkish)

Kohn, L. T., Corrigan, J. M., & Donaldson, M. S. (Eds.). (2000). *To err is human: Building a safer healthcare system.* Washington, DC: National Academy Press.

Matsunaga, M. (2011). How to factor-analyze your data right: Do's, don'ts, and how-to's. *International Journal of Psychological Research, 3*(1), 97–110. https://doi.org/10.21500/20112084.854

McHugh, M. D., & Stimpfel, A. W. (2012). Nurse reported quality of care: A measure of hospital quality. *Research in Nursing & Health, 35*(6), 566–575. https://doi/org/10.1002/nur.21503

Nunnally, J. C., & Bernstein, I. H. (1994). *Psychometric theory* (3rd ed.). New York, NY: McGraw-Hill.

Øvretveit, J. (2000). Total quality management in European healthcare. *International Journal of Health Care Quality Assurance, 13*(2), 74–80. https://doi/org/10.1108/09526860010319523

Pizzi, L. T., Goldfarb, N. I., & Nash, D. B. (2001). Promoting a culture of safety. In K. G. Shojania, B.W. Duncan, K. M. McDonald, & R. W. Wachter (Eds.), *Making health care safer: A critical analysis of patient safety practices. Evidence report/technology assessment.* Retrieved from http://158.132.155.107/posh97/private/culture/promoting-Pizzi.pdf

Schermelleh-Engel, K., Moosbrugger, H., & Müller, H. (2003). Evaluating the fit of structural equation models: Tests of significance and descriptive goodness-of-fit measures. *Online Methods of Psychological Research, 8*(2), 23–74.

Singla, A. K., Kitch, B. T., Weissman, J. S., & Campbell, E. G. (2006). Assessing patient safety culture: A review and synthesis of the measurement tools. *Journal of Patient Safety, 2*(3), 105–115. https://doi/org/10.1097/01.jps.0000235388.39149.5a

Stanton, M. W. (2004). Hospital nurse staffing and quality of care. *Agency for Healthcare Research and Quality, 14*(4-0029), 1–12. Retrieved from https://archive.ahrq.gov/research/findings/factsheets/services/nursestaffing/nursestaff.pdf

Stimpfel, A. W., & Aiken, L. H. (2013). Hospital staff nurses' shift length associated with safety and quality of care. *Journal of Nursing Care Quality, 28*(2), 122–129. https://doi/org/10.1097/NCQ.0b013e3182725f09

Talib, F., Rahman, Z., & Azam, M. (2011). Best practices of total quality management implementation in health care settings. *Health Marketing Quarterly, 28*(3), 232–252. https://doi/org/10.1080/07359683.2011.595643

van Schoten, S., de Blok, C., Spreeuwenberg, P., Groenewegen, P., & Wagner, C. (2016). The EFQM model as a framework for total quality management in healthcare results of a longitudinal quantitative study. *International Journal of Operations & Production Management, 36*(8), 901–922. https://doi/org/10.1108/IJOPM-03-2015-0139

Vogelsmeier, A., & Scott-Cawiezell, J. (2007). A just culture: The role of nursing leadership. *Journal of Nursing Care Quality, 22*(3), 210–212. https://doi/org/10.1097/01.NCQ.0000277776.97276.0b

Wardhani, V., Utarini, A., van Dijk, J. P., Post, D., & Groothoff, J. W. (2009). Determinants of quality management systems implementation in hospitals. *Health Policy, 89*(3), 239–251. https://doi/org/10.1016/j.healthpol.2008.06.008

World Health Organization. (2008). *World alliance for patient safety: Forward programme.* Retrieved from https://apps.who.int/iris/bitstream/handle/10665/70460/WHO_IER_PSP_2008.04_eng.pdf?sequence=1&isAllowed=y

World Health Organization. (2013). *The high 5s project: Interim report.* Retrieved from http://www.who.int/patientsafety/implementation/solutions/high5s/High5_InterimReport.pdf

World Health Organization. (2015). *Patient safety tool kit.* Retrieved from http://applications.emro.who.int/dsaf/EMROPUB_2015_EN_1856.pdf

3

Work-Related Predictors of Sleep Quality in Chinese Nurses: Testing a Path Analysis Model

Yuan LI[1] • Jinbo FANG[2]* • Chunfen ZHOU[3]

ABSTRACT

Background: Good sleep is essential to human health. Insufficient quality sleep may compromise the wellness of nurses and even jeopardize the safety of patients. Although the contributors of sleep quality in nurses have been previously studied, the direct and indirect effects of modifiable work-related predictors remain uncertain.

Purpose: The study was designed to explore the direct and indirect effects of modifiable work-related factors on sleep quality in Chinese nurses.

Methods: A multistage sampling method was employed in this cross-sectional study to recruit 923 participants. An evidence-based predicting model was postulated and then subsequently tested and optimized using path analysis.

Results: The final model fit the data well, with the involved predictors accounting for 34.1% of the variance in sleep quality of the participants. Shift work, job demands, exposure to hazards in work environments, chronic fatigue, and inter-shift recovery were identified as direct predictors, while whereas job satisfaction, job control, support at work, and acute fatigue were identified as indirect predictors.

Conclusions/Implications for Practice: Sleep quality in Chinese nurses is influenced directly and indirectly by various modifiable work-related factors. Interventions such as adjusting work shifts and reducing job burdens should be prioritized by administrative staff to ensure the sleep quality and clinical performance of Chinese nurses and to subsequently improve nursing care quality.

Key Words:
Chinese nurses, path analysis, predicting model, sleep quality, work-related factor.

Introduction

Although "sleep quality" is widely used, this term lacks definitional consensus. A panel of experts that was recently assembled to address this intellectual enquiry drew the conclusion that sleep continuity variables such as sleep latency, length of sleep, and frequency of awakenings as well as sleep efficiency are appropriate indicators of good sleep quality across the human life-span (Ohayon et al., 2017). Adequate quality sleep and feeling well-rested are required to remain healthy and productive. It has been reported that sleep deprivation over the short term negatively impacts mood, vigilance, and rapid response capabilities, whereas sleep deprivation over the long term leads to thought retardation (Han, Yuan, Zhang, & Fu, 2016), chronic fatigue (Fang, Qiu, Xu, & You, 2013), elevated mortality, cardiovascular diseases, and obesity and diabetes (Itani, Jike, Watanabe, & Kaneita, 2017). In addition, sleep challenges may have detrimental psychological consequences such as anxiety and depression. Furthermore, the reciprocal correlation between sleep condition and psychological state has been noted (Kouros & El-Sheikh, 2015). Of particular interest is the finding of a strong U-shaped relationship between sleep duration in employees and socioeconomic loss, with the nadir of the "U" unveiling itself for the recommended 7–8 hours of sleep per night (Burton, Chen, Schultz, & Li, 2017). More frequent healthcare utilization, productivity loss, absenteeism, and presenteeism resulting from poor sleep may contribute to reduced economic outcomes.

The Centers for Diseases Control and Prevention have declared that "sleep is essential for good health; it is a vital necessity, not a luxury." However, inherently involved in intense and hectic work, nurses are always at a high risk of insufficient sleep and sleep disorders (Kunzweiler et al., 2016). In an assessment using the Pittsburgh Sleep Quality Index (PSQI), over 70% of Chinese nurses in a prior study were reported to have experienced poor sleep quality, which is a ratio that is much higher than the 39.4% reported for the general population (Lin, Liao, Chen, & Fan, 2014). Sleep problems in nursing personnel may not only compromise well-being but also impair judgment and performance, which may jeopardize the safety of patients (Eanes, 2015). A recent study conducted to evaluate medical errors made by nurses

[1]Doctoral Candidate, RN, Junior Nurse, West China School of Nursing, Sichuan University, Chengdu City, Sichuan Province, China • [2]PhD, RN, Associate Professor, Nursing Department, West China Hospital, Sichuan University, Chengdu City, Sichuan Province, China • [3]MSN, RN, Junior Nurse, Mental Health Center of West China Hospital, Sichuan University, Chengdu City, Sichuan Province, China.

found that approximately 40% of nurses had committed at least one medical error during their career and that 78.3% of nurses identified sleepiness as a main culprit of nurse medical error (Kahriman & Öztürk, 2016). As patient safety is a priority of healthcare industries, the widely acknowledged relationship between the sleep quality of nurses and patient safety requires more research into this issue. Over the past decade, individual factors, behavioral factors, physical factors, and psychosocial factors have been identified as contributors to poor sleep in nurses (Chung, Liu, Lee, & Hsu, 2013; Han et al., 2016). Nevertheless, most of these factors, for example, age and marital status, are not subject to immediate utilization in related organizational interventions. Although work-related factors are more readily manipulated by administrative staff, few studies have addressed these factors. In addition, most related research has focused on the effects of shift work or on isolated cases only (Caruso, 2014; Lin et al., 2014). Thus, it remains unclear how these proposed factors interrelate with each other and impact sleep quality. Therefore, this study conducted a multiaspect-oriented investigation of modifiable work-related factors that are associated with sleep quality in Chinese nurses and then proposed, tested, and optimized an innovative, evidence-based hypothesized model using path analysis.

After a thorough literature review, an initial model incorporating nine explanatory variables was established (Figure 1). Except for intershift recovery and acute fatigue, the other variables, including shift work, job demands, job control, support at work, exposure to hazards in work environments, job satisfaction, and chronic fatigue, were posited as direct factors. Direct factors are factors that act on the outcome (sleep quality) directly, rather than through other intermediate factors. Furthermore, job satisfaction and chronic fatigue were hypothesized as mediators of the developed model. Specifically, job demands, job control, support at work, and exposure to hazards in work environments were each perceived to affect job satisfaction independently (Zhang et al., 2014) and to act as mediators of sleep quality, whereas chronic fatigue played a mediating role between job demands, job satisfaction, intershift recovery, and acute fatigue and the outcome (Fang et al., 2013). As intershift recovery and acute fatigue were not found to impact the outcome directly, they were presumed to be indirect factors that affect sleep quality through the mediating factor of chronic fatigue.

Shift work was identified repeatedly as one of the significant factors affecting sleep quality in nurses (Lin et al., 2014). Because healthcare services in hospitals must be offered on a 24-hour basis, nursing work is usually arranged in rotation, making it impossible for nurses to rest on a regular schedule. Unfortunately, sleep times misaligned with the endogenous circadian rhythm may trigger difficulties in falling asleep, early awakenings, and disrupted sleep (Caruso, 2014). Recent evidence supports that nurses on night duty are more inclined than their day-shift colleagues to manifest inferior sleep quality (Han et al., 2016). Hence, shift work was assumed to be a direct predictor of sleep quality in this study.

A synthesis of job demands (mainly psychological), job control (decision latitude), and support at work (support

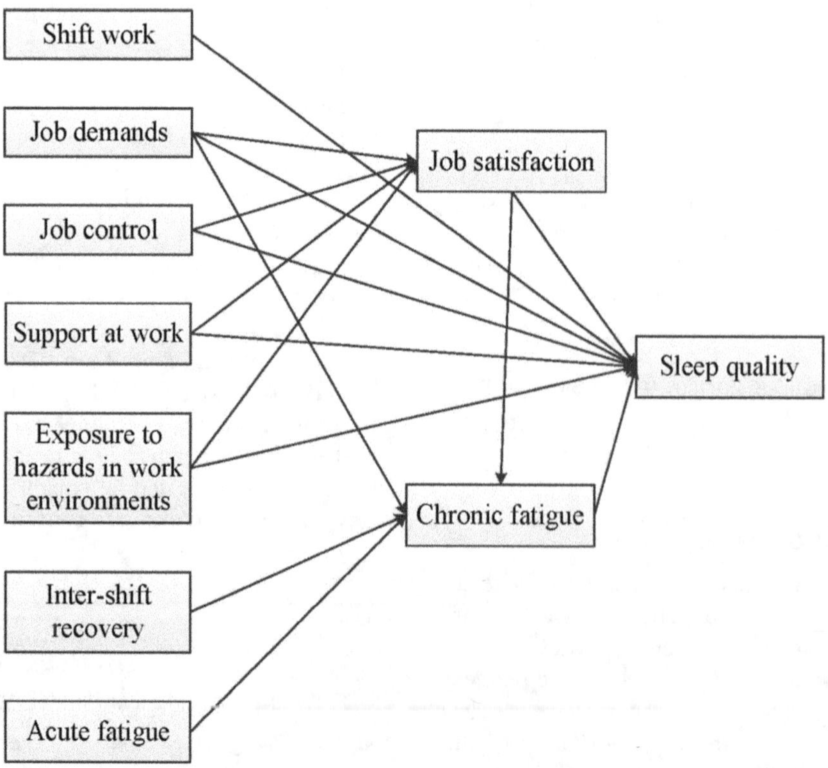

Figure 1. The original hypothesized model for predicting sleep quality in Chinese nurses.

available from coworkers and supervisors) has been shown to credibly predict job strain (Akerstedt, Nordin, Alfredsson, Westerholm, & Kecklund, 2012), which has been documented to relate inversely to sleep quality (Kunzweiler et al., 2016). A recent study of Nigerian nurses suggests that excessive job demands, if not buffered by job control and support, may give rise to mental exhaustion and ill health (van Doorn, van Ruysseveldt, van Dam, Mistiaen, & Nikolova, 2016). Additional studies verifying the links between these three occupational features and sleep quality confirm that high work demands are among the risk factors for sleep quality and that limited control over job and lack of support further elevate these risk factors (Akerstedt et al., 2012; Ruotsalainen, Verbeek, Mariné, & Serra, 2014). Therefore, this study hypothesized that job demands, job control, and support at work should associate directly with quality of sleep in nurses.

Hazardous work environments are presumed to be associated with an elevated risk of physical injury and a lowered degree of safety support, and the cumulative effects of prolonged exposure to these environments carry a higher risk of adverse impacts. A recent literature review (Caddick, Gregory, Arsintescu, & Flynn-Evans, 2018) on the environmental parameters of good sleep concluded that artificial light, ambient noise, ambient temperature, and air quality are crucial environmental factors affecting sleep deprivation. In addition, cross-sectional research on organic solvents and electromagnetic field exposures (Liu et al., 2014) ascertained that these factors affected sleep quality negatively in various study subgroups. Accordingly, exposure to hazards in work environments was incorporated into this study as a direct predictor of sleep quality.

Job satisfaction is a noteworthy construct, especially in the realm of administration, that may predict work behaviors such as organizational citizenship and withdrawal behaviors such as absenteeism and turnover. The effects of poor job satisfaction may be so far-reaching that the overall feelings from one's job experience may even affect everyday (non-job-related) life activities. As reported by Kunzweiler et al. (2016), sleep disruptions are closely related to poor job satisfaction and sleep quality decreases proportionally with job dissatisfaction. A multisite research in China found that nearly half of Chinese nurses were dissatisfied with their current jobs, that a supportive work environment (support at work) may play an alleviating role, that perceived high job demands (job demands) and limited job autonomy (job control) may intensify dissatisfaction, and that an unfavorable practice environment with continual security threat (exposure to hazards in work environments) may aggravate dissatisfaction even further (Zhang et al., 2014). Thus, this study assumed that job satisfaction both impacts sleep quality directly and mediates the relationships between job demands, job control, support at work, and exposure to hazards in work environments and quality of sleep in Chinese nurses.

Fatigue in nursing staffs is a long-standing problem that comprises both chronic (long-term) and acute (short-term) aspects. Numerous studies have validated the significant correlation between employee fatigue and sleep quality (Han et al., 2016; Korompeli, Chara, Chrysoula, & Sourtzi, 2013). Korompeli et al. (2013) revealed a positive connection between chronic fatigue and all sleep scales and summarized that the population of nurses with elevated chronic fatigue levels overlapped closely with those experiencing relatively severe sleep disturbance. Empirical studies have verified that chronic fatigue evolves from the persistent failure to recover from acute fatigue and that intershift recovery may help counteract the onset of this type of fatigue (Winwood, Bakker, & Winefield, 2007). A well-supported structural equation model (Fang et al., 2013) indicated that, in addition to acute fatigue and intershift recovery, chronic fatigue is also directly influenced by job demands and job satisfaction. In light of the abovementioned evidence, this study included chronic fatigue into the hypothesized model as a direct factor of the outcome and as a mediator between job demands, job satisfaction, intershift recovery, and acute fatigue and sleep quality.

The problem of sleep quality among nurses has become a critical issue for healthcare systems because of its high prevalence, negative effects on individual health and patient care quality, and associated costs. The modifiable work-related factors that impinge on sleep quality in nurses merit further exploration to evaluate and enhance the current situation. This study was designed to explore and describe the modifiable work-related factors that are capable of predicting sleep quality in Chinese nurses, to differentiate the direct and indirect effects of these identified factors, and to provide research-based evidence to help guide the future development of strategies to improve the sleep quality of nurses.

Methods

Sample and Setting

This cross-sectional design study was conducted in Chengdu, China. The inclusion criteria for participants were (a) working in inpatient departments, (b) providing direct patient care, and (c) working 8-hour/night shifts, whereas exclusion criteria were otherwise qualified nurses who were currently on maternity leave, had physical/mental diseases, or were taking medications during the data collection period. The sample size of the path analysis was determined using the formula: $N = L/f^2 + k + 1$ (Cohen, Cohen, West, & Aiken, 2003), where N = number of sample, L = noncentrality parameter, f^2 = effect size for regression statistics (calculated using $f^2 = R^2/1\text{-}R^2$), and k = the number of predictors for multiple correlation testing. When Type I error = 0.05 and power = 0.8, the L value was found to be 15.65 (Cohen et al., 2003). According to previous studies (Chung et al., 2013; Kunzweiler et al., 2016) on sleep quality, the R^2 ranges from $.130^2$ to $.785^2$. To maximize the statistical power, $.130^2$ was adopted to calculate the effect size (f^2). Taking the number of variables and nonresponse rate into consideration, 1,071 nurses were invited to participate in this study.

A multistage sampling process was implemented to recruit participants. First, one general hospital was selected from each of the five districts in Chengdu by simple, random sampling. Second, we collected the lists of all eligible nurses from the selected hospitals and randomly sequenced each nurse by computer. Then, the nurses who would be invited to participate were selected from this list using systematic sampling.

Data Collection

Ethical approval was obtained before commencing the study from the Institutional Review Board for Clinical Trials and Biomedical Research at the West China Hospital, Sichuan University (No. 2008SCU086). Official permission was granted by the targeted nursing departments, and written informed consent was obtained from all of the participants. Permissions from the original authors who had developed the scales that were used in this study were obtained by e-mail. The questionnaires used in this study contained no identifiable information. Data were analyzed at an aggregated level, and the authors were not able to identify the data of individual participants during or after data collection. Questionnaires were distributed by trained staff from each nursing department between December 2012 and April 2013. Upon distributing, every participant was informed about the study objectives and given detailed instructions. They were required to take his or her own time to complete and then seal the questionnaire and then to submit the sealed questionnaire within 3 days to the box outside their wards. One thousand nineteen completed questionnaires were returned, of which 923 were considered valid, giving an overall effective response rate of 86.18% (923/1,071).

Instruments

Demographic form

Demographics including age, marital status, education, professional and position title, years of working as a nurse, working unit, and number of night/evening shifts per month were collected.

Pittsburgh Sleep Quality Index

The PSQI is a psychometrically sound instrument that is widely used to quantify the subjective sleep quality of respondents over the immediately preceding 1-month period. The Chinese version, validated by Tsai et al. (2005), was applied here to estimate sleep quality in Chinese nurses. Seven components comprising 19 items constitute this self-report questionnaire. The component scores are summed to obtain a single, global score, which has a total possible range of 0–21, with higher points indicating worse sleep condition. According to Tsai et al., using 5 as the cutoff point for poor sleep gives the instrument a sensitivity and a specificity of 98% and 55%, respectively, and the Chinese PSQI showed an adequate reliability coefficient of .83. In this study, the reliability test for the Chinese PSQI yielded a Cronbach's alpha of .73.

Job Content Questionnaire

The Job Content Questionnaire, developed by Karasek (1985), was intended to measure the psychosocial characteristics of jobs. The verified Chinese version was adopted in our study. The Job Demands Subscale, Job Control Subscale, and Support at Work Subscale are the core components of the Job Content Questionnaire, which are each assessed using a 4-point Likert scale, with 1 indicating "*strongly disagree*" and 4 indicating "*strongly agree.*" In this study, the Cronbach's alpha for the three subscales were .76, .68, and .90, respectively.

Exposure to Hazards in Hospital Work Environments scale

The Exposure to Hazards in Hospital Work Environments scale is our modified Chinese version of the Hospital Occupational Hazards Scale (Gillmore, 1990), which was constructed to assess how frequent nurses in hospital work environments are exposed to physical, chemical, and biological hazards. This 20-item tool is scored using a Likert-type 5-point scale (1 = *never*, 5 = *always*). This study presented good internal consistency (Cronbach's alpha = .82) and test–retest reliability (.76 within a 2-week period), and the content validity index was rated at .87.

Job Satisfaction Scale

The Job Satisfaction Scale (Karasek, 1985) was designed to evaluate overall feelings about one's job. The verified Chinese version (Cheng, Luh, & Guo, 2003) with five self-report items was employed in this study. The weighted item scores add up to a total score that ranges from 0 to100, with higher scores representing higher levels of job satisfaction (Karasek, 1985). In this study, the Cronbach's alpha was .76 for this instrument.

Occupational Fatigue Exhaustion Recovery scale

The Occupational Fatigue Exhaustion Recovery scale (Winwood, Lushington, & Winefield, 2006), originally developed based on nursing populations, is the only instrument that is currently able to differentiate between chronic and acute fatigue states and to measure effective fatigue recovery between shifts. The Chronic Fatigue Subscale and Acute Fatigue Subscale measure the subjective feeling of fatigue, whereas the Intershift Recovery Subscale measures the feeling of recovery between work shifts. The English questionnaire was translated into Chinese and then back-translated into English by two bilingual experts until complete consent was achieved. The accuracy and consistency of meaning were scrutinized by a nursing professor. Occupational Fatigue Exhaustion Recovery items are scored on a 7-point Likert scale (0 = *strongly disagree*, 6 = *strongly agree*). The Cronbach's alphas were .81 and .82 for the Chronic and Acute Fatigue Subscales, respectively, and .86 for the Intershift Recovery Subscale.

Statistical Analysis

Data were analyzed using SPSS Version 23.0 and Amos Version 23.0 (IBM Corp., Armonk, NY, USA). Considering the different scales used by each instrument, all of the data, with the exception of demographic information, were transformed into a 0–100 ranking scale. Descriptive analyses were then used to delineate the sample characteristics. Pearson correlation analyses were first conducted to test if the associations among the variables met the prerequisites for performing path analysis. Next, path analysis was applied to test and modify the model. The model-data fit was evaluated using χ^2, χ^2/df, root mean square error of approximation (RMSEA), normed fit index (NFI), comparative fit index (CFI), and goodness of fit index (GFI). A nonsignificant χ^2 and χ^2/df remaining in between 1 and 2 indicate an acceptable model fit, and the RMSEA should be less than .05. With regard to NFI, CFI, and GFI, values no less than .90 indicate a good model fit, whereas values above .95 indicate an excellent fit (Cohen et al., 2003). The bootstrap resampling technique, especially appropriate for nonnormal data, was employed in this study to test the significance of direct and indirect variable effects (MacKinnon, Lockwood, & Williams, 2004). Typically, the resampling process should be repeated at least 1,000 times during analysis as a means of mimicking the original sampling process to generate a more reliable confidence interval (MacKinnon et al., 2004). This study set 1,000-times bootstrapping as recommended to yield a 95% confidence interval. Moreover, the squared multiple regression correlation coefficient (R^2) was estimated to identify the variance in sleep quality that was explained by proposed factors.

Results

Sample Characteristics

The participants had a mean age of 29.73 years; most were married (62.3%); 70.6% held an associate degree, and 17.5% held a baccalaureate or higher degree; nearly half were junior nurses (49.2%); and the overwhelming majority (92.6%) were staff nurses. The median year of professional nursing experience was 8.00. Nearly half (44.6%) of the participants worked more than eight night/evening shifts per month, and the largest percentages worked in the medical department (32.1%) and surgical department (27.5%; Table 1).

Modification of the Original Model

Pearson correlation analyses were initially used to examine the bivariate correlations among the variables (Table 2). The proposed associations between job control and sleep quality (r = .000, p = .991) failed to reach statistical significance. Thus, this pathway was ruled out in the following analyses, as per the prerequisite of conducting path analysis. Next, path analysis was performed to test, trim, and modify the hypothesized model. On the basis of theoretical reasoning and modification indices, three pathways (intershift recovery and job satisfaction/intershift recovery and sleep quality/acute fatigue and job satisfaction) were added to generate a much improved fit, whereas two nonsignificant pathways (support at work and sleep quality/job satisfaction and sleep quality) were

TABLE 1.

Demographic Characteristics of Participants (N = 923)

Characteristic	*n*	%
Age (years; *M* and *SD*)	29.73	6.91
20–29	532	57.6
30–39	290	31.4
40–55	101	11.0
Marital status		
Never married	320	34.7
Married	575	62.3
Divorced	27	2.9
Widowed or separated	1	0.1
Educational level		
Secondary technical certificate	110	11.9
Associate degree	652	70.6
Bachelor degree	159	17.3
Master degree and above	2	0.2
Professional title		
Junior nurse	454	49.2
Senior nurse	301	32.6
Assistant advanced nurse	153	16.6
Associate advanced nurse or advanced nurses	15	1.6
Present title of position		
Staff nurse	855	92.6
Head nurse	60	6.5
General head nurse	6	0.7
Director of nursing	2	0.2
Years of working experience in nursing profession[a] (*M* and *SD*)	9.73	7.36
1–9	528	57.2
10–19	282	30.6
20–39	113	12.2
Shift work[b]		
0	149	16.2
1–4	170	18.4
5–7	192	20.8
≥ 8	412	44.6
Work unit		
Medical	296	32.1
Surgical	254	27.5
Pediatrics	90	9.8
Obstetrics and gynecology	87	9.4
Ophthalmology and otorhinolaryngology	88	9.5
Psychiatric	22	2.4
Oncology	16	1.7
ICU	45	4.9
Others	25	2.7

Note. Age ranges from 20 to 55 years. Working experience year ranges from 1 to 39 years. ICU = intensive care unit.

[a]Median = 8.00, Q1 = 4.00, Q3 = 15.00 (The data did not conform to the normal distribution, so it is represented by the interquartile range. Q1 = the first quartile; Q3 = the third quartile). [b]Number of night/evening shifts per month.

TABLE 2.

Correlation Matrix of Study Variables (N = 923)

Variable	1	2	3	4	5	6	7	8	9	10
1. Shift work	1									
2. Job demands	.106**	1								
3. Job control	−.077*	.290**	1							
4. Support at work	−.031	.091**	.210**	1						
5. Exposure to hazards in work environments	.012	.332**	.290	−.153**	1					
6. Intershift recovery	−.198**	−.345**	.095**	.244**	−.397**	1				
7. Acute fatigue	.140**	.389**	−.017	−.201**	.449**	−.685**	1			
8. Chronic fatigue	.161**	.391**	−.003	−.155**	.409**	−.625**	.705**	1		
9. Job satisfaction	−.127**	−.308**	.131**	.305**	−.435**	.534**	−.507**	−.551**	1	
10. Sleep quality	.157**	.313**	.000	−.111**	.361**	−.498**	.503**	.522**	−.392**	1

$^{*}p < .05$. $^{**}p < .01$.

removed to guarantee the parsimony of the final model. Multiple tests were conducted to compare the modified models, which yielded the best data-fit model (χ^2 = 17.645, χ^2/df = 1.961, RMSEA = .032, NFI = .994, CFI = .997, GFI = .996; Figure 2).

Predictors of Sleep Quality in Chinese Nurses

The final model accounted for 34.1% of the variance in the outcome of interest. Shift work, job demands, exposure to hazards in work environments, and chronic fatigue were found to affect sleep quality in Chinese nurses directly (total effect [TE] = .056, p = .041; TE = .108, p = .002; TE = .138, p = .002; and TE = .288, p = .002, respectively), which echoed our stated hypotheses. In addition, the mediating role of chronic fatigue was confirmed. Contrary to our initial expectation, intershift recovery was also found to exert a direct influence over sleep quality (TE = −.299, p = .004). Job satisfaction, the only indirect predictor of outcome that was identified (indirect effect [IE] = −.058, p = .001), should thus be regarded as a distal mediator. Contrary to our initial assumption, job control and support at work were found to have an indirect influence on sleep quality (IE = −.007, p = .001, and IE = −.010, p = .001, respectively), whereas, in line with our initial assumption, the effect of acute fatigue (IE = .136,

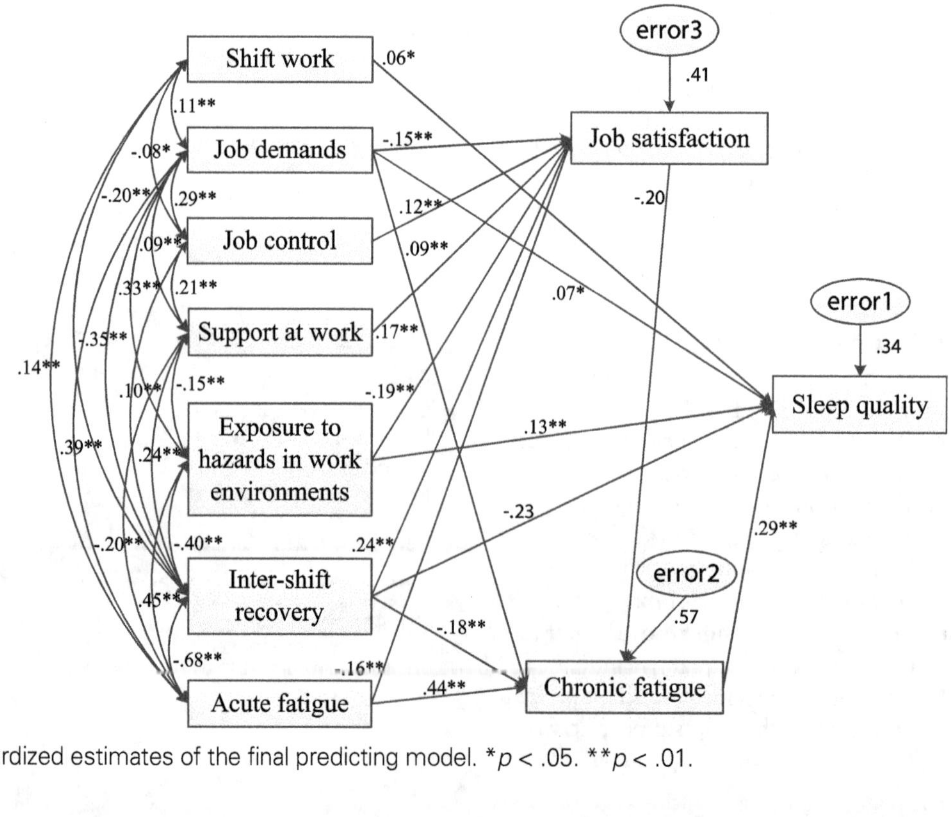

Figure 2. Standardized estimates of the final predicting model. $^{*}p < .05$. $^{**}p < .01$.

TABLE 3.
Direct, Indirect, and Total Effects of Causal Variables on the Outcome (N = 923)

			Bootstrap (B = 1000)	
Effect of Causal Variable	Point Estimate (β)	*SE*	Bias-Corrected 95% CI	Percentile 95% CI
1. Shift work				
TE	0.056*	0.027	[0.004, 0.110]	[0.004, 0.110]
DE	0.056*	0.027	[0.004, 0.110]	[0.004, 0.110]
IE	—	—	—	—
2. Job demands				
TE	0.108**	0.033	[0.046, 0.177]	[0.045, 0.177]
DE	0.073*	0.031	[0.014, 0.140]	[0.013, 0.139]
IE	0.036**	0.008	[0.021, 0.055]	[0.020, 0.054]
3. Job control				
TE	−0.007**	0.002	[−0.012, −0.004]	[−0.011, −0.003]
DE	—	—	—	—
IE	−0.007**	0.002	[−0.012, −0.004]	[−0.011, −0.003]
4. Support at work				
TE	−0.010**	0.002	[−0.016, −0.006]	[−0.015, −0.006]
DE	—	—	—	—
IE	−0.010**	0.002	[−0.016, −0.006]	[−0.015, −0.006]
5. Exposure to hazards in work environments				
TE	0.138**	0.033	[0.075, 0.201]	[0.076, 0.201]
DE	0.127**	0.034	[0.064, 0.191]	[0.064, 0.192]
IE	0.011**	0.003	[0.007, 0.019]	[0.006, 0.017]
6. Intershift recovery				
TE	−0.299**	0.034	[−0.358, −0.225]	[−0.366, −0.230]
DE	−0.232**	0.038	[−0.305, −0.151]	[−0.308, −0.155]
IE	−0.067**	0.013	[−0.092, −0.043]	[−0.092, −0.043]
7. Acute fatigue				
TE	0.136**	0.021	[0.095, 0.179]	[0.093, 0.176]
DE	—	—	—	—
IE	0.136**	0.021	[0.095, 0.179]	[0.093, 0.176]
8. Chronic fatigue				
TE	0.288**	0.041	[0.204, 0.367]	[0.203, 0.366]
DE	0.288**	0.041	[0.204, 0.367]	[0.203, 0.366]
IE	—	—	—	—
9. Job satisfaction				
TE	−0.058**	0.011	[−0.082, −0.037]	[−0.080, −.036]
DE	—	—	—	—
IE	−0.058**	0.011	[−0.082, −0.037]	[−0.080, −.036]

Note. All the estimates provided here are standardized estimates. TE = total effect; DE = direct effect; IE = indirect effect; SE = standard error; CI = confidence interval.
$^*p < .05$. $^{**}p < .01$.

p = .001) was found to be fully indirect. In addition, statistical significance was approached by all of the direct and indirect effects of sleep quality on the grounds of bootstrapping results (Table 3).

Discussion

Poor sleep quality in nurses is known not only to adversely affect their physical and mental health but also to cascade into other undesirable outcomes such as medical errors, degraded work performance, and even involvement in malpractice lawsuits (Eanes, 2015). This study prospectively examined the direct and indirect effects of modifiable work-related predictors of sleep quality in Chinese nurses using a path analysis model. The findings indicate that predictors included in the final model could explain 34.1% of the variance in sleep quality. According to Cohen et al. (2003), this result represents a medium-sized effect. Considering that only variables that were easily manipulated and related to work were proposed, 34.1% represents a relatively large proportion.

These results indicate that countermeasures that target the factors in the developed model could play important roles in ameliorating poor sleep quality in Chinese nurses.

Direct Predictors

The final model focuses on shift work, job demands, exposure to hazards in work environments, and chronic fatigue as direct predictors, which reflects both the original model and the findings of previous studies (Han et al., 2016; Hope, Øverland, Brun, & Matthiesen, 2010; Sandberg et al., 2016). More frequent night-shift work, implying more artificial light exposure and daytime sleep, negatively affects the normal circadian system, which regulates human sleep, suppresses daytime sleep, and promotes the secretion of melatonin (Korompeli et al., 2013). Enforced night-shift work may help explain why night-shift nurses face a high risk of poor sleep quality. There is scholarly consensus that more demanding work schedules increase the risk of sleep problems (Sandberg et al., 2016; Van Doorn et al., 2016). Excessive demands put employees at a greater risk of psychologically and physiologically exhaustion, which are known to impair normal sleep patterns. In addition, exposure to hazards in work environments, an intrinsic trait of certain professions, has been directly associated with sleep quality. Parallel evidence was found in a study of offshore personnel working on the Norwegian continental shelf (Hope et al., 2010). The nursing profession is unique in that it combines the regular threats of physical, mental, and chemical hazards with potential exposure to contaminated biological wastes. As a result, detrimental effects may occur spontaneously and be continuously aggravated for long periods afterward. Chronic fatigue, regarded as an illness or as a long-term condition, reduces overall health, of which sleep quality is a component. The mediating role of chronic fatigue between job satisfaction, job demands, intershift recovery, and acute fatigue and sleep quality was confirmed in this study, echoing the study of Fang et al. (2013).

Intershift recovery, in addition to its anticipated indirect effect, was found to act directly on sleep quality. Winwood et al. (2007) found that respondents who had a more fulfilling recovery between work shifts reported distinctly better sleep. Although humans are perceived to be well adapted to facing demanding environments, the capacity of the interrelated systems (e.g., physiological mechanisms) that underpin this resilience is not unlimited (Winwood et al., 2007). Persistent environmental stressors may destabilize the neuro-psycho-endocrine mechanism functions that regulate the stress response and result in maladaptive health outcomes, including sleep disturbance, if no timely, ameliorative interventions are implemented.

Taken together, systemic changes that address the fundamental issues underlying work arrangement, job intensity, and optimizing workplace conditions should be earnestly taken into account to offset the deleterious effects exerted by the direct, negative predictors of sleep quality. Likewise, sufficiently long nonworking periods should be included in work shift schedules by nursing supervisors to maximize the recovery of nurses from their late work-shift strain and to minimize cumulative fatigue.

Indirect Predictors

Job satisfaction, job control, and support at work were found to act indirectly on sleep quality, which was inconsistent with our hypothesis. Perhaps, this discrepancy is because of differences between the sample in this study and those in the reference studies used. Job satisfaction, referring to how employees feel about their work, was concluded to be an indirect factor, exerting influence on nurse sleep quality through the function of chronic fatigue. Hence, this study interpreted job satisfaction as a distal mediator. The indirect effect of the proposed factors on sleep quality was found to be mediated first by job satisfaction and then chronic fatigue. Similar findings were presented by Kunzweiler et al. (2016), who explored the factors that influenced sleep quality in German nurses. Employees perceiving their job to be below the satisfactory threshold may exhibit declining interest or involvement and express feelings of being unvalued and depressed. Such a negative mental status tends to increase fatigue, undermine their overall fitness, and ultimately disturb sleep rhythm. Insufficient rewards and benefits as well as heavy workloads and responsibilities have been identified as the major job-dissatisfaction complaints among Chinese nurses (Chen & Fang, 2016). Job control and support at work were found to exert indirect, positive effects on sleep quality. The association between low control, as measured by repetitive work plus limited autonomy, and poor sleep quality was previously confirmed in a systematic review (Ruotsalainen et al., 2014). In addition, lacking support at work was found to be correlated with the increased reporting of sleep problems (Akerstedt et al., 2012). As illustrated by the demand–control model, job strain in workers that results from overwhelming demands and limited control coupled with little support in turn affects their physical and mental health (Sandberg et al., 2016).

Corresponding to our initial hypothesis, acute fatigue was identified as an indirect predictor of sleep quality. The progression from acute fatigue to chronic fatigue has been widely reported in other studies as well (Fang et al., 2013; Winwood et al., 2006). Only when promptly ameliorated can acute or transient fatigue become adaptive rather than stressful (Winwood et al., 2006).

To decrease emotional exhaustion and enhance sleep quality among Chinese nurses, organizational interventions should be implemented that target indirect as well as direct predictors. Implementing countermeasures to brighten nursing career prospects, enforcing empowerment strategies to improve decision latitude, and dissolving worksite apathy are all approaches that are recommended for implementation by nursing managers. Furthermore, recovery activities that prevent acute fatigue from progressing into chronic fatigue or even burnout should be actively provided.

Limitations

The target population in this study included only nurses who were employed at general hospitals in urban areas of China. Therefore, the generalizability of findings may be limited. Because of the cross-sectional research design employed, inferences of causality cannot be drawn with certainty. Therefore, longitudinal or experimental designs are recommended in future studies of this topic. Moreover, all of the variables were measured using retrospective, self-report means. Thus, the influence of common method variance and self-report bias cannot be ruled out. Future research on this topic may include real-time assessments by using an experience sampling or a daily diary design. Moreover, path analysis is a structural equation model that is used in confirmatory rather than exploratory analysis. Thus, the thoroughness of the literature review and the construction of the original model impact the whole process significantly.

Conclusions and Implications for Nursing

Sleep is necessary for good health, as individual wellness and occupational safety for nurses relate strongly to the quality of patient care. Therefore, joint efforts and systematic changes should be taken by policy makers, hospital administrators, and nursing managers to relieve sleep problems in nurses. Direct, modifiable work-related predictors as well as indirect predictors of sleep quality in Chinese nurses were revealed in this empirical study. Programs to effectively improve the significant adjustable factors to help nurses recognize and improve their sleep condition should be prioritized in organizational strategies.

Future research on improving quality of sleep in nursing personnel should focus on (a) appropriately arranging work shifts and human resource allocations, (b) utilizing effective tactics to alleviate stress and reverse fatigue, and (c) optimizing the physical and psychosocial work environment.

Acknowledgments

We are grateful to participants for their participation and to Bechu Shelley Mathew for assisting with editing the English in this article.

References

Akerstedt, T., Nordin, M., Alfredsson, L., Westerholm, P., & Kecklund, G. (2012). Predicting changes in sleep complaints from baseline values and changes in work demands, work control, and work preoccupation—The WOLF-project. *Sleep Medicine, 13*(1), 73–80. https://doi.org/10.1016/j.sleep.2011.04.015

Burton, W. N., Chen, C. Y., Schultz, A. B., & Li, X. (2017). Association between employee sleep with workplace health and economic outcomes. *Journal Occupational and Environmental Medicine, 59*(2), 177–183. https://doi.org/10.1097/JOM.0000000000000934

Caddick, Z. A., Gregory, K., Arsintescu, L., & Flynn-Evans, E. E. (2018). A review of the environmental parameters necessary for an optimal sleep environment. *Building and Environment, 132*(1), 11–20. https://doi.org/10.1016/j.buildenv.2018.01.020

Caruso, C. C. (2014). Negative impacts of shiftwork and long work hours. *Rehabilitation Nursing, 39*(1), 16–25. https://doi.org/10.1002/rnj.107

Chen, Y. M., & Fang, J. B. (2016). Correlation between nursing work environment and nurse burnout, job satisfaction, and turnover intention in the western region of mainland China. *The Journal of Nursing, 63*(1), 87–98. https://doi.org/10.6224/JN.63.1.87 (Original work published in Chinese)

Cheng, Y., Luh, W. M., & Guo, Y. L. (2003). Reliability and validity of the Chinese version of the job content questionnaire in Taiwanese workers. *International Journal of Behavioral Medicine, 10*(1), 15–30. https://doi.org/10.1207/S15327558IJBM1001_02

Chung, M. H., Liu, W. I., Lee, H. L., & Hsu, N. (2013). Selected neurophysiological, psychological, and behavioral influences on subjective sleep quality in nurses: A structure equation model. *PLoS One, 8*(11), e79529. https://doi.org/10.1371/journal.pone.0079529

Cohen, J., Cohen, P., West, S. G., & Aiken, L. S. (2003). *Applied multiple regression/correlation analysis for the behavioral sciences* (3rd ed.). Mahwah, NJ: Lawrence Erlbaum Associates.

Eanes, L. (2015). CE: The potential effects of sleep loss on a nurse's health. *American Journal of Nursing, 115*(4), 34–40. https://doi.org/10.1097/01.NAJ.0000463025.42388.10

Fang, J., Qiu, C., Xu, H., & You, G. (2013). A model for predicting acute and chronic fatigue in Chinese nurses. *Journal of Advanced Nursing, 69*(3), 546–558. https://doi.org/10.1111/j.1365-2648.2012.06029.x

Gillmore, V. L. (1990). *Workplace variables and experienced occupational hazards as predictors of health of specialty nurses* (Unpublished doctoral dissertation). University of Maryland, Baltimore, MD, USA.

Han, Y., Yuan, Y., Zhang, L., & Fu, Y. (2016). Sleep disorder status of nurses in general hospitals and its influencing factors. *Psychiatria Danubina, 28*(2), 176–183.

Hope, S., Øverland, S., Brun, W., & Matthiesen, S. B. (2010). Associations between sleep, risk and safety climate: A study of offshore personnel on the Norwegian continental shelf. *Safety Science, 48*(4), 469–477. https://doi.org/10.1016/j.ssci.2009.12.006

Itani, O., Jike, M., Watanabe, N., & Kaneita, Y. (2017). Short sleep duration and health outcomes: A systematic review, meta-analysis, and meta-regression. *Sleep Medicine, 32*, 246–256. https://doi.org/10.1016/j.sleep.2016.08.006

Kahriman, İ., & Öztürk, H. (2016). Evaluating medical errors made by nurses during their diagnosis, treatment and care practices. *Journal of Nursing Management, 25*(19–20), 2884–2894. https://doi.org/10.1111/jocn.13341

Karasek, R. A. (1985). *Job content questionnaire uses' guide.* Los Angeles, CA: University of Southern California.

Korompeli, A., Chara, T., Chrysoula, L., & Sourtzi, P. (2013). Sleep disturbance in nursing personnel working shifts. *Nursing Forum, 48*(1), 45–53. https://doi.org/10.1111/nuf.12005

Kouros, C. D., & El-Sheikh, M. (2015). Daily mood and sleep: Reciprocal relations and links with adjustment problems. *Journal of Sleep Research, 24*(1), 24–31. https://doi.org/10.1111/jsr.12226

Kunzweiler, K., Voigt, K., Kugler, J., Hirsch, K., Bergmann, A., & Riemenschneider, H. (2016). Factors influencing sleep quality among nursing staff: Results of a cross sectional study. *Applied Nursing Research, 32*, 241–244. https://doi.org/10.1016/j.apnr.2016.08.007

Lin, S. H., Liao, W. C., Chen, M. Y., & Fan, J. Y. (2014). The impact of shift work on nurses' job stress, sleep quality and self-perceived health status. *Journal of Nursing Management, 22*(5), 604–612. https://doi.org/10.1111/jonm.12020

Liu, H., Chen, G., Pan, Y., Chen, Z., Jin, W., Sun, C., ... Yu, Y. (2014). Occupational electromagnetic field exposures associated with sleep quality: A cross-sectional study. *PLoS One, 9*(10), e110825. https://doi.org/10.1371/journal.pone.0110825

MacKinnon, D. P., Lockwood, C. M., & Williams, J. (2004). Confidence limits for the indirect effect: Distribution of the product and resampling methods. *Multivariate Behavioral Research, 39*(1), 99–128. https://doi.org/10.1207/s15327906mbr3901_4

Ohayon, M., Wickwire, E. M., Hirshkowitz, M., Albert, S. M., Avidan, A., Daly, F. J., ... Vitiello, M. V. (2017). National Sleep Foundation's sleep quality recommendations: First report. *Sleep Health, 3*(1), 6–19. https://doi.org/10.1016/j.sleh.2016.11.006

Ruotsalainen, J. H., Verbeek, J. H., Mariné, A., & Serra, C. (2014). Preventing occupational stress in healthcare workers. *Cochrane Database of Systematic Reviews, 2014*(12), CD002892. https://doi.org/10.1002/14651858.CD002892.pub4

Sandberg, J. C., Nguyen, H. T., Quandt, S. A., Chen, H., Summers, P., Walker, F. O., & Arcury, T. A. (2016). Sleep quality among Latino farmworkers in North Carolina: Examination of the job Control-Demand-Support model. *Journal of Immigrant and Minority Health, 18*(3), 532–541. https://doi.org/10.1007/s10903-015-0248-3

Tsai, P. S., Wang, S. Y., Wang, M. Y., Su, C. T., Yang, T. T., Huang, C. J., & Fang, S. C. (2005). Psychometric evaluation of the Chinese version of the Pittsburgh Sleep Quality Index (CPSQI) in primary insomnia and control subjects. *Quality of Life Research, 14*(8), 1943–1952. https://doi.org/10.1007/s11136-005-4346-x

van Doorn, Y., van Ruysseveldt, J., van Dam, K., Mistiaen, W., & Nikolova, I. (2016). Understanding well-being and learning of Nigerian nurses: A job demand control support model approach. *Journal of Nursing Management, 24*(7), 915–922. https://doi.org/10.1111/jonm.12397

Winwood, P. C., Bakker, A. B., & Winefield, A. H. (2007). An investigation of the role of non-work-time behavior in buffering the effects of work strain. *Journal of Occupational and Environmental Medicine, 49*(8), 862–871. https://doi.org/10.1097/JOM.0b013e318124a8dc

Winwood, P. C., Lushington, K., & Winefield, A. H. (2006). Further development and validation of the Occupational Fatigue Exhaustion Recovery (OFER) scale. *Journal of Occupational and Environmental Medicine, 48*(4), 381–389. https://doi.org/10.1097/01.jom.0000194164.14081.06

Zhang, L. F., You, L. M., Liu, K., Zheng, J., Fang, J. B., Lu, M. M., ... Bu, X. Q. (2014). The association of Chinese hospital work environment with nurse burnout, job satisfaction, and intention to leave. *Nursing Outlook, 62*(2), 128–137. https://doi.org/10.1016/j.outlook.2013.10.010

4

The Current Status of the Administrative Dispositions of Nurses: A Nationwide Survey in South Korea

Suyoung KIM[1] • Sanghee KIM[2]*

ABSTRACT

Background: In South Korea, the professional role of nurse has been redefined from "assistant to" to "partner of" doctors as part of an overall national health promotion strategy.

Purpose: This descriptive survey was designed to describe the current status of administrative dispositions related to nurses in South Korea.

Methods: Data were collected between January 2014 and December 2018. The raw data were obtained from 3,553 public health centers nationwide after a request for the disclosure of information related to the administrative disposition of nurses in each city and province. The data included details on administrative dispositions, laws related to administrative dispositions, violations, and standards for administrative dispositions.

Results: Most of the nurses affected by administrative dispositions worked for primary and secondary healthcare providers. The most common type of administrative disposition was license suspension (n = 66, 80.5%), and most violations for administrative disposition involved unlicensed medical practice (n = 38, 46.3%). Nurses who had more-specific standards provided as evidence of the disposition faced longer periods of license suspension (p = .035).

Conclusions/Implications for Practice: Nurses should avoid providing nursing care to patients that is not in compliance with medical laws because the administrative action may vary depending on the violation and the severity of their legal infractions. This study was the first to examine administrative actions specifically affecting nurses in South Korea. The administrative actions of medical personnel were found to depend on the number and degree of violations. Nurses must understand the details of nurse-related administrative dispositions to avoid violating medical laws.

KEY WORDS:
administrative dispositions, violation, nurse, nursing action, medical law.

Introduction

The Medical Act was first established in South Korea in 1973 to standardize the medical services provided by healthcare providers and related institutions and to protect and promote public health. The medical law of South Korea addresses the issues necessary for all people to have medical benefits (Hong et al., 2018; S. Kim & Choi, 2015). Under the medical law, medical practice by healthcare providers entails certain rights and responsibilities. Although nursing behaviors were previously considered as part of medical treatment in South Korea, this has recently changed as nursing-care-related liabilities are being imposed on nurses rather than doctors because of changes in nurses' self-perceptions of their behaviors (Oh, 2018). Medical law has social law characteristics because it incorporates many acts regarding survival guarantees and public welfare to safeguard the public interest, although medical law has both civil and administrative law characteristics because it includes organizations, procedures, and contents for the actualization of social law (Dronina et al., 2016). In South Korea, default-related medical contracts and compensation associated with illegal acts deal with the civil code as substantive law, including compensation and issues such as the administrative proceedings (mostly insurance fees) of medical institutes, healthcare provider licensing, and sales-related dispositions, which are handled administratively (Heo, 2014). In addition, medical law is connected with criminal law in several important aspects, including medical accidents, medical care insurance law, and the civil and criminal procedural codes (M. Lee, Yoon, & Lee, 2018). Thus, nurses who violate medical law may receive a criminal penalty with a fine, whereas those who fail in their duties may face disqualification or revocation of their license (S. Shin et al., 2020). Nurses who violate their obligations under medical law may receive a criminal penalty as well as administrative disposition. Practicing without a license, distributing false/exaggerated advertising, and practicing outside of approved venues may all result in criminal prosecution (Choi et al., 2019; E. Lee, 2017). Administrative dispositions for nurses may involve

[1]MHS, RN, Public Officer in Charge, Public Health Center, Uijeongbu-si, Gyeonggi-do, Republic of Korea • [2]PhD, RN, Assistant Professor, College of Nursing, Keimyung University, Daegu, Republic of Korea.

the revocation of their license, the suspension of their qualifications, a correction order, a warning, and/or a fine (K. K. Kim et al., 2014). The standards for administrative disposition are described in the administrative rules for violators, with the framework consisting of both common and specific standards. The common standards mainly define general administrative disposition criteria of punitive or reductive disposition regarding an offense and repeat offenses. The specific standards define the duration of license suspension, the revocation of licenses, and warnings regarding offenses and repeat offenses (M. Lee, 2019; W. Lee, Kim, et al., 2018). Depending on the specific standards, a nurse who performs an illegal act such as false charting may be penalized with a fine, warning, or license suspension, with penalty severity depending on the severity of the illegal act and the degree of patient-related damage inflicted.

Although healthcare providers were once the sole decision makers in medical settings, patients are now playing an increasingly important role in medical decision making in South Korea (Oh, 2018). Therefore, legal cases have increased the role of nurses in terms of recognizing their collaborative relationship with physicians for health promotion, with nurses no longer seen as simply doctors' assistants (W. Lee, Kim, et al., 2018). Medical accidents are closely related to nursing care, and related legal violations have increased because nurses are not aware of actions that are prohibited under medical law. In addition, nurses in clinical settings face a higher risk of involvement in legal suits because the scope of nursing tasks has become diversified and specialized, whereas the burden of proof on patients has been eased in medical dispute cases (Jang et al., 2018; Yi, 2018). Therefore, it is necessary to clearly understand the scope of the norms that nurses should follow as caregivers and the administrative standards associated with these norms and to use data to guide and educate nurses on proper decision making. However, there is a lack of research into the scale of administrative measures and the extent of medical law violations by nurses.

This study was performed to identify the current situation of administrative disposition among nurses in South Korea. The specific purposes of this study were the following:

(1) Identify the scale of administrative disposition among nurses in South Korea.
(2) Identify the administrative-disposition violations and their related penalties.
(3) Identify the relationship between the act and standards for administrative disposition.
(4) Develop a plan to reduce the incidence of administrative disposition among nurses.

Methods

Design

A descriptive survey was used in this study to identify the current situation of administrative disposition among nurses in South Korea. This study used raw national data for sampling, tools, and variable selection.

Participants

All of the participants were licensed nurses who were currently practicing nursing in South Korea.

Procedure

The data for this study were collected from January 2014 to December 2018 from 3,553 public health centers after freedom of information requests relating to the administrative disposition of nurses in each city and province (one capital city, six metropolitan cities, eight provinces, and one autonomous city). The collected data consisted of details and standards related to the violation-related administrative dispositions, judgments, acts, and characterizations.

Sample Size

The sample size required for this study was calculated using G*Power software Version 3.1.9.2 (University of Kiel, Kiel, Germany), with an effect size = .3, alpha = .05, and power = 0.90. The calculated sample size for this study was 75. Data were gathered from 3,553 public health centers, and data from the 82 qualified cases with administrative dispositions were included in the analysis.

Study Variables

Details on administrative disposition

Data on administrative dispositions consisted of the nature of the violation, results of the administrative disposition, periods, organizations' requests for a disposition, and judgments on administrative dispositions. Judging administrative dispositions is a governmental power held by administrative agencies, with enforcement measures depending on the specific nature of the violation.

Related law of administrative dispositions

The related law provides rational evidence for administrative dispositions and violations of the law by nurses.

Violations

The violation details for administrative disposition provide the specific reason for a disposition.

Standards of administrative dispositions

The standards of administrative dispositions are the rules governing violations.

Statistical Analysis

The data were analyzed using IBM SPSS Statistics Version 25.0 (IBM Inc., Armonk, NY, USA). Descriptive statistics were used to analyze the general characteristics, details of administrative dispositions, relevant laws, and relevant standards for the dispositions of the participants. Kendall's tau-b correlation analysis for nonparametric data was performed to analyze the relationships among the relevant laws,

Table 1

General Characteristics of the Subjects (N = 82)

Characteristic	*n*	%
Gender		
Male	2	2.4
Female	80	97.6
Age group (years; *M* and *SD*)	49.5	10.2
24–29	3	3.6
30–39	13	15.9
40–49	22	26.8
50–59	29	35.4
Over 60	15	18.3
Workplace		
Capital city	10	12.2
Metropolitan city	19	23.2
Province	51	62.2
Special autonomous city	2	2.4
Hospital type		
Tertiary hospital	0	0.0
General hospital	11	13.4
Hospital	17	20.7
Long-term care hospital	33	40.2
Clinic	21	25.7

standards, and administrative dispositions, with p values of less than .05 considered significant.

Ethical Considerations

The data for this study were collected using freedom of information requests to city and provincial health centers. In some cases, a notice of exemption from research proposals was sent to the lead researcher's associated institutional review board (IRB no.: I-1901/3218).

Results

General Characteristics of the Study Participants

The general characteristics of the study subjects are presented in Table 1. Eighty-two cases of administrative disposition of nurses were identified during the study period (January 2014 to December 2018). Nearly all cases (n = 80, 97.6%) involved female nurses. The most common age group placed on administrative disposition was 50s (n = 29, 35.4%), followed by 60s (n = 15, 18.3%), 30s (n = 13, 15.9%), and 20s (n = 3, 3.6%). The most common work region of suspended nurses in administrative districts in South Korea was provinces (n = 51, 62.2%), followed by metropolitan cities (n = 19, 23.2%), the capital city (n = 10, 12.2%), and the autonomous city (n = 2, 2.4%). The most common hospital type affected by nurse suspensions was long-term care hospitals (n = 33, 40.2%), followed by clinics with 30 beds (n = 21, 25.7%), hospitals with fewer than 100 beds (n = 17, 20.7%), and general hospitals with over 100 but below 300 beds (n = 11, 13.4%). There were no cases of suspended nurses in tertiary hospitals. Most nurses affected by administrative dispositions worked for primary and secondary healthcare providers.

Types of Administrative Dispositions and Nature of Violations

The types of administrative dispositions and the nature of violations found in this study are shown in Table 2. The most common type of administrative disposition given was suspension of license (n = 66, 80.5%), followed by a warning (n = 13, 15.9%) and revocation of license (n = 3, 3.7%). Most license suspensions were "more than 1 month but less than 3 months" (n = 31, 47.0%). The most frequent client requesting a disposition was the National Police Agency (n = 39,

Table 2

Types of Administrative Disposition and Nature of Violation for Administrative Dispositions of Nurses in South Korea (N = 82)

Variable	*n*	%
Administrative disposition		
Suspension of license (month) [a]	66	80.5
< 1	15	22.7
1–3	31	47.0
> 3	20	30.3
Warning	13	15.9
Revocation of license	3	3.7
Administrative clients		
Head of a health center	5	6.1
National Health Insurance Corporation	2	2.4
City mayor or governor	35	42.7
National Police Agency	39	47.6
Ministry of Health and Welfare	1	1.2
Court decision		
Fine (US $) [b]	40	48.8
< 1,000	22	55.0
1,000–2,500	13	32.5
> 2,500	5	12.5
Probation	37	45.1
Imprisonment	2	2.4
Suspension of prosecution	2	2.4
No charge	1	1.3
Violation		
Unlicensed medical practice	38	46.3
False charting	24	29.3
Medical practice by nonmedical practitioner	6	7.3
Not recording	4	4.9
Luring patient with valuables	2	2.4
Lending license	2	2.4
Immoral medical practice	2	2.4
Other	4	4.9

[a] Mean = 1.49 (*SD* = 1.12). [b] Average is USD$1,512.

47.6%), followed by city mayors/governors (n = 35, 42.7%). The most common court decision was a fine (n = 40, 47.7%), and the average fine was USD$1,512. The next most-common court decision was probation (n = 37, 45.1%). The nature of the violations leading to administrative disposition was as follows: unlicensed medical practice (n = 38, 46.3%), false charting (n = 24, 29.3%), medical practice by a nonmedical practitioner (n = 6, 7.3%), failure to make proper records (n = 4, 4.9%), luring patients by providing valuables (n = 2, 2.4%), license lending (n = 2, 2.4%), immoral medical practice (n = 2, 2.4%), and other (n = 4, 4.9%). "Other" included one nurse who was diagnosed with schizophrenia, one nurse who ordered false medical records to be made, and two nurses who used expired medications.

Fines and License Suspension Periods According to the Number and Standards of Violated Laws

The fines and periods of license suspension are presented in Table 3, organized by the number of laws violated and related standards. No significant relationship was found between fines and periods of license suspension according to the number of violations by nurses. Although the fine amounts did not differ significantly, the duration of license suspension (p = .035) differed significantly by number of specific standards involved, with nurses who had higher numbers of specific standards provided as evidence for their disposition facing longer periods of license suspension.

Discussion

The medical laws in South Korea are designed to regulate the direction of the country's health policy and are thus considered administrative laws (Hong et al., 2018; S. Kim & Choi, 2015; Oh, 2018). South Korea's medical laws regulate nurses (Choi et al., 2019; Oh, 2018). Nurses who fail in their duties may face relevant legal penalties (S. Shin et al., 2020). Healthcare providers who violate their duty under the medical law may face license suspension or revocation based on the severity of their violation. In this descriptive study, the status of administrative dispositions of nurses in South Korea was identified and the specific reasons and standards for administrative dispositions were analyzed.

On the basis of the findings of this study, the number of administrative disposition cases involving nurses numbered approximately 80 cases over a 4-year period. However, accurately estimating the total number of these cases in South Korea is difficult because no data on the number of dispositions by job group are publicly available. However, it is notable that nurses facing administrative dispositions were most likely to be in their 50s, work in nonurban settings (provinces), and work in a long-term care hospital.

It is widely presumed that several administrative measures are used mainly against new nurses because of their lack of experience. However, in this study, most of the administrative measures were used against experienced nurses. In this study, cases of administrative disposition for nurses were most common in the age groups associated with experienced nurses, which raises an interesting question that may be examined in future studies: How do experienced nurses understand the nursing practice in the context of current medical laws? Several nursing studies in South Korea have been conducted on newly graduated and novice nurses with the goal of enhancing the clinical performance of young nurses (Choi et al., 2019; Oh, 2018). However, few studies have addressed the working conditions and abilities of experienced nurses. Therefore, the results of this study suggest that it is necessary to determine whether experienced nurses fully understand the scope of their work and operate within the standards set by medical law.

Distribution inequality exists among medical institutions in South Korea, as most tertiary hospitals in the country are concentrated in metropolitan areas, whereas provincial

Table 3

Degree of Fine and License Suspension According to the Number of Violated Laws and Specific Standards (N = 82)

Variable	No.	n	%	Fine ($)		Period of License Suspension (Months)	
				r	p	r	p
Number of violated laws	1	14	17.1	−.248	.087	−.097	.187
	2	65	79.3				
	3	2	2.4				
	4	1	1.2				
Number of specific standards	0	13	15.9	.068	.356	.201[a]	.035
	1	65	79.2				
	2	4	4.9				

[a] Kendall's tau-b nonparametric correlation analysis.

areas are predominantly the sites of long-term care hospitals and clinics. The main users of long-term care hospitals are older adults. Moreover, the number of long-term care hospitals is expected to continue increasing because of South Korea's rapidly aging society (second only to Japan among the Organisation for Economic Co-operation and Development countries). Long-term care hospitals more often experience shortages of nurses and insufficient patient safety education (Jang et al., 2018). Furthermore, these hospitals maintain vague regulations regarding general nursing practices, and their quality control has been discussed in several studies (J. H. Shin & Hyun, 2015). Thus, on the basis of the results of this study, investigating the status of the scope of delegation of other nonmedical people in nursing practice is necessary to determine whether relevant guidance and supervision are being implemented in accordance with the Medical Act in long-term care hospitals.

The period of license suspension was found to differ based on the severity and extent of the legal violations. In 2018, doctors found guilty of reporting false medical records, ghost surgery, or immoral behavior toward patients such as sexual assault received a license suspension of 1 month (Hong et al., 2018; Jung et al., 2018). Furthermore, doctors who failed to keep medical records, did not sign their records, or formed a medical practice with nonmedical practitioners received a license suspension of more than 3 months (Jung et al., 2018). As doctors and nurses have different duties to perform in clinical settings, it is difficult to compare their punishments in terms of the degree of administrative disposition, but the suspension period for nursing licenses in this study was 1–3 months, and the average fine was roughly USD$1,500, which are comparable with the punishments received by doctors. Although punishment varies based on the severity of the infringement, unlicensed doctors who practiced medicine on people in South Korea received fines of roughly USD$2,000–$2,500. Furthermore, given the degree of punishment in most offenses by nurses for administrative disposition such as false charting and allowing nonmedical practitioners to perform in medical practices, nursing performance is no longer considered medical assistance in the legal context. The dispositions of nurses have changed because their acts are now judged as independent decisions and also because nursing records represent important evidence supporting the validity and results of nursing care, making these records a critical tool for protecting nurses from unintended medical accidents. However, determining whether false charting by nurses leads to dispositions is critical. Therefore, nurses must ensure they do not provide ungrounded nursing care to patients and must write correct, fact-based charts in clinical situations. Hospital organizations must implement systems to ensure nursing practices comply with the provisions of the Medical Act and that written results are accurate and well managed.

The process of administrative disposition for violations of medical laws mostly begins with the filing of a civil complaint, and its procedure is divided into administrative restrictions and criminal penalties. In South Korea, the disposition process is commissioned by the Ministry of Health and Welfare, local governments, or the prosecution, and the steps consist of prior notice, submission of opinions, and execution measures (Jeong, 2013). In this study, the clients were mostly the National Police Agency, mayors, and governors, with suspended nurses receiving a fine or probation proceeding to face criminal or civil suits (Cho & Park, 2019). These results show that nursing practice may be covered by civil or criminal law, except for the facts defined in medical laws. The main reason that medical personnel become involved in criminal or civil lawsuits is criminal negligence that involves serious injury to the patient, with the corresponding administrative disposition also imposed upon the court ruling (Jeong, 2013; Jung et al., 2018). A fine is imposed on the violator for the misconduct, and they must pay a certain amount to the state because of a conviction from the prosecutor. If it is a serious crime, the criminal record remains on that person's permanent record (Cho & Park, 2019). In the past, most professional manslaughter charges involved doctors. However, in recent court cases, nursing practice has been treated as a coequal part of the medical practice, which may be interpreted as giving patients significant responsibility for any damage (K. K. Kim et al., 2014; Jang et al., 2018; M. Lee, Yoon, & Lee, 2018). Therefore, nurses must realize that their nursing behavior will no longer be excepted from medical disputes. Moreover, nursing organizations must establish dedicated departments and personnel to provide legal knowledge and continuously check the legality of nursing behavior to prevent/prepare for medical accidents.

In this study, for nurses, the higher the number of specific standards that applied in the administrative dispositions, the more significant the differences in the duration of license suspension. The specific standards for administrative disposition were defined in this study as the specific criteria for disposal according to the degree of violation, with the more violations and evidential Acts applied, the more standards for the dispositions applied, which may be interpreted as influencing the outcome of the disposal (Heo, 2014; Y. Kim et al., 2019). In South Korea, aggravated punishment may be imposed upon the reissuance of illegalities via the same act, and many violations of medical laws may result in aggravated punishment (Cho & Park, 2019). In cases of excessive misconduct, the administrative disposition criteria related to the medical law shall follow more severe disposal criteria related to the suspension, and the remainder shall be disposed of by adding one half of each disposal criteria. On the other hand, the administrative disposition criteria are not added as punishment if there are two or more violations in the case of false or unpreserved medical records (Jeong, 2013; J. Lee, 2010). Nurses should be careful not to provide patients with nursing care that is not based on medical law because administrative action may vary depending on the violation of medical laws and severity of the action. Although minor breaches of medical law are subject to redress or warning via administrative action, suspension is possible when repeated violations occur. Therefore, nurses should understand clearly the scope of the norms to be followed to avoid unintentional violations.

The importance of patient safety has increased, and the protection of patients' rights is valued around the world. Demand for revision of the Medical Act in South Korea has grown over time, and efforts by nursing organizations and clinical institutions will be required to guarantee the safety and quality of nursing practice for patients and to help nurses avoid administrative dispositions. New nursing knowledge based on medical acts and patient safety will be developed, and further research using surveys and status analyses will be needed to help decrease the number of administrative disposition violations by nurses. In addition, clinical institutions such as hospitals need to organize education and supervision systems based on the Medical Act for nurses who provide care to patients, and nurses must work to gain full legal knowledge so they may avoid administrative dispositions because of unintentional violations of medical laws.

Conclusions and Implications

In this study, administrative dispositions of nurses were most frequently encountered in long-term care hospitals, with the main reasons for these dispositions including unlicensed medical practice and false charting. Moreover, having a higher number of specific standards related to an offense was found to be associated with a significantly longer period of license suspension. The results of this study suggest that nursing behaviors must be based on medical laws and that nurses must maintain correct nursing records. Furthermore, nurses must work to acquire knowledge related not only to medical laws but also to administrative laws, because administrative action may vary depending on the violation of medical law and the severity of the action. This study was the first to use raw, nationwide data to assess the administrative actions taken on nurses who committed illegal medical practices in South Korea. However, as the research data in this study were not obtained using structured questionnaires, the reliability and validity of these data are uncertain. Further research may use in-depth interviews with nurses to determine the reasons behind the illegal actions or decisions taken. On the basis of the findings of this study, future studies should extend the study period or incorporate larger sample populations to assess potential differences related to region, hospital type, career, or level of nurse experience. Because this study was conducted on Korean nurses, it should be easier to interpret the meaning of the findings by comparing each country's medical laws with the disposal of each country's violations and its criteria.

The administrative actions of medical personnel depend on the number and severity of violations. The findings of this study suggest that nurses must understand the details of relevant administrative dispositions to avoid violating medical laws.

Acknowledgment

We thank the people who managed the administrative dispositions of nurses in each city and province.

Author Contributions

Study conception and design: KSH
Data collection: KSY
Data analysis and interpretation: KSH
Drafting of the article: KSH, KSY
Critical revision of the article: KSH, KSY

References

Cho, J. T., & Park, J. (2019). Multi-level analysis of disorder policing and fear of crime in South Korea. *Asian Journal of Criminology, 14*(2), 113–127. https://doi.org/10.1007/s11417-019-9282-8

Choi, S., Jang, S. G., & Lee, W. (2019). The scope of practice for registered nurses in 64 South Korean laws. *Journal of Korean Academy of Nursing, 49*(6), 760–770. https://doi.org/10.4040/jkan.2019.49.6.760

Dronina, Y., Yoon, Y. M., Sakamaki, H., & Nam, E. W. (2016). Health system development and performance in Korea and Japan: A comparative study of 2000–2013. *American Journal of Lifestyle Medicine, 6*(1), 16–26. https://doi.org/10.15280/jlm.2016.6.1.16

Heo, S. W. (2014). The codification of administrative law in South Korea. In W. Y. Wang (Ed.), *Ius comparatum: Global studies in comparative law* (pp. 161–165). https://doi.org/10.1007/978-3-319-03446-1_14

Hong, S. E., Hong, M. K., Park, B. Y., Woo, K. J., & Kang, S. R. (2018). Is the "ghost surgery" the subject of legal punishment in Korea? *Annals of Surgical Treatment and Research, 94*(4), 167–173. https://doi.org/10.4174/astr.2018.94.4.167

Jang, B. Y., Kang, D. M., Kim, Y. K., Kim, S. Y., & Ko, K. S. (2018). The roles of doctors, nurses, and industrial hygienists in the healthcare management services in Korea: A comparison of the opinions of specialized health management institutions and entrusted enterprises. *Annals of Occupational and Environmental Medicine, 30*(1), Article 50. https://doi.org/10.1186/s40557-018-0261-9

Jeong, H. (2013). The role of administrative law in economic development and democracy in Korea. In Korea Legislation Research Institute (Ed.), *Introduction to Korean law* (pp. 85–112). Springer.

Jung, J. Y., Kim, S. Y., Kim, D. G., Kim, C. B., Chi, K.-C., Kang, W. K., & Lee, W. (2018). Analysis of lawsuit cases in the department of surgery in Korea. *Annals of Surgical Treatment and Research, 94*(3), 113_117. https://doi.org/10.4174/astr.2018.94.3.113

Kim, K. K., Kjervik, D. K., & Foster, B. (2014). Quality indicators for initial licensure and discipline in nursing laws in South Korea and North Carolina. *International Nursing Review, 61*(1), 35–43. https://doi.org/10.1111/inr.12069

Kim, S., & Choi, S. (2015). The medical professionalism of Korean physicians: Present and future. *BMC Medical Ethics, 16*, Article 56. https://doi.org/10.1186/s12910-015-0051-7

Kim, Y., Kim, J., & Shin, S. A. (2019). Relationship between the legal nurse staffing standard and patient survival after perioperative cardiac arrest: A cross-sectional analysis of Korean administrative data. *International Journal of Nursing Studies, 89*, 104–111. https://doi.org/10.1016/j.ijnurstu.2018.09.012

Lee, E. (2017). Reporting of medication administration errors by nurses in South Korean hospitals. *International Society for Quality in Health Care, 29*(5), 728–734. https://doi.org/10.1093/intqhc/mzx096

Lee, J. (2010). State control of medicine through legislation and revision of the Medical Law: Licensed and unlicensed medical practices in the 1950s–60s. *Ŭi Sahak, 19*(2), 85–431.

Lee, M. (2019). The effects of criminal punishment on medical practices in the medical environment. *International Journal of Environmental Research and Public Health, 16*(4), Article 604. https://doi.org/10.3390/ijerph16040604

Lee, M., Yoon, K., & Lee, K.-S. (2018). Social network analysis in the legislative process in the Korean medical device industry. *Inquiry, 55*, Article 46958018791858. https://doi.org/10.1177/0046958018791858

Lee, W., Kim, S. Y., Lee, S. I., Lee, S. G., Kim, H. C., & Kim, I. (2018). Barriers to reporting of patient safety incidents in tertiary hospitals: A qualitative study of nurses and resident physicians in South Korea. *International Journal of Health Planning and Management, 33*(4), 1178–1188. https://doi.org/10.1002/hpm.2616

Oh, E. G. (2018). Women's leadership and nursing profession in South Korea. *Asian Pacific Island Nursing Journal, 3*(2), 65–72. https://doi.org/10.31372/20180302.1085

Shin, J. H., & Hyun, T. K. (2015). Nurse staffing and quality of care of nursing home residents in Korea. *Journal of Nursing Scholarship, 47*(6), 555–564. https://doi.org/10.1111/jnu.12166

Shin, S., Park, J. D., & Shin, J. H. (2020). Improvement plan of nurse staffing standards in Korea. *Asian Nursing Research, 14*(2), 57–65. https://doi.org/10.1016/j.anr.2020.03.004

Yi, M. (2018). Leadership in nursing in Korea. *Asian Pacific Island Nursing Journal, 3*(2), 56–64. https://doi.org/10.31372/20180302.1082

5

The Impact of Nurse-Led Cardiac Rehabilitation on Quality of Life and Biophysiological Parameters in Patients With Heart Failure

Porkodi ARJUNAN[1]* • Ramakrishnan Venkatakrishnan TRICHUR[2]

ABSTRACT

Background: Cardiovascular diseases are the leading cause of mortality in the Indian subcontinent, accounting for 38% of deaths annually. One cardiovascular disease in particular, heart failure, is a growing public health problem both in India and worldwide.

Purpose: Heart failure is a chronic, progressive disease with increasing rates of incidence and prevalence. This study was conducted to determine the influence of a nurse-led cardiac rehabilitation program on quality of life and biophysiological parameters in patients with chronic heart failure. In this study, it was hypothesized that participants in the cardiac rehabilitation program would report significantly more-positive changes in quality of life and biophysiological parameters than their peers who did not participate in this program.

Methods: In this randomized controlled trial, the participants were patients with chronic heart failure who had been admitted to a tertiary care hospital in India. The participants assigned to the intervention group received both nurse-led cardiac rehabilitation and routine care. In addition, intervention group participants received a booklet on cardiac rehabilitation, *Healthy Way to Healthy Heart,* at discharge and fortnightly telephone reminders about good cardiac rehabilitation practices. A standard questionnaire was used to collect targeted information on participants' general and disease-specific quality of life at 1 and 3 months postintervention. Biophysiological parameters such as body mass index, blood pressure, and serum cholesterol values were also measured.

Results: Two thirds of the participants in each group (65% in the intervention group and 66% in the control group) were between 51 and 70 years old. The mean score for the mental component summary of generic quality of life steadily decreased in the control group and steadily increased in the intervention group at the first and second posttests.

Conclusions/Implications for Practice: Nurses working in cardiology units play a pivotal role in educating and managing the health status of patients with heart failure. Providing cardiac rehabilitation to patients with heart failure benefits the quality of life of these patients. Nurses working in cardiology units should encourage patients with heart failure to practice cardiac rehabilitation for a longer period to further improve their quality of life.

KEY WORDS:
biophysiological parameters, heart failure, nurse-led cardiac rehabilitation, quality of life, patients with chronic disease.

Introduction

Cardiovascular diseases (CVDs) are the leading cause of death worldwide, and in Southeast Asia, 38% of all deaths occur before the age of 70 years (World Health Organization, 2015). Heart failure (HF) is a CVD that is a growing public health problem both in India and worldwide (Nagai et al., 2016). Globally, HF affects approximately 26 million people (Ambrosy et al., 2014). In India, it has been reported that HF affects 1.3–4.6 million individuals, with an annual incidence of 0.5–1.8 million (Population Division, Department of Economic and Social Affairs, United Nations, 2013). In addition, over 5.1 million people live with HF in developed countries such as the United States of America (Hobbs et al., 2016), and this number is expected to increase to more than eight million by 2030 (Heidenreich et al., 2011).

HF is a syndrome of many CVDs, including coronary artery disease, hypertensive heart disease, dilated cardiomyopathy, and valvular heart disease (Felker et al., 2003). Therefore, the rising incidence of cardiac diseases that cause HF is increasing the rates of chronic HF (CHF) mortality and morbidity (Heart Failure Society of America, 2010). The effective management of HF depends on the related underlying cause. Hence, there are multiple combinations of treatments for HF, including medical, surgical, and supportive management (Shaffer & Maurer, 2015).

[1]PhD, RN, Reader, Faculty of Nursing, Sri Ramachandra Institute of Higher Education & Research (DU), Chennai, India • [2]MD, Professor, Department of Emergency Medicine, Sri Ramachandra Institute of Higher Education & Research (DU), Chennai, India.

Quality of life (QoL) is an important outcome indicator for patients with CVD (Amedro et al., 2016; Teixeira et al., 2011). Most patients with HF experience changes in functional abilities that negatively affect QoL (Hong, 2015). Thus, it is important that these patients adapt to the chronic nature of their condition by having thorough knowledge about this disease and its management. The common factors that affect QoL in patients with HF include attitudes toward following cardiac rehabilitation (CR), knowledge about the disease, and the current stage of the disease (Evangelista et al., 2010; Nesbitt et al., 2014).

The effective management of CHF also requires controlling the risk factors and lifestyle habits that are known to worsen the disease. For instance, decreased level of high-density lipoproteins (HDL) is a risk factor for cardiovascular events (Forti & Diament, 2006). A significant association between increased cholesterol level and poor outcomes in patients with CHF has been highlighted in prior studies (Kalantar-Zadeh et al., 2004). Furthermore, poor prognosis has been reported in patients with CHF because of decreased serum sodium level (Rusinaru et al., 2012), decreased hemoglobin level in the blood, and low ejection fraction (Ezekowitz et al., 2003; Tang & Katz, 2006). In addition, other physiological parameters such as decreased body mass index (BMI) have been associated with increased mortality in patients with CHF (Pocock et al., 2005).

CR is a major component of the critical management required by patients with CHF. Therefore, it is important to teach patients with CHF regarding the nature of this disease and the associated behavioral and lifestyle modifications necessary to achieve effective management. Educating patients with CHF is most effective when it is tailored to patient age group and disease status (Schopfer & Forman, 2016). CR has been reported in many studies to have a positive effect on QoL in patients with HF (Conway, 2015). On the basis of the literature, topics such as etiology, pathophysiology, signs and symptoms, pharmacological treatment, lifestyle modification, diet and exercise, sexual activity, sleep and breathing disorders, adherence, psychosocial aspects, and disease prognosis (McMurray et al., 2012) should be included in educational programs designed for patients with HF.

The objective of this study was to evaluate the effect of a nurse-led CR program on QoL and biophysiological parameters in patients with HF.

Methods

Study Design and Participants

This randomized controlled trial study was conducted at one tertiary care hospital in India. Two hundred patients hospitalized with HF and between 31 and 88 years old were enrolled and randomly assigned into either the intervention or control group using computer-generated block randomization. The English alphabet letters "A" (intervention group) and "B" (control group) were affixed to 10 blocks each. The resultant 20 blocks were sealed individually in sequentially numbered, opaque envelopes and locked in the principal investigator's office cupboard. The sample size for this study was calculated based on a previous study (Austin et al., 2005). Considering QoL as the primary outcome, the estimated sample size was 180, which achieved a power of 80% at a level of significance at .05. A 10% attrition rate was estimated. Thus, a sample size of 200 was recruited, with 100 in each group. The study participants were blinded to group assignment. Inclusion criteria included > 31 years old, a medical diagnosis of HF with ejection fraction less than 40%, and dyspnea Grades II and III based on the New York Heart Association classification. Exclusion criteria included having undergone surgery as a part of the treatment for HF; experiencing complications such as arrhythmias, peripheral vascular disease, cerebrovascular accident, and end-stage renal disease; having a history of congenital heart disease; and having a treatment plan that involves ventricular assistive devices.

Measurement

The demographic variables of the participants were assessed using a structured questionnaire. General QoL and disease-specific QoL were assessed using the following standard questionnaires: Medical Outcomes Study Questionnaire Short Form 36 Health Survey (SF-36) and the Minnesota Living with Heart Failure Questionnaire (MLHFQ). The SF-36 was used to assess functional health and well-being scores as well as physical and mental health summary measures. This tool comprises 36 items that are each scored using a 5-point Likert scale. The physical component summary of the SF-36 includes the four domains of physical functioning, role functioning physical, bodily pain, and general health perceptions, whereas the mental component summary includes the four domains of vitality, social functioning, role functioning emotional, and mental health. A higher total score on the SF-36 indicates better QoL. The reliability of the SF-36 was previously measured as .90.

Disease-specific QoL was measured using the MLHFQ. This tool includes 21 items covering HF-related physical, psychological, and social impairments in three domains, including physical (eight items), emotional (five items), and global (all 21 items). Each item is rated on a scale of 0–5, with higher scores indicating poorer QoL. The reliability of the MLHFQ was previously measured as .87. The biophysiological measures considered in this study included BMI, systolic and diastolic blood pressure (BP), lipid profile, hemoglobin, random blood sugar, serum sodium, and potassium.

Intervention

After conducting the pretest, the nurse-led CR program, consisting of structured teaching about the disease condition, diet, exercise, medication, home care instruction, smoking cessation, and lifestyle modification, was administered on a one-to-one basis in three different sessions at the bedside of the intervention group. The intervention group was further required to participate in a 6-minute walk test. A booklet, *Healthy Way to Healthy Heart*, was provided to the intervention group on the day of discharge. In addition, telephone calls were made to each intervention group participant once every 2 weeks over the 3-month posttest period. Posttest 1 data were collected 1 month after the intervention, and Posttest 2 data were collected 3 months after the intervention. The participants in the control group received routine care only (e.g., physician's visits, nursing care, physiotherapy) and received the booklet *Healthy Way to Healthy Life* after providing Posttest 2 data.

Data Collection Procedures

The data were collected from January 8, 2011, to October 2, 2014. The institutional review board of Sri Ramachandra Medical College & Research Institute (Deemed University) approved this study (IEC[NI]/07/Nov/01/03). The principal investigator explained to the participants the risks and benefits of the study and the confidentiality of the data as well as answered questions before obtaining informed consent. The demographic variables of the study participants were collected via one-to-one interviews and medical records. QoL information was collected from the participants using the two questionnaires (SF-36 V2 and MLHFQ), and biophysiological parameters were collected from medical records. After confirming appointments with intervention group participants, the investigator visited them at their bedside and taught them CR for 3 consecutive days using a laptop. The booklet *Healthy Way to Healthy Life* was given to intervention group participants at discharge, and they were contacted by the investigator once every 2 weeks over the 3-month posttest period as part of the reinforcement process. The pretest data collection was conducted on the second day of hospital admission. Posttest 1 was conducted 30 days after completion of the intervention, with completed questionnaires collected by the investigator at each participant's 1-month follow-up clinical visit. Posttest 2 was conducted 90 days after completion of the intervention, with completed questionnaires collected by the investigator at each participant's 3-month follow-up clinical visit (Figure 1).

Figure 1

A Flowchart: Data Collection Procedure

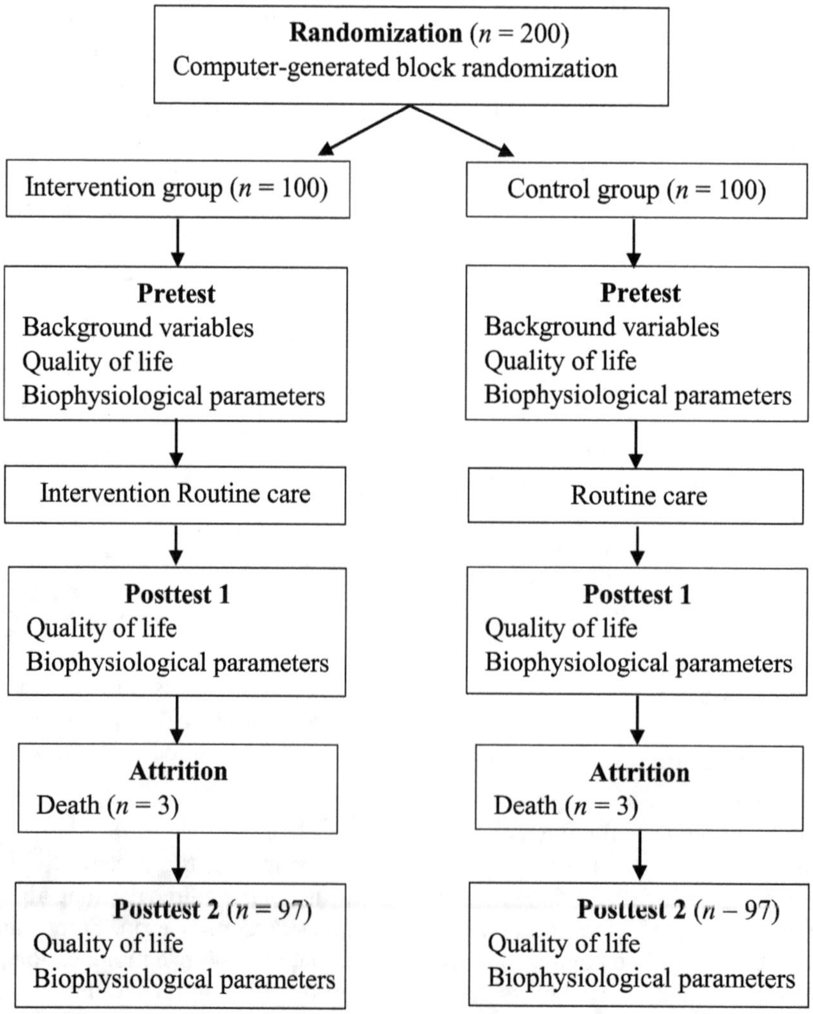

Statistical Analysis

Continuous variables are presented in this study as mean and standard deviation, whereas categorical variables are presented as frequencies and percentages. A paired t test was conducted to identify the effect of the structured teaching program on QoL and biophysiological parameters. An independent t test was conducted to compare differences in variable values between the intervention and control groups. A nonparametric test such as the Wilcoxon signed ranks test and Mann–Whitney test was conducted when a nonnormal distribution of a mean value greater than 2 times of the standard deviation was observed. Repeated-measures analysis of variance was used to compare the intervention effect among pretest, Posttest 1, and Posttest 2. For all of the statistical tests, a p value of < .05 was considered significant. All of the statistical analyses were performed using SPSS Version 22.0 (IBM, Inc., Armonk, NY, USA).

Results

Demographics of the Study Participants

Two hundred patients with HF were included as participants in this study. As shown in Table 1, most of the participants were in the 51- to 70-year age range in both the intervention group (65%) and the control group (66%), and over three quarters of the participants were male in both the intervention group (78%) and the control group (79%). Furthermore, no significant differences were identified between the two groups in terms of demographic characteristics, with the exception of monthly total family income (p = .028).

Intergroup Comparison of Biophysiological Parameters at Pretest

The biophysiological parameter data for the two groups at pretest are shown in Table 2. The mean scores for BMI were within the normal range for both groups, and the mean values for low-density lipoprotein values were at the optimal level for both groups. The HDL mean scores for the intervention group (33.91) and control group (35.12) indicate a high risk for heart disease. Random blood sugar level was above normal for both groups. Other biophysiological parameters, including systolic and diastolic BP, sodium, potassium, and hemoglobin, were within normal limits for both groups. Furthermore, no significant differences in biophysiological parameters were identified between the two groups at pretest.

Intergroup Comparison of Biophysiological Parameters at Posttest 2

The results summarized in Table 3 show significant differences in diastolic BP (t = 3.86, p < .001), HDL (t = 8.43, p < .001), hemoglobin (t = 2.31, p = .02), random blood sugar (t = 2.55, p = .01), sodium (t = 3.93, p < .001), and potassium (t = 5.01, p < .001) levels between the intervention and control groups after the intervention, with the intervention group showing significantly lower mean levels than the control group.

Impact on Quality of Life

The results presented in Table 4 show at Posttest 2 a significant improvement in the physical component (t = 2.23, p = .02), mental component (t = 11.17, p < .001), and disease-specific (t = 5.92, p < .001) QoL of the participants in the intervention group in comparison with the control group. Moreover, disease-specific QoL (t = 2.19, p = .02) improved more significantly in the intervention group than in the control group at Posttest 1.

Result of Repeated Measure on Quality of Life

The results in Table 5 describe the changes from baseline in the physical, mental, and disease-specific QoL of the participants, indicating that significant interactions have a more favorable effect on the physical (M = 46.53, SD = 3.72), mental (M = 45.93, SD = 6.70), and disease-specific (M = 33.24, SD = 9.18) QoL in the intervention group than in the control group. The intervention group exhibited an increase in QoL during the second posttest.

Discussion

The results of this study show that the CR educational program, which focused on improving disease knowledge, exercise, medication, and lifestyle habits, effectively improved QoL in the intervention group. The physical component of the generic QoL in the intervention group gradually increased from baseline through the second posttest. This suggests that following the rehabilitation program for a minimum of 3 months should improve physical QoL in patients with HF. The patients who received only routine care in the control group experienced a gradual decrease in the physical component of the generic QoL from baseline through the second posttest. These findings are consistent with Hasanpour-Dehkordi et al. (2016), who found that training, caring, and consultative nursing interventions improve QoL in patients with CHF.

In addition, the findings of this study indicate that this nurse-led CR program significantly and rapidly (within 1 month postintervention) improves the mental health components of QoL such as vitality, social functioning, role functioning emotional, and mental health. This suggests that there is a need to enhance physical care for problems common among patients with HF such as body pain and measures to improve self-care. It also further substantiates that receiving adequate knowledge regarding disease condition and lifestyle modification enhances the confidence of patients with HF to live a healthy life, thereby improving their functional abilities.

Table 1

Participants' Demographic Characteristics (N = 200)

Demographic Variable	Intervention (*n* = 100)		Control Group (*n* = 100)		χ^2	*p*
	n	%	*n*	%		
Age (years; mean = 59.57, *SD* = 11.16)					1.18	.550
31–50	22	22	17	17		
51–70	65	65	66	66		
> 70	13	13	17	17		
Gender					0.03	.863
Male	78	78	79	79		
Female	22	22	21	21		
Level of education					0.88	.820
Nonliterate	14	14	10	10		
Primary school	23	23	22	22		
High school	45	45	49	49		
College	18	18	19	19		
Occupation					0.04	.980
Skilled	44	44	45	45		
Professional	21	21	20	20		
Retired	35	35	35	35		
Marital status					4.80	.187
Married	96	96	96	96		
Unmarried	4	4	1	1		
Separated/widowed	0	0	3	3		
Religion					2.63	.269
Hindu	91	91	90	90		
Christian	4	4	8	8		
Muslim	5	5	2	2		
Residence					1.85	.397
Urban	50	50	41	41		
Rural	19	19	25	25		
Semiurban	31	31	34	34		
Monthly total family income (USD)					9.08	.028*
≤ 59.35	41	41	22	22		
59.36–89.02	21	21	23	23		
89.03–118.70	13	13	21	21		
> 118.70	25	25	34	34		
Type of family					0.33	.565
Extended family	57	57	61	61		
Nuclear	43	43	39	39		
Tobacco use					0.99	.321
Yes	21	21	27	27		
No	79	79	73	73		

The baseline disease-specific QoL for both groups in this study was nearly equivalent, whereas the first and second posttest scores for disease-specific QoL improved significantly in the intervention group and decreased significantly in the control group. CR education, exercise, and improved 6-minute walk functional ability may contribute to the identified improvements in QoL in the intervention group. Cajanding (2016) reported similar findings in Filipino patients with HF who underwent cognitive behavioral therapy and reported significant improvements in QoL, self-esteem, and mood scores compared with the control (standard care) group.

Biophysiological Parameters

Regarding the impact of the nurse-led CR on BMI, no significant difference was found between the two groups from pretest through the second posttest. The average BMI from pretest to the second posttest had increased in both the

Table 2

Biophysiological Parameters of the Intervention and Control Groups at Pretest (N = 200)

Biophysiological Parameter	Intervention Group (*n* = 100)		Control Group (*n* = 100)		Mean Difference	*t*	*p*
	Mean	*SD*	Mean	*SD*			
BMI (kg/m^2)	24.29	3.02	24.94	3.92	0.65	1.31	.18
Systolic BP (mmHg)	124.22	22.10	125.12	16.47	0.90	0.32	.74
Diastolic BP (mmHg)	78.88	11.95	80.14	9.31	1.26	0.83	.40
LDL (mg/dL)	99.84	40.82	94.26	37.92	5.58	0.89	.37
HDL (mg/dL)	33.91	15.03	35.12	10.51	1.21	0.59	.55
Triglyceride (mg/dL)	121.08	73.53	132.72	72.62	11.64	1.35	.17
Hemoglobin (gm/dL)	12.28	2.33	12.27	2.07	0.01	0.03	.97
RBS (mg/dL)	174.20	97.09	176.70	107.97	2.49	0.40	.68
Serum sodium (mEq/L)	134.46	6.05	134.26	5.35	0.20	0.24	.80
Serum potassium (mEq/L)	4.17	0.77	4.10	0.73	0.07	0.72	.46

Note. BMI = body mass index; BP = blood pressure; LDL = low-density lipoprotein; HDL = high-density lipoprotein; RBS = random blood sugar.

groups with a mean difference of 0.59, which, although not statistically significant, had clinical significance because the intervention group was within normal BMI whereas the BMI of the control group had increased. This may be attributable to dietary habit changes made after reading the booklet and to routine care by the dietician who visited both of the groups and discussed the diet plan.

The results showed no significant differences in biophysiological parameters such as BMI, BP, hemoglobin, random blood sugar, and serum electrolytes between the two groups during pretest. Moreover, diastolic BP level was within normal when compared with the control group. Therefore, the changes observed in diastolic BP occurred within the normal level. The 3-month follow-up period may not be sufficient to show significant changes in patients with HF, and it is possible that the mortality rate in the control group would increase. However, Tuomilehto et al. (1998) indicated that low diastolic BP is a significant predictor of cardiovascular mortality in the older adult (> 50 years old) population and that the risk of death from low diastolic BP and high systolic BP is higher in patients with CHF. These findings were not in agreement with this study.

Table 3

Changes in Biophysiological Parameters Between the Intervention and Control Groups After the Intervention: Posttest 2 (N = 200)

Biophysiological Parameter	Intervention Group		Control Group		Mean Difference	*t*	*p*
	Mean	*SD*	Mean	*SD*			
BMI (kg/m^2)	24.54	2.99	25.13	3.67	0.59	1.23	.22
Systolic BP (mmHg)	123.96	9.09	126.74	9.41	2.78	2.09	.38
Diastolic BP (mmHg)	80.39	5.77	83.63	5.88	3.23	3.86	< .001***
LDL (mg/dL)	90.24	6.07	87.62	23.36	2.61	1.06	.28
HDL (mg/dL)	49.46	6.18	41.00	7.71	8.46	8.43	< .001***
Triglyceride (mg/dL)	109.29	23.90	118.56	42.91	9.26	1.85	.06
Hemoglobin (gm/dL)	12.15	1.73	11.61	1.52	0.54	2.31	.02*
RBS (mg/dL)	137.71	34.74	153.67	5.67	15.95	2.55	.01**
Serum sodium (mEq/L)	139.90	3.90	137.91	3.09	1.99	3.93	< .001***
Serum potassium (mEq/L)	4.32	0.51	4.02	0.28	0.29	5.01	< .001***

Note. BMI = body mass index; BP = blood pressure; LDL = low-density lipoprotein; HDL = high-density lipoprotein; RBS = random blood sugar.
**p* < .05. ***p* < .01. ****p* < .001.

Table 4

Changes From Baseline in Quality of Life Between the Intervention and Control Groups at Posttests 1 and 2 (N = 200)

Variable	Intervention Group (*n* = 100)		Control Group (*n* = 100)		Mean Difference	*t*	*p*
	Mean	*SD*	Mean	*SD*			
Physical component QoL							
Pretest	33.69	7.68	35.47	5.87	1.78	1.84	.06
Posttest 1	43.67	6.85	42.92	8.05	0.75	0.71	.47
Posttest 2	46.53	3.72	44.87	6.30	1.66	2.23	.02*
Mental component QoL							
Pretest	38.64	11.67	41.87	12.32	3.22	1.90	.05
Posttest 1	38.85	7.45	39.64	10.28	0.79	0.62	.53
Posttest 2	45.93	6.70	34.87	7.07	11.05	11.17	< .001***
Disease-specific QoL							
Pretest	48.51	24.30	43.70	20.99	4.81	1.49	.13
Posttest 1	35.37	14.47	40.12	16.07	4.75	2.19	.02*
Posttest 2	33.24	9.18	43.33	14.03	10.09	5.92	< .001***

Note. QOL = quality of life.
$^{*}p < .05$. $^{***}p < .001$.

Dyslipidemia significantly affected the control group, whereas posttest HDL levels were significantly improved in the intervention group. Potočnjak et al. (2016) found an association between low HDL cholesterol and increased risk for hospital mortality in acute patients with HF. BMI was calculated using the standard equation and expressed as kilograms per square meter (kg/m^2). The results of this study indicate that CR education has minimal/no effect on BMI. However, Tevik et al. (2015) found that poor nutritional status almost doubled the risk of early mortality, independent of age and HF severity. The mean scores for BMI, systolic BP, low-density lipoproteins, and triglycerides for both groups indicate that biophysiological parameters fell within normal ranges. These findings are similar to Miller et al. (2011), who found that participants with a normal BMI (< 25 kg/m^2) were more likely to have triglyceride levels < 150 mg/dl (43%) and < 200 mg/dl (39%).

Implications for Practice

Nurses working in cardiology units should encourage patients with HF to practice CR for longer periods to improve their QoL. CR programs should be incorporated into the management plans for patients with HF to enhance QoL.

Table 5

Repeated-Measures ANOVA on Quality of Life at Different Periods of Time Among the Intervention and Control Groups (N = 200)

Quality of Life	Pretest		Posttest 1		Posttest 2		*F*	*p*
	Mean	*SD*	Mean	*SD*	Mean	*SD*		
PCS							5.35	.020*
Intervention group	33.72	7.74	43.84	6.77	46.53	3.72		
Control group	35.61	5.78	43.27	7.88	44.87	6.31		
MCS							42.65	< .001***
Intervention group	38.60	11.59	38.93	7.02	45.93	6.70		
Control group	42.01	12.42	40.09	9.99	34.87	7.07		
Disease specific							12.26	.001***
Intervention group	48.09	24.46	34.86	13.62	33.24	9.18		
Control group	43.60	21.20	39.67	16.07	43.33	14.03		

Note. ANOVA = analysis of variance; PCS = physical component summary; MCS = mental component summary.
$^{*}p < .05$. $^{***}p < .001$.

Nurses may adopt telenursing strategies to overcome the physical problems that typically impeded postdischarge access to patients with HF. Long-term follow-up studies or cohort studies are necessary to assess the durability of the benefits of rehabilitation interventions in patients with HF.

Limitations

This study was limited to a single center, and thus the generalizability of findings may be affected. Participation was limited to patients diagnosed with HF because of coronary artery disease, dilated cardiomyopathy, or hypertensive heart disease and with ejection fractions below 40%. Diagnoses of myocardial infarction and valvular heart disease leading to HF were excluded because the mode of treatment for these conditions is surgery.

Conclusions

CHF affects the QoL of patients, with the most significant impacts affecting physical aspects such as physical functioning, role functioning physical, bodily pain, and general health perceptions and less significantly affecting mental health aspects such as vitality, social functioning, role functioning emotional, and mental health. Nurses involved in CR should focus on improving the physical functioning of patients with CHF.

Author Contributions

Study conception and design: PA, RVT
Data collection: PA
Data analysis and interpretation: PA
Drafting of the article: PA
Critical revision of the article: RVT

References

Ambrosy, A. P., Fonarow, G. C., Butler, J., Chioncel, O., Greene, S. J., Vaduganathan, M., Nodari, S., Lam, C. S. P., Sato, N., Shah, A. N., & Gheorghiade, M. (2014). The global health and economic burden of hospitalizations for heart failure: Lessons learned from hospitalized heart failure registries. *Journal of the American College of Cardiology, 63*(12), 1123–1133. https://doi.org/10.1016/j.jacc.2013.11.053

Amedro, P., Picot, M. C., Moniotte, S., Dorka, R., Bertet, H., Guillaumont, S., Barrea, C., Vincenti, M., De La Villeon, G., Bredy, C., Soulatges, C., Voisin, M., Matecki, S., & Auquier, P. (2016). Correlation between cardio-pulmonary exercise test variables and health-related quality of life among children with congenital heart diseases. *International Journal of Cardiology, 203*, 1052–1060. https://doi.org/10.1016/j.ijcard.2015.11.028

Austin, J., Williams, R., Ross, L., Moseley, L., & Hutchison, S. (2005). Randomised controlled trial of cardiac rehabilitation in elderly patients with heart failure. *European Journal of Heart Failure, 7*(3), 411–417. https://doi.org/10.1016/j.ejheart.2004.10.004

Cajanding, R. J. M. (2016). The effectiveness of a nurse-led cognitive–behavioral therapy on the quality of life, self-esteem and mood among Filipino patients living with heart failure: A randomized controlled trial. *Applied Nursing Research, 31*, 86–93. https://doi.org/10.1016/j.apnr.2016.01.002

Conway, B. (2015). Rehabilitation for patients with heart failure. *Practice Nursing, 26*(4), 168–171. https://doi.org/10.12968/pnur.2015.26.4.168

Evangelista, L. S., Rasmusson, K. D., Laramee, A. S., Barr, J., Ammon, S. E., Dunbar, S., Ziesche, S., Patterson, J. H., & Yancy, C. W. (2010). Health literacy and the patient with heart failure—Implications for patient care and research: A consensus statement of the Heart Failure Society of America. *Journal of Cardiac Failure, 16*(1), 9–16. https://doi.org/10.1016/j.cardfail.2009.10.026

Ezekowitz, J. A., McAlister, F. A., & Armstrong, P. W. (2003). Anemia is common in heart failure and is associated with poor outcomes: Insights from a cohort of 12 065 patients with new-onset heart failure. *Circulation, 107*(2), 223–225. https://doi.org/10.1161/01.CIR.0000052622.51963.FC

Felker, G. M., Adams, K. F. Jr., Konstam, M. A., O'connor, C. M., & Gheorghiade, M. (2003). The problem of decompensated heart failure: Nomenclature, classification, and risk stratification. *American Heart Journal, 145*(2), S18–S25. https://doi.org/10.1067/mhj.2003.150

Forti, N., & Diament, J. (2006). High-density lipoproteins: Metabolic, clinical, epidemiological and therapeutic intervention aspects. An update for clinicians. *Arquivos Brasileiros de Cardiologia (Brazilian Archives of Cardiology), 87*(5), 671–679. https://doi.org/10.1590/S0066-782x2006001800019 (Original work published in Portuguese)

Hasanpour-Dehkordi, A., Khaledi-Far, A., Khaledi-Far, B., & Salehi-Tali, S. (2016). The effect of family training and support on the quality of life and cost of hospital readmissions in congestive heart failure patients in Iran. *Applied Nursing Research, 31*, 165–169. https://doi.org/10.1016/j.apnr.2016.03.005

Heart Failure Society of America. (2010). Executive summary: HFSA 2010 comprehensive heart failure practice guideline. *Journal of Cardiac Failure, 16*(6), 475–539. https://doi.org/10.1016/j.cardfail.2010.04.005

Heidenreich, P. A., Trogdon, J. G., Khavjou, O. A., Butler, J., Dracup, K., Ezekowitz, M. D., Finkelstein, E. A., Hong, Y., Johnston, S. C., Khera, A., Lloyd-Jones, D. M., Nelson, S. A., Nichol, G., Orenstein, D., Wilson, P. W., Woo, Y. J., & American Heart Association Advocacy Coordinating Committee; Stroke Council; Council on Cardiovascular Radiology and Intervention; Council on Clinical Cardiology; Council on Epidemiology and Prevention; Council on Arteriosclerosis; Thrombosis and Vascular Biology; Council on Cardiopulmonary; Critical Care; Perioperative and Resuscitation; Council on Cardiovascular Nursing; Council on the Kidney in Cardiovascular Disease; Council on Cardiovascular Surgery and Anesthesia, and Interdisciplinary Council on Quality of Care and Outcomes Research (2011). Forecasting the future of cardiovascular disease in the

United States: A policy statement from the American Heart Association. *Circulation, 123*(8), 933–944. https://doi.org/10.1161/CIR.0b013e31820a55f5

Hobbs, J. K., Escutia, D., Harrison, H., Moore, A., & Sarpong, E. (2016). Reducing hospital readmission rates in patients with heart failure. *Medsurg Nursing, 25*(3), 145–152.

Hong, E. (2015). Health-related quality of life and health condition of community-dwelling populations with cancer, stroke, and cardiovascular disease. *Journal of Physical Therapy Science, 27*(8), 2521–2524. https://doi.org/10.1589/jpts.27.2521

Kalantar-Zadeh, K., Block, G., Horwich, T., & Fonarow, G. C. (2004). Reverse epidemiology of conventional cardiovascular risk factors in patients with chronic heart failure. *Journal of the American College of Cardiology, 43*(8), 1439–1444. https://doi.org/10.1016/j.jacc.2003.11.039

McMurray, J. J., Adamopoulos, S., Anker, S. D., Auricchio, A., Böhm, M., Dickstein, K., Falk, V., Filippatos, G., Fonseca, C., Gomez-Sanchez, M. A., Jaarsma, T., Køber, L., Lip, G. Y., Maggioni, A. P., Parkhomenko, A., Pieske, B. M., Popescu, B. A., Rønnevik, P. K., Rutten, F. H., ... Zeiher, A., & ESC Committee for Practice Guidelines. (2012). ESC guidelines for the diagnosis and treatment of acute and chronic heart failure 2012: The Task force for the diagnosis and treatment of acute and chronic heart failure 2012 of the European Society of Cardiology. Developed in collaboration with the Heart Failure Association (HFA) of the ESC. *European Heart Journal, 33*(14), 1787–1847. https://doi.org/10.1093/eurheartj/ehs104

Miller, M., Stone, N. J., Ballantyne, C., Bittner, V., Criqui, M. H., Ginsberg, H. N., Goldberg, A. C., Howard, W. J., Jacobson, M. S., Kris-Etherton, P. M., Lennie, T. A., Levi, M., Mazzone, T., Pennathur, S., & American Heart Association Clinical Lipidology, Thrombosis, and Prevention Committee of the Council on Nutrition, Physical Activity, and Metabolism; Council on Arteriosclerosis, Thrombosis and Vascular Biology; Council on Cardiovascular Nursing; Council on the Kidney in Cardiovascular Disease. (2011). Triglycerides and cardiovascular disease: A scientific statement from the American Heart Association. *Circulation, 123*(20), 2292–2333. https://doi.org/10.1161/CIR.0b013e3182160726

Nagai, T., Honda, Y., Sugano, Y., Nishimura, K., Nakai, M., Honda, S., Iwakami, N., Okada, A., Asaumi, Y., Aiba, T., Noguchi, T., Kusano, K., Ogawa, H., Yasuda, S., Anzai, T., & NaDEF Investigators. (2016). Circulating omega-6, but not omega-3 polyunsaturated fatty acids, are associated with clinical outcomes in patients with acute decompensated heart failure. *PLOS ONE, 11*(11), Article e0165841. https://doi.org/10.1371/journal.pone.0165841

Nesbitt, T., Doctorvaladan, S., Southard, J. A., Singh, S., Fekete, A., Marie, K., Moser, D. K., Pelter, M. M., Robinson, S., Wilson, M. D., Cooper, L., & Dracup, K. (2014). Correlates of quality of life in rural patients with heart failure. *Circulation: Heart Failure, 7*(6), 882–887. https://doi.org/10.1161/CIRCHEARTFAILURE.113.000577

Pocock, S. J., Wang, D., Pfeffer, M. A., Yusuf, S., McMurray, J. J., Swedberg, K. B., Ostergren, J., Michelson, E. L., Pieper, K. S., & Granger, C. B. (2005). Predictors of mortality and morbidity in patients with chronic heart failure. *European Heart Journal, 27*(1), 65–75. https://doi.org/10.1093/eurheartj/ehi555

Population Division, Department of Economic and Social Affairs, United Nations. (2013). *World population prospects: The 2012 revision, highlights and advance tables.* Working Paper No. ESA/P/WP.228.

Potočnjak, I., Degoricija, V., Trbušić, M., Terešak, S. D., Radulović, B., Pregartner, G., Berghold, A., Tiran, B., Marsche, G., & Frank, S. (2016). Metrics of high-density lipoprotein function and hospital mortality in acute heart failure patients. *PLOS ONE, 11*(6), Article e0157507. https://doi.org/10.1371/journal.pone.0157507

Rusinaru, D., Tribouilloy, C., Berry, C., Richards, A. M., Whalley, G. A., Earle, N., Poppe, K. K., Guazzi, M., Macin, S. M., Komajda, M., & Doughty, R. N. (2012). Relationship of serum sodium concentration to mortality in a wide spectrum of heart failure patients with preserved and with reduced ejection fraction: An individual patient data meta-analysis†: Meta-Analysis Global Group in Chronic heart failure (MAGGIC). *European Journal of Heart Failure, 14*(10), 1139–1146. https://doi.org/10.1093/eurjhf/hfs099

Schopfer, D. W., & Forman, D. E. (2016). Growing relevance of cardiac rehabilitation for an older population with heart failure. *Journal of Cardiac Failure, 22*(12), 1015–1022. https://doi.org/10.1016/j.cardfail.2016.10.010

Shaffer, J. A., & Maurer, M. S. (2015). Multiple chronic conditions and heart failure: Overlooking the obvious? *JACC: Heart Failure, 3*(7), 551–553. https://doi.org/10.1016/j.jchf.2015.04.005

Tang, Y. D., & Katz, S. D. (2006). Anemia in chronic heart failure: Prevalence, etiology, clinical correlates, and treatment options. *Circulation, 113*(20), 2454–2461. https://doi.org/10.1161/CIRCULATIONAHA.105.583666

Teixeira, F. M., Coelho, R. M., Proença, C., Silva, A. M., Vieira, D., Vaz, C., Moura, C., Viana, V., Areias, J. C., & Areias, M. E. (2011). Quality of life experienced by adolescents and young adults with congenital heart disease. *Pediatric Cardiology, 32* (8), 1132–1138. https://doi.org/10.1007/s00246-011-0039

Tevik, K., Thürmer, H., Husby, M. I., de Soysa, A. K., & Helvik, A. S. (2015). Nutritional risk screening in hospitalized patients with heart failure. *Clinical Nutrition, 34*(2), 257–264. https://doi.org/10.1016/j.clnu.2014.03.014

Tuomilehto, J., Ryynänen, O. P., Koistinen, A., Rastenyte, D., Nissinen, A., & Puska, P. (1998). Low diastolic blood pressure and mortality in a population-based cohort of 16 913 hypertensive patients in North Karelia, Finland. *Journal of Hypertension, 16*(9), 1235–1242.

World Health Organization. (2015). *Cardiovascular diseases (CVDs): Fact sheet.* http://www.searo.who.int/india/topics/cardiovascular_diseases/factsheet_cvd_2015.pdf

6

The Relationship Between Nursing Workload, Quality of Care and Nursing Payment in Intensive Care Units

Li-Yin CHANG[1] • Hsiu-Hui YU[2] • Yann-Fen C. CHAO[3]*

ABSTRACT

Background: Nursing workload is highly associated with patient safety. It has been argued that the imbalance between nursing payment and nursing workload in Taiwan National Health Insurance (NHI)-covered intensive care units (ICUs) has resulted in the inadequate allocation of nursing manpower. However, limited empirical data are currently available to support this argument.

Purpose: The aim of this study was to investigate the correlation between nursing workload, quality of care, and NHI-covered nursing payments in ICU settings.

Methods: This macrodata analysis study retrieved data from the existing ICU patient classification system, nursing quality monitoring system, and infection control monitoring system of a medical center in central Taiwan. Data on the Therapeutic Intervention Scoring System-28 (TISS-28) and non-TISS-28 scores, nursing hours, and nursing labor utilization rate were retrieved for the 23-month period beginning in January 2013 and ending in November 2014. The indices of care quality used in this study included incidence of falls, pressure sore density, incidence of restraint use, incidence of tube self-extraction, and infection density.

Results: A total of 92,442 data sets were collected from eight ICUs, with 61% of the direct ICU nursing hours categorized as TISS-28 and 39% categorized as non-TISS-28. Mean nursing hours totaled 12.5 hours. The direct nursing hours, the total nursing hours, the bed occupancy rate, the nursing hours calculated by patient classification system, and the nursing hours calculated by nurse–patient ratio were statistically, significantly correlated respectively with all of the care quality indices except for incidence of falls. The number of items of patient care in the patient classification records was greater than that of NHI-covered nursing payments. The NHI-covered nursing payment for every patient accounted for only 4.77% of the total medical expenses in the ICU.

Conclusions/Implications for Practice: Data from the patient classification database, quality monitoring database, and medical cost database indicate excessive nursing workload and underpayment from the Taiwan NHI program. Current nursing workload was significantly associated with care quality. This study provides empirical data for administrators to consider when revising nursing staffing and NHI payment policies.

Key Words:
nursing workload, care quality, nursing payment, patient classification system.

Introduction

The intensive care unit (ICU) workload affects care quality and mortality (Aiken et al., 2011; Cho et al., 2015; Cho, Hwang, & Kim, 2008; Cho & Yun, 2009; Miranda, de Rijk, & Schaufeli, 1996; Padilha et al., 2007). Care quality is negatively influenced by factors including patient falls, pressure sores, infections, and other adverse events. A systematic literature review investigating resources and adverse outcomes in nursing ICUs indicated that, of 15 studies (1989–2002), only two found a statistical correlation among nursing resources and adverse events, only one found a correlation between nursing resources and mortality, seven found no statistical correlation between nursing resources and mortality, and 10 found a correlation between nursing resources and adverse events, although no statistical tests were performed (West, Mays, Rafferty, Rowan, & Sanderson, 2009). Miranda et al. (1996) developed the Therapeutic Intervention Scoring System-28 (TISS-28) to reclassify and simplify the 76 items of the TISS into 28 items. They also performed an investigation on nursing activities and divided these into six major categories, with TISS-28 as one of the categories. TISS-28 may also be used to predict the therapeutic costs and work assignments of nursing personnel (Goj, Knapik, Kucewicz-Czech, & Lubon, 2009) as the basis for the workloads of different ICU nursing

[1]*PhD, RN, Director, Department of Nursing, China Medical University Hospital, and Adjunct Assistant Professor, Department of Nursing, China Medical University* • [2]*MSN, RN, Department of Nursing, Taichung Veterans General Hospital* • [3]*PhD, RN, Chair Professor, College of Nursing, Hungkuang University.*

personnel (Padilha et al., 2007). Furthermore, recent studies in Taiwan investigating the correlation between nursing workload and patient safety have shown a correlation between hours of overtime and patient safety indices. In addition, when the patient–nurse ratio exceeds 7, the risks associated with indices such as falls, decubitus, the incidence of tube self-extraction, nosocomial pneumonia, and urinary tract infection increase (Liu, Lee, Chia, Chi, & Yin, 2012). Moreover, the findings of some studies indicate that increasing daily nursing hours by 1 hour decreases the number of patients with infection in wards by 0.02%, decreases the number of patients receiving cardiopulmonary resuscitation in wards by 0.18%, and increases the number of emergency patient success rate of resuscitation by 0.17% (Liang et al., 2010).

Despite the high average number of hours spent by nurses on caring for ICU patients, the Taiwan National Health Insurance (NHI) Administration (formerly the Bureau of NHI) approved payments averaging only NT$16,883 per nurse per month. This amount accounts for less than 40% of the average personnel costs of nursing personnel (NT$47,000). Moreover, the 42 specific NHI-covered diagnosis/treatment items fully implemented by nursing personnel accounted for only 1% of the overall items of NHI. In addition to "ward nursing payments," many items covering direct or indirect participation of nursing personnel are included in the coverage points of various diagnosis and treatment items and are paid in a package (nonitemized) format (Ministry of Health and Welfare, Taiwan, ROC, 2012).

In summary, whereas nursing workloads are known to be negatively associated with patient safety, the NHI-covered ICU nursing payments are low and not proportional to workload. Therefore, it is important to acquire empirical data on the correlations among ICU workload, patient safety, and NHI-covered nursing payments. The purpose of this study was to examine the correlation between ICU nursing workload and care quality and between ICU nursing workload and NHI-covered nursing payments.

Methods

Research Design

This was a macrodata analysis of data retrieved from the existing ICU patient classification system (PCS), nursing quality monitoring system, and infection control monitoring system of a medical center in central Taiwan. Data from January 2013 to November 2014, a total of 23 months, were analyzed. Data of interest included TISS-28 scores, total nursing hours, utility index of nursing manpower (UINM), mortality, relevant care quality data, and NHI-covered nursing payments.

Subjects

Nursing personnel and patients of the eight ICUs (136 beds in total) at the targeted medical center contributed the data. The main data collected from the patient classification information system included indices of nursing workload such as TISS-28 and non-TISS-28 scores, average daily total nursing hours of units, nursing hours by PCS, and UINM. Moreover, this study analyzed nursing hours, which were calculated according to the nurse–patient ratio (NPR) of number of nursing personnel taking care of patients per day and the bed occupancy rate. Care quality data were collected from the hospital nursing quality monitoring system. Data on incidence of falls, incidence density of pressure sores, incidence of patient restraint, incidence of tube self-extraction, and incidence density of infection for analysis were also collected. NHI-covered nursing payment items from the PCS and NHI-nursing payment items under application, as extracted from hospital patient expense files, were also retrieved.

TABLE 1.
Direct Nursing Hours, TISS-28

Unit	Day	Bed	Basic Care		Ventilation Support Care		Cardiovascular Support Care	
			Mean	*SD*	Mean	*SD*	Mean	*SD*
CCU	698	16	37.5	6.8	15.9	4.5	4.5	2.9
MICU	698	17	47.4	5.5	44.8	5.1	4.5	1.6
NSCU	698	16	39.7	4.7	29.3	5.4	3.1	1.3
NICU	697	14	22.9	4.4	27.6	5.8	2.9	1.5
PICU	698	15	24.4	7.0	19.7	6.0	1.6	1.7
RICU	696	24	46.6	7.8	44.5	8.0	3.7	1.7
SICU	698	22	61.9	8.7	49.6	7.4	10.5	2.9
TNCU	698	12	24.4	5.9	17.8	4.8	0.9	0.5
Total	5,581	136	38.1	6.4	31.1	5.9	3.9	1.8

Note. TISS-28 = Therapeutic Intervention Scoring System 28; CCU = coronary care unit; MICU = medical intensive care unit; NSCU = neurosurgical care unit; NICU = neonatal intensive care unit; PICU = pediatric intensive care unit; RICU = respiratory intensive care unit; SICU = surgical intensive care unit; TNCU = trauma-neuro care unit.

Definitions of Terms

1. Nursing activities: activities of ICU nurses, including direct nursing, indirect nursing, relevant nursing, and personal activities.
2. Direct nursing: direct nursing care and services received by patients, including the preparation stage, operational stage, and utensil arrangement stage. This study included direct nursing activities belonging to TISS-28 and direct nursing activities not belonging to TISS-28.
3. Care quality: Mortality and relevant care quality data, including incidence of falls, incidence density of pressure sores, incidence of patient restraint, incidence of tube self-extraction, and incidence density of infection, were collected from a hospital information system.
4. Nursing workload: Direct nursing of TISS-28 and non-TISS-28, nursing hours by PCS (PCS nursing hour), and nursing hours by NPR (NPR nursing hour) [(number of nursing personnel in three shifts × 8) / (number of beds × bed occupancy rate)] were used to calculate nursing workload.
5. The statistical formula used for patient classification is described below (Chang, Lin, Lu, Wang, & Chang, 2002):

Calculation of PCS nursing hours

Total nursing hours/patient/day (minutes) = direct nursing time (minutes) + indirect nursing time (174.9 minutes) + relevant nursing time (28.8 minutes)

Total nursing hours/unit = [direct nursing time (minutes) of all the patients + number of patients × 203.7 minutes] / 60 minutes

Calculation of the utility index of nursing manpower

Day Shift Utility Index (D-UINM), Evening Shift Utility Index (E-UINM), and Night Shift Utility Index (N-UINM) were calculated as follows: shift ideal nursing care unit / shift actual nursing care unit × 100

6. NHI-covered nursing payment items: in compliance with the version of "The National Health Insurance Pharmaceutical Benefits and Reimbursement Schedule," as implemented on July 1, 2014, covering 44 diagnosis and treatments items that are mainly offered by nursing personnel.

Data Collection

After receiving institutional review board approval (No. CE13311), the ICU patient classification information system, nursing quality monitoring system, and infection control system were accessed to extract data, which were then categorized by NHI-covered nursing payment items. Next, the data were arranged and inspected, with items of data that did not meet the exclusion criterion deleted. Finally, definition coding and statistical analysis were performed. Data covering the period from January 2013 to November 2014 were used in the analysis.

Results

Analysis on Intensive Care Unit Direct Nursing Hours

This study collected 5,581 days of patient classification data from eight ICUs covering a period of 23 months (698 days). As shown in Table 1, most of the nursing hours were spent on basic care (38.1 ± 6.4), ventilation support care (31.1 ± 5.9), and metabolic support care (5.9 ± 1.5). The proportions of various items also varied with the characteristics of the various ICUs.

Table 2 lists the average daily direct nursing hours provided by the ICUs that were not related to TISS-28 (i.e., were non-TISS-28). Most of the nursing hours in this category were

Renal Support Care		Neurological Support Care		Metabolic Support Care		Special Interventional Treatment or Procedure	
Mean	*SD*	Mean	*SD*	Mean	*SD*	Mean	*SD*
1.9	1.3	0.0	0.1	4.3	0.9	4.4	2.7
2.6	1.4	0.1	0.3	6.7	0.9	2.5	1.4
1.2	0.5	3.0	1.6	5.1	1.0	1.5	1.1
0.4	0.4	0.0	0.0	10.6	4.5	0.9	0.8
1.0	1.0	0.1	0.3	3.8	1.1	1.2	1.3
2.6	1.1	0.1	0.2	8.5	1.3	1.8	1.2
4.1	1.5	0.1	0.2	6.8	1.3	1.9	1.5
0.4	0.3	2.5	1.4	3.4	1.0	0.8	0.8
1.8	0.9	0.7	0.5	5.9	1.5	1.9	1.3

TABLE 2.
Direct Nursing Hours, Non-TISS-28

Unit	Day	Support		Communication		Safety		Comfortable		Hygiene	
		Mean	*SD*	Mean	*SD*	Mean	*SD*	Mean	*SD*	Mean	*SD*
CCU	698	7.1	2.6	14.8	4.9	0.5	0.3	1.4	0.7	18.8	3.4
MICU	698	0.9	0.8	9.4	4.0	0.9	0.4	0.9	0.4	22.5	2.6
NSCU	698	0.4	0.6	3.1	1.7	0.8	0.5	0.8	0.4	15.1	2.2
NICU	697	1.2	1.5	6.0	7.2	4.2	3.8	3.2	0.9	15.6	3.5
PICU	698	2.4	1.4	10.4	4.1	0.4	0.3	1.4	0.6	16.6	4.2
RICU	696	2.3	1.5	12.6	4.0	1.2	0.7	1.0	0.4	26.2	4.0
SICU	698	7.5	2.7	14.9	3.7	1.8	0.7	1.8	0.7	21.9	2.9
TNCU	698	0.3	0.4	3.4	1.5	0.3	0.4	0.5	0.2	10.4	2.7
Total	5,581	2.8	1.4	9.3	3.9	1.3	0.9	1.4	0.5	18.4	3.2

Note. TISS = Therapeutic Intervention Scoring System; CCU = coronary care unit; MICU = medical intensive care unit; NSCU = neurosurgical care unit; NICU = neonatal intensive care unit; PICU = pediatric intensive care unit; RICU = respiratory intensive care unit; SICU = surgical intensive care unit; TNCU = trauma-neuro care unit.

spent on hygiene (18.4 ± 3.2), activities (17.8 ± 2.6), and communication (9.3 ± 3.9). The average daily direct nursing hours provided by each ICU was 137.6 ± 20.8, with 83.7 ± 13.8 hours categorized as TISS-28 (61%) and 53.9 ± 9.4 hours categorized as non-TISS-28 (39%).

Intensive Care Unit Nursing Hours and Utility Index of Nursing Manpower

As shown in Table 3, subjects received an average of 12.49 nursing hours per day per ICU; the average number of nursing hours was 12.39 at adult ICUs and 12.81 at pediatric ICUs. In terms of UINM, the night-shift UINM was 114.78% ± 16.41%, the day-shift UINM was 113.66% ± 18.89%, and the evening-shift UINM was 108.8% ± 16.83%, indicating that the UINM of night and day shifts was higher. In other words, there was a relative lack of manpower and significant work overloading.

Correlation Between Intensive Care Unit Nursing Workload and Care Quality

As shown in Table 4, the average Acute Physiology and Chronic Health Evaluation (APACHE) II score of the five adult ICUs was 20.57 ± 3.21. The APACHE II scores of the medical and respiratory ICUs were higher. In terms of care quality, only four patients at the cardiac ICU experienced falls, whereas other patients did not experience any

TABLE 3.
Nursing Hours and Utility Index of Nursing Manpower

Unit	Day	Bed	Mean Patient Number/ Day	Total Nursing Hour		N-UINM		D-UINM		E-UINM		Nursing Hour by PCS
				Mean	*SD*	Mean	*SD*	Mean	*SD*	Mean	*SD*	
CCU	698	16	13.60	178.19	30.02	117.35	15.59	129.08	26.47	121.29	20.42	13.18
MICU	698	17	15.97	221.34	18.70	122.91	15.46	118.19	14.87	113.05	13.95	13.88
NSCU	698	16	15.26	175.87	15.79	115.83	12.06	101.19	11.97	108.93	13.05	11.55
NICU	697	14	11.42	142.86	24.14	116.37	19.76	120.85	22.38	112.49	17.61	12.61
PICU	698	15	10.15	131.54	32.14	110.72	17.91	117.66	24.52	113.91	21.62	13.01
RICU	696	24	21.74	252.64	32.05	115.17	15.80	100.60	12.07	100.92	13.89	11.63
SICU	698	22	21.09	288.37	28.81	119.12	(15.98	116.92	16.77	108.85	16.54	13.75
TNCU	698	12	10.63	114.22	23.75	100.78	18.76	104.79	22.05	90.99	17.58	10.33
Total	5,581	136		188.13	25.68	114.78	16.41	113.66	18.89	108.80	16.83	12.49

Note. CCU = coronary care unit; MICU = medical intensive care unit; NSCU = neurosurgical care unit; NICU = neonatal intensive care unit; PICU = pediatric intensive care unit; RICU = respiratory intensive care unit; SICU = surgical intensive care unit; TNCU = trauma-neuro care unit; N-UINM = night-shift utility index of nursing manpower; D-UINM = day-shift utility index of nursing manpower; E-UINM = evening-shift utility index of nursing manpower; PCS = patient classification system.

Activities		Movement		Assistance		Subtotal TISS-28		Subtotal Non-TISS-28		Total TISS	
Mean	*SD*	Mean	*SD*	Mean	*SD*	Mean	*SD*	Mean	*SD*	Mean	*SD*
16.3	3.1	4.5	2.3	1.1	1.4	68.5	13.9	64.5	12.9	133.0	24.3
21.5	1.6	1.4	0.9	1.5	1.0	108.6	11.2	59.0	7.2	167.6	15.9
19.6	1.7	1.0	0.8	0.9	0.7	82.8	11.0	41.6	4.4	124.4	13.3
7.7	2.6	0.8	0.6	0.3	0.4	65.3	12.5	39.0	11.0	104.3	18.3
12.0	3.1	1.1	0.8	0.6	0.5	51.9	14.3	44.9	11.7	96.8	24.6
24.6	3.0	1.2	0.7	2.6	2.5	107.7	17.6	71.8	10.5	179.5	25.8
28.9	3.2	2.2	1.0	4.0	1.7	134.9	18.2	82.9	10.7	217.8	26.5
12.2	2.8	0.5	0.5	0.3	0.3	50.0	11.9	27.8	6.6	77.8	17.8
17.8	2.6	1.6	1.0	1.4	1.0	83.7	13.8	53.9	9.4	137.6	20.8

falls. The incidence density of pressure sores was 0.18% (range = 0.14%–0.24%), the average incidence of patient restraint was 5.24% (range = 0%–8.35%), the average incidence of tube self-extraction was 0.29% (range = 0.11%–0.87%), the average incidence density of infection was 8.29% (range = 3.97%–12.36%), and the average mortality rate was 10.35% ± 8.21% (range = 3.21%–22.15%). Examined using Pearson correlation, the variable PCS nursing hours was positively correlated with NPR nursing hours ($r = .51$, $p < .01$), the incidence of patient restraint was significantly correlated with higher APACHE II scores ($r = .63$, $p < .01$), and the incidence of self-extubation was significantly negatively correlated with incidence of patient restraint ($r = -.25$, $p < .01$). In terms of bed occupancy rate, direct nursing hours, total nursing hours, NPR nursing hours, the incidence of patient restraint, and APACHE II scores were positively correlated with mortality rate. However, the incidence density of infection was negatively correlated with higher nursing hours (Table 5).

Correlation Between Intensive Care Unit Nursing Workload and National-Health-Insurance-Covered Nursing Payment

A total of 92,442 items of data from daily ICU patient classification records were collected. The results showed that the number of PCS-covered items was significantly higher than the number of NHI-covered nursing payment items. The five items with the greatest disparities included respiratory tract suction (times), perineal rinsing, nasogastric tube feeding, nursing care surveillance fee of physical restraint days, and use of a heat lamp. The top five NHI-covered nursing payment items were feeding pump (days), a small amount or retention of enemas, 24-hour ECG monitor, ice blanket (within 12 hours), and drug sensitivity tests. Twelve NHI-covered nursing payment items were not recorded (27.3%; 12/44 = 27.3%). The average NHI-covered ICU payment was NT$186,141. However, an average of only NT$7,246 was paid under NHI-covered nursing payments. Approximately 2% of the patients (210 patients) did not apply for NHI-covered nursing payment items. The NHI-covered nursing payment of every patient accounted for an average of 4.77% of the total ICU medical expenses.

Discussion

Intensive Care Unit Workload

The average daily total direct nursing hours provided by each ICU were 61% TISS-28 and 39% non-TISS-28. This result is consistent with the results of prior research (Chang, Lin, Yu, Lu, & Chang, 2009; Chang, Yu, Shih, & Pong, 2013) and reflects the stability of this PCS. For ICU nursing hours, Yeh and Chao (2010) conducted a focus group. In their study, the nursing supervisors suggested that the ideal nursing hours of ICU should be >12 hours. A questionnaire survey of the Taiwan Union of Nurses Association in December 2010 showed that the average patient–bed ratio for ICUs in 17 medical centers was 2.51 and that the average nursing hours were 12.66 (Foundation of Medical Professionals Alliance in Taiwan, 2010). This study showed that the average number of nursing hours in the eight ICUs based on patient classification was 12.49. This finding indicates that increasing nursing manpower remains an issue awaiting effective resolution. In terms of UINM, night-shift UINM, day-shift UINM, and evening-shift UINM were 114.78% ± 16.41%, 113.66% ± 18.89%, and 108.8% ± 16.83%, respectively, which improved significantly compared

Nursing Workload and Care Quality Indices of the Eight ICUs

Item	CCU (*n* = 16)		MICU (*n* = 17)		NSCU (*n* = 16)		NICU (*n* = 14)	
	Mean	*SD*	Mean	*SD*	Mean	*SD*	Mean	*SD*
Indices of nursing workload								
Bed occupancy rate	0.85	0.06	0.94	0.03	0.95	0.04	0.82	0.10
Total direct nursing hours	133.08	11.64	167.56	9.32	124.48	7.98	104.31	10.64
Total nursing hours/unit	178.27	14.35	221.36	10.26	175.94	9.55	142.97	14.40
Nursing hours by PCS	13.18	0.51	13.88	0.49	11.55	0.36	12.61	0.95
Nursing hours by NPR	10.72	0.45	11.81	0.55	10.72	0.38	10.86	0.82
APACHE II			25.00	1.28	19.96	1.22		
Indices of care quality								
Incidence density of pressure sores (%)	0.24	0.24	0.17	0.17	0.22	0.21	0.21	0.26
Incidence of patient restraint (%)	4.96	1.27	8.35	1.70	5.47	1.37	0.00	0.00
Incidence of falls (%)	0.04	0.10	0.00		0.00		0.00	
Incidence of tube self-extraction (%)	0.24	0.48	0.19	0.21	0.12	0.20	0.87	1.53
Incidence density of infection (‰)	4.83	3.15	8.58	3.58	10.59	4.37	3.97	4.04
Mortality rate (%)	3.21	1.33	20.13	5.43	7.63	4.32	6.79	6.04

Note. PCS = patient classification system; NPR = nurse–patient ratio; APACHE II = Acute Physiology and Chronic Health Evaluation II.

with the night-shift UINM, day-shift UINM, and evening-shift UINM (128.04%, 128.34%, and 121.78%, respectively), as analyzed based on the research team's patient classification in 2012 (Chang et al., 2013). However, the use of patient classification to calculate nursing hours precisely to reflect nursing workload showed that the appropriate UINM is 90%–110%. Therefore, it is still necessary to increase manpower.

Intensive Care Unit Nursing Workload and Care Quality

The research results showed that the bed occupancy rate, the direct nursing hours, and the nursing hours as calculated by both NRP and APACHE II were statistically significantly correlated with mortality rate, showing positive correlations between both higher occupancy rates and patient severity and the rate of mortality. This result is similar

TABLE 5.

Correlations Between Nursing Workload and Care Quality (N = 5,581)

Variable	①	②	③	④	⑤
①Bed occupancy rate	1				
②Total direct nursing hours	.490**	1			
③Total nursing hours/unit	.523**	.995**	1		
④Nursing hours by PCS	−.180*	.530**	.455**	1	
⑤Nursing hours by NPR	−.290**	.322**	.298**	.514**	1
⑥APACHE II	−.113	.275**	.267**	.389**	.240**
⑦Incidence density of pressure sores	.010	−.085	−.091	−.001	−.149*
⑧Incidence of patient restraint	.242**	.413**	.430**	.079	.252**
⑨Incidence of falls	−.086	−.027	−.039	.091	−.040
⑩Incidence of tube self-extraction	−.214**	−.142	−.158*	.109	−.042
⑪Incidence density of infection	.349**	.119	.128	−.198**	−.133
⑫Mortality rate	.293**	.517**	.536**	.107	.214**

Note. PCS = patient classification system; NPR = nurse–patient ratio; APACHE II = Acute Physiology and Chronic Health Evaluation II.
a = Cannot be computed because at least one of the variables is constant.
**p* < .05. ***p* < .01.

PICU (n = 15)		RICU (n = 24)		SICU (n = 22)		TNCU (n = 12)		Total (N = 136)	
Mean	*SD*	Mean	*SD*	Mean	*SD*	Mean	*SD*	Mean	*SD*
0.67	0.11	0.91	0.06	0.96	0.02	0.93	0.07	0.88	0.11
96.76	14.53	179.62	16.44	217.87	15.20	77.85	13.71	137.69	46.07
131.44	19.56	252.71	20.88	288.45	16.23	114.27	19.16	188.18	59.60
13.01	0.49	11.63	0.36	13.75	0.63	10.33	0.99	12.49	1.31
11.53	0.75	11.06	0.31	11.96	0.25	10.41	1.56	11.13	0.90
		22.43	1.08	18.43	1.04	17.96	1.55	20.57	3.21
0.14	0.20	0.14	0.15	0.14	0.12	0.21	0.24	0.18	0.20
4.96	1.50	8.01	1.55	5.22	1.20	4.93	1.27	5.24	2.71
0.00		0.00		0.00		0.00		0.01	0.10
0.55	0.89	0.11	0.18	0.15	0.19	0.11	0.26	0.29	0.70
6.83	2.53	7.44	2.93	11.71	3.69	12.36	6.22	8.29	4.85
4.45	3.31	22.15	6.02	11.52	5.16	6.95	5.53	10.35	8.21

to that of West et al. (2009), which correlated higher occupancy rates and lower nursing hours with higher infection densities. The outcomes of this study are also similar to those of Liu et al. (2012). The further finding of this study that the incidence density of pressure sores in patients rose with lower nursing hours suggests that better staffing is beneficial to pressure sore prevention. This is consistent with the result of the systematic literature review of West et al. A recent study in Taiwan investigated the correlation between nursing workload and patient safety, where nurses used a diary to record personal working conditions for 2 weeks. The results showed that, when the NPR exceeds 7, the risks of indices such as falls, decubitus, intubation tube slippage, posthospitalization infection of pneumonia, and urinary tract infections increase (Liu et al., 2012). However, Liu et al.'s subjects were primarily patients in general wards,

⑥	⑦	⑧	⑨	⑩	⑪	⑫
1						
−.065						
.631**	−.036	1				
a	.070	−.029	1			
.031	.055	−.249**	.027	1		
−.302**	.046	.178*	−.126	−.092	1	
.651**	−.090	.480**	−.119	−.105	.042	1

and data were collected over a short period by nursing personnel. Conversely, the disease severity and risk of rapid changes in the disease conditions of ICU patients are typically greater than those of general ward patients. In addition, our study highlighted a statistically significant correlation between nursing hours and all of the care quality indices except for the incidence of falls (Tables 4 and 5). This provides further support to address the importance of maintaining an appropriate NPR and equitable nursing hours to maintain the quality of patient care.

Intensive Care Unit Nursing Workload and National-Health-Insurance-Covered Nursing Payment

The present research results showed that the number of patients in patient classification records was greater than that of patients receiving NHI-covered nursing services. As five items, including respiratory tract suction (times), perineal rinsing, nursing care surveillance fee of physical restraints, and use of a heat lamp, are packaged in ICU nursing payments and as various items are capped by a maximum number of applications per hospitalization, these data are largely inconsistent with data obtained from patient classification records. Twelve NHI-covered nursing payment items were not recorded (27.3%). Some of these items are not used in the ICUs, whereas others are seldom used (e.g., alcohol swab bath and warm water cleaning). This study found that that the NHI-covered nursing payment for each patient accounted for 4.77% of the total ICU medical expenses. Compared with ICU patient classification items, there were more direct nursing items and fewer NHI-covered nursing items. The nursing hours in the ICU were high. However, NHI-covered ICU nursing payments averaged 3,840 points/bed per day. NHI-covered nursing payments to hospitals total approximately NT$19.9–20.3 billion annually. According to calculations, approximately 87,750 nursing personnel take care of inpatients in medical institutions. The NHI Administration covered an average of NT$16,883 per nurse per month, which accounts for less than 40% of the average cost of nursing personnel (NT$47,000), indicating that NHI coverage for nursing care is notoriously low (Foundation of Medical Professionals Alliance in Taiwan, 2010). Thus, either ICU nursing payments should be increased to conform to the actual costs of patient care or NHI-covered nursing payment items should be increased to calculate the proportional distribution of nursing contributions according to treatment items and thus accentuate the importance of nursing.

Conclusions

Data from a patient classification database, a quality monitoring database, and a medical cost database support that nurses are saddled with significant work overloading under the current NHI payment system. In addition, nursing workload was shown to be significantly associated with care quality. This study was limited by the short, 2-year history of the PCS, which restricted data collection to a 2-year period only. In the future, we suggest that research should increase the time span of data collection. This study represents only a preliminary survey of the shortfall in NIH-covered nursing fee items and should be used as a reference to elicit further evidence-based data. This study provides empirical data for administrators to consider when revising nursing staffing and NHI payment policies.

Acknowledgments

The authors express thanks to all of the nursing personnel at the participating ICUs for their cooperation and to the Taiwan Nurses Association for funding this project (TWNA-1032013).

References

Aiken, L. H., Cimiotti, J. P., Sloane, D. M., Smith, H. L., Flynn, L., & Neff, D. F. (2011). Effects of nurse staffing and nurse education on patient deaths in hospitals with different nurse work environments. *Medical Care, 49*(12), 1047–1053. https://doi.org/10.1097/MLR.0b013e3182330b6e

Chang, L. Y., Lin, L. Y., Lu, S. J., Wang, M. H., & Chang, M. Y. (2002). Exploring ICU nursing activities with TISS-28. *VGH Nursing, 19*(3), 254–263. https://doi.org/10.6142/VGHN.19.3.254 (Original work published in Chinese)

Chang, L. Y., Lin, L. Y., Yu, H. C., Lu, S. J., & Chang, M. Y. (2009). Establishing a patient classification system in intensive care units: Based on the therapeutic intervention scoring system-28. *VGH Nursing, 26*(4), 324–335. https://doi.org/10.6142/VGHN.26.4.324

Chang, L. Y., Yu, H. H., Shih, S. J., & Pong, S. C. (2013). Establishing the TISS-28 based patient classification informatic system in intensive care units. *VGH Nursing, 30*(3), 308–319. https://doi.org/10.6142/VGHN.30.3.308

Cho, E., Sloane, D. M., Kim, E. Y., Kim, S., Choi, M., Yoo, I. Y., … Aiken, L. H. (2015). Effects of nurse staffing, work environments, and education on patient mortality: An observational study. *International Journal of Nursing Studies, 52*(2), 535–542. https://doi.org/10.1016/j.ijnurstu.2014.08.006

Cho, S. H., Hwang, J. H., & Kim, J. (2008). Nurse staffing and patient mortality in intensive care units. *Nursing Research, 57*(5), 322–330. https://doi.org/10.1097/01.NNR.0000313498.17777.71

Cho, S. H., & Yun, S. C. (2009). Bed-to-nurse ratios, provision of basic nursing care, and in-hospital and 30-day mortality among acute stroke patients admitted to an intensive care unit: Cross-sectional analysis of survey and administrative data. *International Journal of Nursing Studies, 46*(8), 1092–1101. https://doi.org/10.1016/j.ijnurstu.2009.02.001

Foundation of Medical Professionals Alliance in Taiwan. (2010). *2010 forum on estimating manpower needs—Report on recommendations in each category.* Retrieved from https://www.mohw.gov.tw/dl-21290-961ffcea-bb35-4f2e-9833-df70d8f049a1.html (Original work published in Chinese)

Goj, K., Knapik, P., Kucewicz-Czech, E., & Lubon, D. (2009). The Therapeutic Intervention Scoring System (TISS-28) for assessment of cardiac surgical postoperative intensive care. *Anaesthesiology Intensive Therapy, 41*(1), 34–37.

Liang, Y. W., Huang, L. C., Yin, Y. C., Chen, W. Y., Chuang, C. L., & Lee, J. L. (2010). Effect of nurse staffing on patient outcomes: A review of the literature. *The Journal of Nursing, 57*(5), 77–82. https://doi.org/10.6224/JN.57.5.77 (Original work published in Chinese)

Liu, L. F., Lee, S., Chia, P. F., Chi, S. C., & Yin, Y. C. (2012). Exploring the association between nurse workload and nurse-sensitive patient safety outcome indicators. *The Journal of Nursing Research, 20*(4), 300–309. https://doi.org/10.1097/jnr.0b013e3182736363

Ministry of Health and Welfare, Taiwan, ROC. (2012). *Clarifying healthcare coverage items, quality-of-hospital-care awards, and other related expenditure applications.* Retrieved from http://blog.xuite.net/edesk9/twblog/147749040-%E6%BE%84%E6%B8%85%E5%A0%B1%E8%BC%89%E5%81%A5%E4%BF%9D%E8%AD%B7%E7%90%86%E7%B5%A6%E4%BB%98%E5%8D%A0%E7%8E%87%E5%8F%8A%E4%BD%8F%E9%99%A2%E8%AD%B7%E7%90%86%E7%85%A7%E8%AD%B7%E5%93%81%E8%B3%AA%E7%8D%8E%E5%8B%B5%E7%AD%89%E6%94%AF%E5%87%BA%E6%87%89%E7%94%A8%E6%83%85%E5%BD%A2 (Original work published in Chinese)

Miranda, D. R., de Rijk, A., & Schaufeli, W. (1996). Simplified therapeutic intervention scoring system: The TISS-28 items—Results from a multicenter study. *Critical Care Medicine, 24*(1), 64–73. https://doi.org/10.1097/00003246-199601000-00012

Padilha, K. G., Sousa, R. M., Kimura, M., Miyadahira, A. M., da Cruz, D. A., Vattimo Mde, F., ... Mayor, E. R. (2007). Nursing workload in intensive care units: A study using the Therapeutic Intervention Scoring System-28 (TISS-28). *Intensive and Critial Care Nursing, 23*(3), 162–169. https://doi.org/10.1016/j.iccn.2006.07.004

West, E., Mays, N., Rafferty, A. M., Rowan, K., & Sanderson, C. (2009). Nursing resources and patient outcomes in intensive care: A systematic review of the literature. *International Journal of Nursing Studies, 46*(7), 993–1011. http://dx.doi.org/10.1016/j.ijnurstu.2007.07.011

Yeh, M. C., & Chao, Y. M. (2010). *Nurse workforce and nurse practitioner system: Vision and challenges.* Miaoli County, Taiwan, ROC: National Health Research Institutes. (Original work published in Chinese)

7

Exploration of the Association Between Religious Affiliation and Attitude Toward Spiritual Care in Clinical Nurses

Yi-Chien CHIANG[1] • Hsiang-Chun LEE[2] • Tsung-Lan CHU[3] • Chin-Yen HAN[4] • Ya-Chu HSIAO[5]*

ABSTRACT

Background: Religion is an important cultural asset that is known to affect the thoughts, behaviors, and lifestyles of individuals. However, the impact of religious affiliation, religious activities, and religious beliefs on the attitudes of nurses toward providing spiritual care to their patients is an issue that has been inadequately explored.

Purposes: The aim of this study was to explore the relationship between religion (including religious affiliation, religious activities, and religious beliefs) and attitude toward spiritual care in clinical nurses.

Methods: This study used a cross-sectional correlation study design. Six hundred nineteen nurses were included as participants. The measurements used included a questionnaire on religious affiliation, religious activities, and religious beliefs; the Spiritual Health Scale-Short Form; the Spiritual Care Attitude Scale; and a sociodemographic datasheet. The study employed hierarchical regression modeling to establish the relationships between the aspects and degrees of religious belief and practice as well as the attitudes of participants toward spiritual care.

Results: Most of the participants participated infrequently in religious activities. After controlling for demographic variables and spiritual health, religious belief was found to be an important factor impacting participants' attitudes toward providing spiritual care.

Conclusions/Implications for Practice: The findings indicate that religious belief is an important factor impacting the attitudes of nurses toward providing spiritual care and that the religious/spiritual beliefs of nurses may impact on their fitness to provide spiritual care to patients. Education on religion may be needed to improve the attitude of nurses toward providing spiritual care.

Key Words:
religion, spirituality, nurse.

Introduction

Religion is an important cultural characteristic that is known to affect the thoughts, behaviors, and lifestyles of individuals. Around 90% of people worldwide are involved in some form of religious activities (Grim, Johnson, Skirbekk, & Zurlo, 2015). Previous studies have shown religious beliefs and practices to be associated with health conditions and to potentially assist people to cope with stress (Bonelli & Koenig, 2013; Medved Kendrick, 2017).

The hospital palliative care regulation issued by the Taiwanese legislature in 2000 emphasizes the importance of providing spiritual care to patients. The healthcare systems in Taiwan have started integrating the spiritual needs of patients into religious/spiritual cares. The hospital palliative care regulation requires hospitals to establish related facilities and provide mandated services. However, to date, only 50% of the hospitals in Taiwan have met these requirements (Liu & Wu, 2008; Tzeng & Yin, 2006). Nurses, who comprise the highest proportion of healthcare providers in Taiwan, will likely be the key providers of spiritual care in clinical practice settings.

Taiwan is home to more than 22 distinct religious faith traditions (Ministry of the Interior, Taiwan, ROC, 2018). Therefore, healthcare providers are frequently challenged to tend to the spiritual needs of patients of different religious faiths. The spiritual care training and personal religious/spiritual beliefs of healthcare providers potentially impact their ability to provide effective spiritual care. For example, one study found that nurses who were more spiritual provided better spiritual care to their patients than their less-spiritual peers (Chan, 2010; Wu & Hsiao, 2009).

Patients hope that healthcare providers will address their spiritual needs and desire to receive spiritual care during the healthcare process (Borneman, Ferrell, & Puchalski, 2010).

[1]PhD, RN, Associate Professor, Department of Nursing, Chang Gung University of Science and Technology, and Associate Research Fellow, Department of Pediatrics, Chang Gung Memorial Hospital at Linkou • [2]MSN, RN, Assistant Professor, Department of Nursing, Chang Gung University of Science and Technology • [3]MSN, RN, Director, Administration Center of Quality Management Department, Chang Gung Medical Foundation, and Assistant Professor, Department of Nursing, Chang Gung University of Science and Technology • [4]PhD, RN, Associate Professor, Department of Nursing, Chang Gung University of Science and Technology, and Associate Research Fellow, Department of Nursing, Chang Gung Memorial Hospital at Linkou • [5]EdD, RN, Professor, Department of Nursing, Chang Gung University of Science and Technology, and Research Fellow, Department of Nursing, Chang Gung Memorial Hospital at Linkou.

However, health professionals do not generally concern themselves with the religious/spiritual issues of their patients (Best, Butow, & Olver, 2016). It remains unclear whether the religious beliefs of healthcare providers affect their professional sensitivities in assessing the spiritual needs of their patients or in providing spiritual care. Moreover, it is particularly important that nurses in Taiwan be aware of patients' spiritual needs. Therefore, the aims of this study were to explore the association between religion (including religious affiliation, religious activities, and religious beliefs) and attitudes toward spiritual care among clinical nurses.

Literature Review

The meanings of spirituality and religion

Spirituality is the value system and worldview of an individual. Spirituality may be explained by the association between the self with the self as well as with others, nature, and God. When the relationships with the self, others, God, and nature are in communion and harmony, the individual has a rich, meaningful, peaceful, and hopeful love of life (Lin, Liou, & Chen, 2008; McSherry & Jamieson, 2011). Spirituality shares similarities with religion. For example, religion is usually viewed as an important way for people to express their spirituality (Burkhart & Solari-Twadell, 2001; Edwards, Pang, Shiu, & Chan, 2010). In the Oxford Dictionary, religion is defined as "the belief in and worship of a superhuman controlling power, especially a personal God or gods" (Soanes & Stevenson, 2006, p. 1487). Therefore, although similar, spirituality and religion are still different concepts. Religion is more objective and external and may involve ritual practices that one performs in a community, which guide an individual's behaviors, whereas spirituality is the subjective, internal, and unique experience of an individual with a super-being that imbues life with meaning (Barber, 2012).

Taiwan is a society of multiple religious faiths. Some Taiwanese do not clearly associate with a specific religious affiliation, although they participate in certain religious activities (Hsiao, Chiang, Lee, & Han, 2013). Religion has been defined as the belief in and awareness of a super-being (Koenig, King, & Carson, 2012). Several instruments are available that measure organized and private religious activities, motivation, involvement, belief, commitment, attitude, coping, affiliation, and faith development (Hall, Meador, & Koenig, 2008; Hill & Hood, 1999). These instruments may be classified into the three categories of religious affiliation, religious activities, and religious beliefs (Chiang, Lee, Chu, Han, & Hsiao, 2017; Hall et al., 2008; Koenig et al., 2012) and are typically used to assess people belonging to a specific religious faith such as Catholicism, Judaism, Taoism, or Buddhism. Religious activities may be defined as attending public or private religious activities, typified by variables such as church attendance, scripture reading, and praying. Religious beliefs may refer to the perception of the importance of religion and religious beliefs. Therefore, religious affiliation, religious activities, and religious beliefs may be applied as observable variables for religion. Moreover, as spirituality has been defined as an individual's inner force and resource for giving unique meaning to life, spiritual health may be assessed using the Spiritual Health Scale (Hsiao et al., 2013).

Spiritual care and its characteristics

Activities that are intended to satisfy the spiritual needs of patients may be incorporated under spiritual care. Spiritual care has been defined as the care provided by nurses to help patients gain a harmonious connection with the self, others, nature, and higher beings (Lin et al., 2008). The content of spiritual care may include a healing presence, the therapeutic use of self, the intuitive sense, exploration of the spiritual perspective, patient-centeredness, meaning-centered therapeutic interventions, and the creation of a spiritually nurturing environment (Ramezani, Ahmadi, Mohammadi, & Kazemnejad, 2014). From the experience of clinical practice, patients who are ill or in the terminal stages of disease typically have greater spiritual needs. In one study, almost 80% of patients with advanced cancer relied on religion to cope with their illness (Phelps et al., 2009). Religious support helps patients who are diagnosed with advanced cancer feel hope and peace and may equip them to better face death (Hsiao, Gau, Ingleton, Ryan, & Shih, 2011). Moreover, satisfying the spiritual needs of patients may influence their medical decision making and quality of life at the end of their life. For example, Balboni et al. (2010) reported that patients who received spiritual support from their healthcare provider had a better quality of life at the end of life than those who did not.

Both environmental and personal factors affect the provision by nurses of spiritual care to their patients. Related environmental factors include hospital policy, ward space, and nursing education and training (Edwards et al., 2010; Noble & Jones, 2010), whereas personal factors include demographic profile, self-spirituality, and perception of spiritual care. For example, Chan (2010) indicated that nurses holding religious beliefs who were married, had past hospitalization experiences, and had worked in obstetrics and gynecology departments tended to be more willing to provide spiritual care to their patients. Finally, previous studies indicate that the spirituality, interpretation of spiritual care, and attitudes toward spiritual care of nurses affect their provision of spiritual care (Chan, 2010; Edwards et al., 2010).

Methods

Design

A cross-sectional survey study design was used in this study, and data were drawn from the Survey of Religion, Spirituality, and Nursing (SRSN) study. The SRSN was a comprehensive study that was designed to explore the relationship between the spirituality and professional performance of nurses. The first part of the study was focused on instrument development, and the second part was focused on exploring the predictors of spiritual care and professional behaviors. The data for the SRSN study were collected in 2012. Only the results of the SRSN related to religion and attitude toward spiritual care were adopted and used in this article.

Participants

A convenience sampling method was used to recruit 619 nurses from three teaching hospitals in Taiwan. The inclusion criteria were nurses who (a) were full-time workers at a hospital, (b) had over 6 months of nursing experience, and (c) agreed to complete the questionnaire. The exclusion criteria were nurses who were not direct-care providers.

The major purpose of this study was to explore the association between religion and attitude toward spiritual care in nurses. Calculating the desired sample size for this study was difficult (Cohen, 1988) because of the lack of existing studies on this topic. Therefore, the authors assumed a small effect size for the association between religion and attitude toward spiritual care, resulting in a partial R^2 (increased R^2) of .0196. Given an alpha level of 5% and a power of 95%, a minimum required sample size of 652 was estimated and an additional 5% was added to compensate for the expected risk of participants dropping out before the end of the study. Six hundred ninety participants were initially invited, with 71 either declining to participate or failing to complete the questionnaires. Thus, the data for 619 participants were available for analysis (response rate: 89.71%).

Data Collection

The rules set by the hospital's institutional review board for the protection of participants' confidentiality (approval number: 98-4001B) were strictly followed for this study. All of the participants provided informed consent to participate in this study after receiving oral and written explanations of the study and its procedures. Data were collected using a self-administrated questionnaire in six parts that covered the following: information on religious affiliation, religious activities, religious beliefs, the Spiritual Health Scale-Short Form (SHS-SF), the Spiritual Care Attitude Scale (SCAS), and sociodemographic details.

Religious affiliation

This scale, established by Chang and Lin (1992), distinguishes between the three religious affiliation categories of primary, secondary, and atheist. Participants proclaiming a belief in a higher spiritual power or god and who identified themselves as having a very clear perception of their religious affiliation and of the religion they practiced were categorized as "primary." Participants who did not assert a firm religious affiliation but did claim belief in a higher spiritual power or god and participated in some religious activities were categorized as "secondary." Finally, participants who did not believe in a god or higher spiritual power and who were not involved in any religious activities were categorized as "atheist."

Religious activities

Religious activities were assessed using a five-item instrument that was developed by the research team of this study using a review literature and in-depth interviews with clinical nurses. Initially, seven original items of the instrument were assessed by seven specialists (including one PhD in religion, two nursing faculty members with PhD degrees, one head nurse, and three senior nurses currently working in hospitals). The content validity index of this instrument was .96, indicating it to have acceptable validity (Polit & Beck, 2006). This instrument is scored using a 4-point Likert scale ranging from 1 = *never* to 4 = *often*. Participants were asked to recall the frequency of involvement in religious activities over the past 6 months. The validity of this instrument was established by performing exploratory factor analysis on a calibration sample (n = 310), with the one extracted factor explaining 48.0% of the variance. In addition, the data from the exploratory factor analysis showed that all of the factor loadings were greater than .50, indicating good convergent validity (Hair, Black, Babin, Anderson, & Tatham, 2006). Furthermore, the research team used a validation sample (n = 309) to conduct a confirmatory factor analysis (CFA) to verify the validity of the factor structure. The results of the CFA revealed that the religious activities instrument had an acceptable construct validity with the model fit indices after the deletion of two items ($\chi^2/df = 6.47$, nonnormed fit index = .88, comparative fit index = .94, standardized root mean square residual = .045, and root mean square error of approximation = .133; Bentler, 1992). Therefore, the final instrument included five items, including participating in religion-related events, praying, reading the bible/religious texts, meditating on religious incantations, and seeking religious guidance to make decisions.

Religious beliefs scale

The Religious Beliefs Scale (RBS) was developed by Chiang et al. (2017) and was derived from in-depth interviews, a literature review, and expert recommendations. The 17 items of the RBS comprise four subscales, including "religious effects," "divine," "religious query," and "religious stress," which explain a combined 64.1% of the total variance. A 5-point Likert scale is used for scoring, with 5 indicating "strongly agree" and 1 indicating "strongly disagree." Chiang et al. (2017) established the acceptable reliability and validity of RBS, calculated a Cronbach's alpha of .87, and used CFA to establish construct validity with acceptable model fit indices. The Cronbach's alpha of the RBS was .89 for this study.

Spiritual care attitude scale

The 15-item SCAS, developed by Chiang, Chiang, Lee, Han, and Hsiao (2014), is a Likert-type scale (1 = *strongly disagree* to 5 = *strongly agree*) encompassing the three subscales of spiritual growth, spiritual core concepts, and spiritual nursing. Chiang et al. (2014) indicated that the three subscales of the SCAS explained 71.06% of the total variance. The reliability of the SCAS was established with a Cronbach's alpha of .96,

TABLE 1.
Sociodemographic Characteristics of Participants (N = 619)

Variable	n	%
Age (years; *M* and *SD*)	30.1	5.6
Seniority (years; *M* and *SD*)	7.9	5.6
Educational level		
Baccalaureate	458	74.0
Associate degree	156	25.2
Missing	5	0.8
Religious affiliation		
Primary	425	68.7
Secondary	160	25.8
Atheist	34	5.5
Marital status		
Single	418	67.5
Married	201	32.5
Job position		
Nurse	552	89.2
Supervisor	65	10.5
Missing	2	0.3

Note. Range of age is from 20 to 60 years; range of seniority is from 0.5 to 28.

and a CFA established its constructed validity (Chiang et al., 2014). The Cronbach's alpha in this study was .94.

Spiritual health scale-short form

The SHS-SF was developed by Hsiao et al. (2013). CFA was used to establish the construct validity of the SHS-SF, with results confirming the model fit indices of the SHS-SF's five-factor model as acceptable. Moreover, analysis showed acceptable reliability with a Cronbach's alpha of .934. The SHS-SF is composed of 24 items in five subscales, including "connection to others" (four items), "meaning derived from living" (six items), "transcendence" (six items), "religious attachment" (four items), and "self-understanding" (four items). A 5-point Likert-type scale was employed for this scale, with scores ranging from "strongly disagree" (1) to "strongly agree" (5). The range of total possible scores was 24–120, with higher scores denoting a higher level of respondent spiritual health (Hsiao et al., 2013). The Cronbach's alpha of the SHS-SF in this study was .93.

Sociodemographic information

This study gathered demographic data on age, marital status, educational status, seniority, and job position.

Data Analysis

The association between independent variables (religious affiliation, religious activities, and religious beliefs) and attitude toward spiritual care was investigated using the hierarchical regression model. Personal information and spiritual health were included in Model 1 and served as control variables. Religious affiliation, religious activities, and religious beliefs were further introduced into Models 2–4, respectively. Finally, the subscales of religious beliefs were incorporated into Model 5 in the presence of the variables included in Model 3. Data analysis was conducted using IBM SPSS Version 22 (IBM, Inc., Armonk, NY, USA).

Results

Sociodemographic Characteristics of Participants

All of the survey participants were female, with a mean age of 30.1 years and an average of 7.9 years of work experience as nurses. Most held bachelor's degrees (74.0%), and 67.5% were single (Table 1).

Descriptive Statistics for Research Variables

Slightly over two thirds (68.7%) of the participants were in the primary religious category (Table 2), with the data in Table 2 showing that primary-category participants earned higher scores for religious activities and religious beliefs than their secondary- and atheist-category peers ($F = 62.36$, $p < .001$ and $F = 40.54$, $p < .001$, respectively). Furthermore, a Pearson correlation found a significant and positive relationship between religious activities and beliefs ($r = .451$, $p < .01$).

Table 3 shows the descriptive data for religious activities, religious beliefs, spiritual health, and attitude toward spiritual care. The mean score for religious activities was 2.07 ($SD = 0.66$), indicating that most participants rarely participated in religious activities. "Seeking religious guidance

TABLE 2.
Differences Among Religious Affiliation, Religious Activities, and Beliefs (N = 619)

			Religious Activity			Religious Belief		
Variable	n	%	M	SD	F/Scheff's test	M	SD	F/Scheff's test
Religious affiliation					62.36*			40.54*
① Primary	425	68.7	2.26	0.65	① > ②, ③	3.33	0.45	① > ②, ③
② Secondary	160	25.8	1.70	0.45		2.97	0.51	
③ Atheist	34	5.5	1.57	0.51		2.99	0.39	

*$p < .001$.

TABLE 3.

Descriptive Statistics for Religious Activities, Religious Beliefs, Spiritual Health, and Spiritual Care Attitude (N = 619)

Scale	No. Items	Mean	*SD*	Possible Range	Actual Range
Religious activities	5	2.07	0.66	1–4	1–4
Participating in religion-related events at religious sites	1	2.01	0.76	1–4	1–4
Praying or asking for help from a higher power	1	2.20	0.95	1–4	1–4
Reading bible/religious texts	1	1.42	0.81	1–4	1–4
Meditating on religious incantations	1	1.97	1.06	1–4	1–4
Seeking religious guidance to make decisions	1	2.76	0.90	1–4	1–4
Religious beliefs	17	3.22	0.49	1–5	1.65–5
Religious effects	9	3.32	0.64	1–5	1.22–5
Divine	3	3.81	0.58	1–5	2.00–5
Religious query	3	2.56	0.72	1–5	1.00–5
Religious stress	2	2.86	0.83	1–5	1.00–5
Spiritual health	24	3.95	0.47	1–5	2.13–5
Connection to others	4	4.35	0.61	1–5	1.00–5
Meaning derived from living	6	4.09	0.57	1–5	2.33–5
Transcendence	6	3.78	0.62	1–5	1.67–5
Religious attachment	4	3.75	0.69	1–5	1.00–5
Self-understanding	4	3.82	0.68	1–5	1.00–5
Spiritual care attitude	15	3.93	0.49	1–5	1.67–5
Spiritual growth	5	3.85	0.60	1–5	1.00–5
Spiritual core concept	4	4.14	0.49	1–5	2.75–5
Spiritual nursing	6	3.85	0.55	1–5	1.33–5

to help me make decisions" ($M = 2.76$, $SD = 0.90$; 61.2%, "sometimes" or "often") was the highest-frequency activity, whereas "reading bible/religious texts" was the lowest-frequency activity ($M = 1.42$, $SD = 0.81$; 72.2%, "never").

The mean score for religious beliefs was 3.22 ($SD = 0.49$), with the subscale "divine" earning the highest score ($M = 3.81$, $SD = 0.58$) and the subscale "religious query" earning the lowest score ($M = 2.56$, $SD = 0.72$). The mean score for spiritual health was 3.95 ($SD = 0.47$), with the subscale "connection to others" earning the highest score and the subscale "religious attachment" earning the lowest score. Finally, the mean score for spiritual care attitude was 3.93 ($SD = 0.49$), with the subscale "spiritual core concept" earning the highest score ($M = 4.14$, $SD = 0.49$).

Predictors of Spiritual Care Attitudes

The results for the predictors of spiritual care attitudes in nurses are shown in Table 4. Model 1 indicates that participants with a longer work experience ($\beta = .18$, $p < .001$) and a higher level of spiritual health ($\beta = .44$, $p < .001$) tended to have higher levels of spiritual care attitude. Models 2 and 3 indicate that religious affiliation and religious activities were not independently associated with spiritual care attitude, after adjustment for the control variables. Model 4 indicates that religious beliefs were positively associated with spiritual care attitudes ($\beta = .16$, $p < .001$). Finally, Model 5 indicates a positive relationship between spiritual care attitudes and the "divine" and "religious stress" subscales ($\beta = .11$, $p < .01$ and $\beta = .11$, $p < .05$, respectively) and a negative relationship between spiritual care attitude and "religious query" ($\beta = -.10$, $p < .01$).

Discussion

This study marks the first investigation of potential associations between the religious beliefs and attitudes toward spiritual care of nurses. The primary findings of this study are that religious beliefs impact the attitudes of nurses toward spiritual care significantly. This study is affected by two notable limitations. First, the results may not be generalizable to all nurses because of the convenience sampling approach used. Second, the theoretical reasoning for this research was limited by the paucity of previous studies on this subject.

The results of this study indicate that around 68.7% of nurses in Taiwan have a religious affiliation and seldom participate in religious activities. In general, the findings are consistent with previous studies conducted in Taiwan (Liu, 2010; Yeager et al., 2006). For example, Yeager et al. (2006) found that, although most of the Taiwanese population had religious affiliations, only 54% rated religious attendance as "never to rarely." In comparison, a large-scale online survey conducted by McSherry and Jamieson ($N = 4,054$) indicated that 84.2% of nurses in Western countries hold a religious affiliation and that 67.2% practice religious activities regularly (McSherry &

TABLE 4.

Hierarchical Regression Model Predicting the Attitude Toward Spiritual Care

	Model				
Block/Variable	Model 1	Model 2	Model 3	Model 4	Model 5
Control variable					
Education (Baccalaureate vs. associate degree)	.07	.07	.06	.07	.07
Marital status (married vs. single)	.05	.05	.05	.04	.03
Seniority (year)	.18***	.19***	.19***	.17***	.17***
Job position (supervisor vs. nurse)	−.02	−.02	−.02	−.01	.005
Spiritual health	.44***	.43***	.42***	.39***	.35***
Independent variable					
Religious affiliation (ref: atheist)					
Primary		.05	.02	.01	−.01
Secondary		−.03	−.03	−.02	−.02
Religious activities			.06	.003	−.04
Religious belief				.16***	–
Religious effects				–	.09
Divine				–	.11**
Religious query				–	−.10**
Religious stress				–	.11*
ΔR^2	.264***	.005	.003	.017***	.040***,[a]
Model summary					
Total R^2	.264	.270	.273	.290	.313
Adjusted R^2	.258	.261	.263	.279	.299

Note. The values in cells not specified were standardized regression coefficients (β). ΔR^2 denotes change in R^2.
[a]Compared with Model 3.
*$p < .05$. **$p < .01$. ***$p < .001$.

Jamieson, 2011). The significantly lower rate of religious activity attendance in Taiwan highlights a cultural difference between East and West that may relate to the traditional Chinese Confucian ideals and the religious culture in Taiwan. First, in Confucianism, "The Master does not speak of prodigies, force, disorder, and gods," with practitioners urged "to keep one's distance from the gods" (Yang & Liu, 2009). Therefore, Taiwanese reticence in accordance with Confucian values to publicly express superstitious and nonscientific beliefs may decrease willingness to participate regularly in religious activities. Second, most Taiwanese (81%) believe in Buddhism, Taoism, and traditional folk religions (Grim et al., 2015). However, many Taiwanese find it difficult to clearly distinguish among these three religious faiths. Furthermore, their doctrines emphasize that individuals who believe in gods will be blessed everywhere and anytime. These religions do not stress the importance of regularly attending religious activities in a specific religious organization, which may result in Taiwanese tending to have relatively weak connections to specific religious organizations and to participate only infrequently in religious activities.

Furthermore, the results of this study show the religious beliefs of the participants to be neutral. This is consistent with Yeagar et al. (2006), who found a neutral religious beliefs score for Taiwanese (M = 5.1; 0–12 scale). This result may relate to the history of the development of the Western medical system in Taiwan, which was heavily influenced during its formative years on missionaries from Western countries. These missionaries helped provide Taiwanese good medical care during the 19th century while promoting Protestant and Catholic religious doctrines. This effort helped foster Taiwan's modern landscape of multiple coexisting religious faiths and the general attitude of respect and acceptance that Taiwanese hold toward most religions.

Ellison and Levin (1998) initiated academic inquiry into the connection between religion and health in the 20th century. The possible mechanism that they proposed as underlying this connection was the improvement effect on individual health of the religious regulation of personal behaviors and lifestyle. Religion may provide coping resources such as praying and worshipping to help reduce perceived stress. In this study, associations were found among the three religious variables of affiliation, activities, and beliefs. The participants in the "primary" religious affiliation category attended religious activities more frequently than their peers in the secondary and atheist categories, and frequency of participation in these activities was shown to relate positively to the strength of religious beliefs ($p < .01$). These findings are similar to previous studies (Neyrinck, Vansteenkiste, Lens, Duriez, & Hutsebaut, 2006). The results of this study identified religious belief, after controlling for the variables of education, marital status, seniority, job position, and spiritual health, as an important factor influencing attitude toward spiritual care and religious affiliation and attendance as having minimal influence on this attitude. Two potential reasons for this finding are suggested. First, a previous study of nurses examining the impact of religiosity on the motivation to provide spiritual care found that the personal philosophies of the subjects, which reflected evangelical Christian religiosity, may have influenced their willingness to provide spiritual care (Taylor, Park, & Pfeiffer, 2014). The religious doctrines of Buddhism and Taoism teach people to view helping others as an opportunity to grow spiritually. This may be a reason why the participants with stronger religious beliefs held more positive attitudes toward spiritual care in this study. Second, the minimal effect of religious affiliation and attendance on the attitude of participants toward spiritual care may relate to the low percentage of participants who self-identified as belonging to a specific religious organization and the high percentage who seldom participated in religious activities.

The results of the hierarchical regression model in Model 5 indicate the need to further examine which subscales impact attitude toward spiritual care in nurses. The divine and religious stress subscales were significantly and positively associated with attitude toward spiritual care, whereas the subscale of religious query was negatively associated with this attitude. This may be a result from the items in the subscale of "religious query" including negative views of religious belief, such as "I feel that God is unfair to me," "I feel that religion is related to superstition," and "the impressions of religion include negative perspectives, passive attitudes, and a tendency to escape from reality." Therefore, the participants with higher scores in the subscale of religious query may exhibit decreased willingness to provide spiritual care. A strong relationship has been identified between religion and spirituality (Balboni, Puchalski, & Peteet, 2014; Rykkje, Eriksson, & Raholm, 2013). A possible reason is that religious query, which conveys a negative aspect of religion that is similar to spiritual struggle, was defined as expressions of conflict, questioning, and doubt regarding matters of faith, God, and religious relationships (Abu-Raiya, Pargament, & Exline, 2015). As the participants who earned higher scores for religious query may be inferring that they are in conflict with gods or think that gods are treating them unfairly during suffering events, they may not perceive serving the spiritual needs of patients as a good way to help.

The spiritual health of nurses was treated in this study as a control variable in the hierarchical regression model predicting attitude toward spiritual care. The reason for this treatment is that previous studies (Chan, 2010; Chiang, Lee, Chu, Han, & Hsiao, 2016; Wu & Hsiao, 2009) have shown results in the Hierarchical Regression Model 1 that also indicate that nurses who exhibit more spirituality tend to have a greater ability to provide spiritual care to patients. Furthermore, van Leeuwen and Cusveller (2004) pointed out that the ability to face their own spirituality is a competency of nurses that is necessary to providing spiritual care. Therefore, the spiritual health of nurses should be regarded as a significant value and a factor that affects the attitude of nurses toward spiritual care and that should be controlled when exploring its predicting factors.

Conclusions

A cross-sectional correlational study design was used in this study to explore the association between religion (including religious affiliation, religious activities, and religious beliefs) and attitude toward spiritual care in clinical nurses. The results found that 68.7% of participants reported having a religious affiliation but participated only rarely in religious activities. In addition, after controlling for education, marital status, seniority, job position, and spiritual health, the religious beliefs of the participants were identified to be an important impact factor of influence on attitudes toward spiritual care. However, their religious affiliation and attendance were shown not to impact these attitudes. The results of this study do not imply that nurses should adopt religious beliefs to provide spiritual care to patients but rather suggest that religious education for nurses may help improve the attitudes of nurses toward spiritual care.

Acknowledgments

This study was supported by grants from the Ministry of Science and Technology Taiwan (NSC 100-2410-H-255-001 and NSC 102-2511-S-255-003-MY2) and the Chang Gung Medical Research Fund (CMRPF1C0081, CMRPF1C0082, BMRP704, and BMRPA63). The authors would like to thank all of the participants for their kind cooperation.

Author Contributions

Study conception and design: All authors
Data collection: YCH, HCL
Data analysis and interpretation: YCH, YCC
Drafting of the article: YCH, YCC
Critical revision of the article: HCL, TLC, CYH

References

Abu-Raiya, H., Pargament, K. I., & Exline, J. J. (2015). Understanding and addressing religious and spiritual struggles in health care. *Health & Social Work, 40*(4), e126–e134. https://doi.org/10.1093/hsw/hlv055

Balboni, M., Puchalski, C., & Peteet, J. (2014). The relationship between medicine, spirituality and religion: Three models for integration. *Journal of Religion & Health, 53*(5), 1586–1598. https://doi.org/10.1007/s10943-014-9901-8

Balboni, T. A., Paulk, M. E., Balboni, M. J., Phelps, A. C., Loggers, E. T., Wright, A. A., ... Prigerson, H. G. (2010). Provision of spiritual care to patients with advanced cancer: Associations with medical care and quality of life near death. *Journal of Clinical Oncology, 28*(3), 445–452. https://doi.org/10.1200/JCO.2009.24.8005

Barber, C. (2012). Spirituality and religion: A brief definition. *British Journal of Healthcare Assistants, 6*(8), 378–381. https://doi.org/10.12968/bjha.2012.6.8.378

Bentler, P. M. (1992). On the fit of models to covariances and methodology to the Bulletin. *Psychological Bulletin, 112*(3), 400–404.

Best, M., Butow, P., & Olver, I. (2016). Doctors discussing religion and spirituality: A systematic literature review. *Palliative Medicine, 30*(4), 327–337. https://doi.org/10.1177/0269216315600912

Bonelli, R. M., & Koenig, H. G. (2013). Mental disorders, religion and spirituality 1990 to 2010: A systematic evidence-based review. *Journal of Religion & Health, 52*(2), 657–673. https://doi.org/10.1007/s10943-013-9691-4

Borneman, T., Ferrell, B., & Puchalski, C. M. (2010). Evaluation of the FICA tool for spiritual assessment. *Journal of Pain & Symptom Management, 40*(2), 163–173. https://doi.org/10.1016/j.jpainsymman.2009.12.019

Burkhart, L., & Solari-Twadell, A. (2001). Spirituality and religiousness: Differentiating the diagnoses through a review of the nursing literature. *Nursing Diagnosis, 12*(2), 45–54. https://doi.org/10.1111/j.1744-618X.2001.tb00118.x

Chan, M. F. (2010). Factors affecting nursing staff in practising spiritual care. *Journal of Clinical Nursing, 19*(15/16), 2128–2136. https://doi.org/10.1111/j.1365-2702.2008.02690.x

Chang, M. K., & Lin, P. H. (1992). The social imaginations of religion: A research problem for sociology of knowledge. *Bulletin of the Institute of Ethnology Academia Sinica, 74,* 95–123.

Chiang, Y. C., Chiang, H. Y., Lee, H. C., Han, C. Y., & Hsiao, Y. C. (2014). The construction and evaluation of a spiritual care attitude scale. *Journal of Nursing and Healthcare Research, 10*(2), 102–112. https://doi.org/10.6225/JNHR.10.2.102 (Original work published in Chinese)

Chiang, Y. C., Lee, H. C., Chu, T. L., Han, C. Y., & Hsiao, Y. C. (2016). The impact of nurses' spiritual health on their attitudes toward spiritual care, professional commitment, and caring. *Nursing Outlook, 64*(3), 215–224. https://doi.org/10.1016/j.outlook.2015.11.012

Chiang, Y. C., Lee, H. C., Chu, T. L., Han, C. Y., & Hsiao, Y. C. (2017). Psychometric testing of a religious belief scale. *The Journal of Nursing Research, 25*(6), 419–428. https://doi.org/10.1097/JNR.0000000000000197

Cohen, J. (1988). *Statistical power analysis for the behavioral sciences* (2nd ed.). Hillsdale, NJ: Lawrence Erlbaum Associates.

Edwards, A., Pang, N., Shiu, V., & Chan, C. (2010). The understanding of spirituality and the potential role of spiritual care in end-of-life and palliative care: A meta-study of qualitative research. *Palliative Medicine, 24*(8), 753–770. https://doi.org/10.1177/0269216310375860

Ellison, C. G., & Levin, J. S. (1998). The religion-health connection: Evidence, theory, and future directions. *Health Education & Behavior, 25*(6), 700–720. https://doi.org/10.1177/109019819802500603

Grim, B. J., Johnson, T. M., Skirbekk, V., & Zurlo, G. A. (2015). *Yearbook of international religious demography 2015.* Leiden, The Netherlands: Brill.

Hair, J. F., Black, W. C., Babin, B. J., Anderson, R. E., & Tatham, R. L. (2006). *Multivariate data analysis* (6th ed.). Upper Saddle River, NJ: Prentice Hall.

Hall, D. E., Meador, K. G., & Koenig, H. G. (2008). Measuring religiousness in health research: Review and critique. *Journal of Religion & Health, 47*(2), 134–163. https://doi.org/10.1007/s10943-008-9165-2

Hill, P. C., & Hood, R. W. Jr. (1999). *Measures of religiosity.* Birmingham, AL: Religious Education Press.

Hsiao, S. M., Gau, M. L., Ingleton, C., Ryan, T., & Shih, F. J. (2011). An exploration of spiritual needs of Taiwanese patients with advanced cancer during the therapeutic processes. *Journal of Clinical Nursing, 20*(7/8), 950–959. https://doi.org/10.1111/j.1365-2702.2010.03278.x

Hsiao, Y. C., Chiang, Y. C., Lee, H. C., & Han, C. Y. (2013). Psychometric testing of the properties of the spiritual health scale short form. *Journal of Clinical Nursing, 22*(21/22), 2981–2990. https://doi.org/10.1111/jocn.12410

Koenig, H. G., King, D. E., & Carson, V. B. (2012). *Handbook of religion and health* (2nd ed.). New York, NY: Oxford University Press.

Lin, Y. H., Liou, S. H., & Chen, C. H. (2008). Spirutal care in nursing practice. *The Journal of Nursing, 55*(3), 69–74. https://doi.org/10.6224/JN.55.3.69 (Original work published in Chinese).

Liu, E. Y. (2010). Are risk-taking persons less religious? Risk preference, religious affiliation, and religious participation in Taiwan. *Journal for the Scientific Study of Religion, 49*(1), 172–178. https://doi.org/10.1111/j.1468-5906.2009.01499.x (Original work published in Chinese)

Liu, Y. J., & Wu, C. S. (2008). Toward a holistic health care: Advocating for hospital chaplain services. *Taiwan Journal of Hospice Palliative Care, 13*(1), 82–100. https://doi.org/10.6537/TJHPC.2008.13(1).7 (Original work published in Chinese)

McSherry, W., & Jamieson, S. (2011). An online survey of nurses' perceptions of spirituality and spiritual care. *Journal of Clinical Nursing, 20*(11/12), 1757–1767. https://doi.org/10.1111/j.1365-2702.2010.03547.x

Medved Kendrick, H. (2017). Are religion and spirituality barriers or facilitators to treatment for HIV: A systematic review of the literature. *AIDS Care, 29*(1), 1–13. https://doi.org/10.1007/s10943-013-9691-4

Ministry of the Interior, Taiwan, ROC. (2018). *Statistics of religious temples, churches profile.* Retrieved from https://www.moi.gov.tw/files/site_stuff/321/2/year/year.html

Neyrinck, B., Vansteenkiste, M., Lens, W., Duriez, B., & Hutsebaut, D. (2006). Cognitive, affective and behavioral correlates of internalization of regulations for religious activities. *Motivation & Emotion, 30*(4), 321–332. https://doi.org/10.1007/s11031-006-9048-3

Noble, A., & Jones, C. (2010). Getting it right: Oncology nurses' understanding of spirituality. *International Journal of Palliative Nursing, 16*(11), 565–569. https://doi.org/10.12968/ijpn.2010.16.11.80022

Phelps, A. C., Maciejewski, P. K., Nilsson, M., Balboni, T. A., Wright, A. A., Paulk, M. E., ... Peteet, J. R. (2009). Religious coping and use of intensive life-prolonging care near death in patients with advanced cancer. *Journal of the American Medical Association, 301*(11), 1140–1147. https://doi.org/10.1001/jama.2009.341

Polit, D. F., & Beck, C. T. (2006). The content validity index: Are you sure you know what's being reported? Critique and recommendations. *Research in Nursing and Health, 29*, 489–497. https://doi.org/10.1002/nur.20147

Ramezani, M., Ahmadi, F., Mohammadi, E., & Kazemnejad, A. (2014). Spiritual care in nursing: A concept analysis. *International Nursing Review, 61*(2), 211–219. https://doi.org/10.1111/inr.12099

Rykkje, L. L., Eriksson, K., & Raholm, M. B. (2013). Spirituality and caring in old age and the significance of religion—A hermeneutical study from Norway. *Scandinavian Journal of Caring Sciences, 27*(2), 275–284. https://doi.org/10.1111/j.1471-6712.2012.01028.x

Soanes, C., & Stevenson, A. (2006). *Oxford dictionary of English*. London, England: Oxford University Press.

Taylor, E. J., Park, C. G., & Pfeiffer, J. B. (2014). Nurse religiosity and spiritual care. *Journal of Advanced Nursing, 70*(11), 2612–2621. https://doi.org/10.1111/jan.12446

Tzeng, H. M., & Yin, C. Y. (2006). Demands for religious care in the Taiwanese health system. *Nursing Ethics, 13*(2), 163–179. https://doi.org/10.1191/0969733006ne835oa

van Leeuwen, R., & Cusveller, B. (2004). Nursing competencies for spiritual care. *Journal of Advanced Nursing, 48*(3), 234–246. https://doi.org/10.1111/j.1365-2702.2006.01643.x

Wu, H. F., & Hsiao, Y. C. (2009). A study of the correlation between the spiritual health status and spiritual care abilities of nurses. *Journal of Nursing and Healthcare Research, 5*(1), 68–78. https://doi.org/10.6225/JNHR.5.1.68 (Original work published in Chinese)

Yang, B. J., & Liu, D. J. (2009). *The analects of Confucius: Chinese-English edition*. Taipei, Taiwan, ROC: Lian-Jing.

Yeager, D. M., Glei, D. A., Au, M., Lin, H. S., Sloan, R. P., & Weinstein, M. (2006). Religious involvement and health outcomes among older persons in Taiwan. *Social Science & Medicine, 63*(8), 2228–2241. https://doi.org/10.1016/j.socscimed.2006.05.007

8

Nursing Staff Characteristics on Resident Outcomes in Nursing Homes

Juh Hyun SHIN

ABSTRACT

Background: The outlook of administrative staff and registered nurses (RNs) plays a critical role in the management of nursing homes. No previous study has compared the outcomes of nursing homes with RNs on staff with those of nursing homes without RNs on staff in Korea.

Purpose: The aim of this study was to investigate the association between nurse-led nursing homes, staff turnover, and resident outcomes in nursing homes in Korea.

Methods: Using a cross-sectional design, 36 nursing homes with 30 or more beds participated. Primary data included 15 quality indicators.

Results: Nursing homes with RNs had statistically significant better resident outcomes. RN turnover related positively to the prevalence of falls ($\beta = 1.68$, $p < .05$) and tube feeding ($\beta = 1.71$, $p < .01$) and negatively to incontinence ($\beta = -1.53$, $p < .01$). Nursing homes with RNs with tenures greater than 1 year had statistically significant lower prevalence of falls ($\beta = -0.47$, $p < .05$), incontinence ($\beta = -0.45$, $p < .05$), weight loss ($\beta = -0.53$ $p < .05$), and bed rest ($\beta = -0.54$, $p < .01$) and increased range of motion ($\beta = 0.51$, $p < .05$). Interestingly, having a nurse as a director for more than 1 year related negatively to the incidence of urinary tract infection ($\beta = -0.56$, $p < .05$) in residents. The rate of RN turnover was found to impact fall prevalence ($\beta = 1.68$, $p < .05$) and tube feeding ($\beta = 1.71$, $p < .01$) positively and to impact incontinence ($\beta = -1.53$, $p < .01$) negatively.

Conclusions: Turnover of nursing home staff and length of tenure may contribute to the more effective management of nursing homes, higher-quality long-term care insurance, and RN-staffing-related laws. Assessing staff characteristics and the tenure of employees promotes the effective management of nursing homes.

KEY WORDS:
nursing home, quality of care, administrator, nursing management.

Introduction

Emphases on quality and cost-effectiveness in the nursing home industry have increased, complicated by providing nursing care with diverse resident demands and limited resources worldwide (McGilton et al., 2016). The population share of older adults in Korea is estimated to rise to 37.4% by 2050 (Statistics Korea, 2013). To facilitate the care of older adults in professional institutions, the Korean government implemented long-term care insurance for older adults in July 2008 (Korean Ministry of Health and Welfare, 2013). However, only 0.1% of registered nurses (RNs) in Korea work in nursing homes (Organisation for Economic Co-operation and Development, 2011). Most nursing homes in Korea employ alternative nurse staffs such as certified nurse aides because of the shortage of nurses and financial reasons. The Korean long-term care law requires nurse staffing as follows: one RN or certified nursing assistant (CNA) per 25 older adults (for nursing homes larger than 30 beds); one RN or CNA, one physical therapist, and one occupational therapist for 10- to 30-bed nursing homes; and one RN or CNA for nursing homes with less than 10 beds (Korean National Health Insurance Corporation, 2013). The scope of responsibilities of certified nurse aides is similar to that of licensed practical nurses (LPNs) in the United States, and the job scope of qualified care workers is equivalent to that of certified nurse aides in the United States (H. Y. Lee, Shin, & Harrington, 2015). The extensive body of literature worldwide on nurse staffing and outcomes includes a number of studies that support the contribution of RNs. However, no research to date has studied the relationship between nursing leadership position on resident outcomes.

Only a few studies have reported that nurse-led specific interventions effectively decreased medication errors (Blozik et al., 2010). In residential settings, nurse practitioners were shown to improve the management of chronic diseases (Neylon, 2015). However, no studies were identified in a search of the literature that addressed the relationship between administrative staff and resident outcomes in Korea.

The outlook of administrative staffs in nursing homes plays a critical role in developing a caring culture (Brannon, Kemper, Heier-Leitzell, & Stott, 2010) and achieving effective financial management (Lerner, Johantgen, Trinkoff, Storr, & Han, 2014). Consistent leadership contributes to efficient staffing and policymaking and the implementation of best nursing practices and high-quality care for residents (Krause,

PhD, RN, Assistant Professor, College of Nursing, Ewha Womans University, Republic of Korea.

2012). The top manager in nursing homes usually includes administrators and directors of nurses (DONs). In the United States, each state has implemented a formal examination system for nursing home administrators (Siegel, Leo, Young, & Castle, 2014). In Korea, administrators are required to hold a social work certificate, in accordance with the Social Welfare Service Law and Medical Law, Article 2 (National Law Information Center, 2015). Nursing home administrators play critical roles in total management, human resource management, collaboration among staffs, providing care for residents with family members, and using community resources. The philosophy, attitudes, and leadership of administrators affect the general management and culture of the nursing home (G. H. Lee & Lee, 2012). Administrators' attitudes regarding culture change in long-term care settings are important. Moreover, the educational background of administrators, their management philosophy and beliefs, their attitudes toward person-centered care, and their perceptions on the importance of the physical environment, financial management, and staffing characteristics were statistically significant in the adoption of unit care in long-term care settings (G. H. Lee & Lee, 2012).

However, about 40% of administrators and DONs in the United States leave their positions within the first year (Executive Search Solutions, 2011). Moreover, the tenure of administrators differs based on proprietorship (profit or not for profit) and chain affiliations (Decker & Castle, 2009; Resnick, Manard, Stone, & Castle, 2009). DONs must have critical thinking skills in the decision-making process on a daily basis to achieve high-quality nursing care with very limited supplies and strict regulations (Siegel, Young, Zysberg, & Santillan, 2015). On the basis of the size of nursing homes, RNs and DONs may be employed in a single position or in two separate positions (Paek, Zhang, Wan, Unruh, & Meemon, 2016). DONs play very important roles in nursing homes because of their position between the structure (administrative role) and process (direct care nurse), as described in Donabedian's structure–process–outcome model (Siegel et al., 2015).

This study examines the importance of nurse staffing and turnover. The turnover of RNs and DONs is another factor that impacts resident outcomes. DON tenure stability has been positively associated with quality ratings (Krause, 2012) and Centers for Medicare and Medicaid's quality indicators (Rantz et al., 2004, 2003) and negatively associated with use of restraints (Anderson, Issel, & McDaniel, 2003) and immobility (Anderson et al., 2003) among residents. The turnover of nursing home administrators was shown to diminish quality outcomes but enhance resident outcomes (Castle & Lin, 2010). Furthermore, high rates of turnover of RNs have been correlated with poor resident outcomes, including increased numbers of residents on antidepressant medications, increased dehydration, and more bed rest (Castle & Anderson, 2011; Shin & Hyun, 2015). In addition, increased turnover of qualified care workers was found to relate positively with a lower prevalence of dehydration and bed rest among residents (Shin & Hyun, 2015). Furthermore, having long-tenured nurses on staff has been correlated with better nursing home resident outcomes (Castle & Engberg, 2007). The increased turnover of DONs was associated with a lower proportion of residents with depression, whereas the high turnover of LPNs and CNAs had no statistically significant effect on resident outcomes in nursing homes (Castle & Anderson, 2011; Castle & Engberg, 2007). More research on the turnover of long-tenured staff in nursing homes is necessary in light of the limited number of relevant studies.

No study in the literature has compared resident outcomes in nursing homes with RNs with those in nursing homes without RNs in Korea. Thus, the purpose of this study was to investigate the association between nurse-led nursing homes, staff turnover, and resident outcomes in nursing homes. The hypotheses follow:

1. Nursing homes led by nurse administrators have better resident outcomes.
2. Nursing homes with RNs have better resident outcomes.
3. Nursing homes with DONs have better resident outcomes.
4. The rate of staff turnover relates to resident outcomes.
5. Tenure in the current position relates to resident outcomes.

Methods

Study Design

We used a descriptive cross-sectional design to evaluate, as dependent variables, the quality outcomes of 15 residents. We contacted by e-mail, by telephone, or in person all of the nursing homes in Korea in operation between 2014 and 2016 to invite their participation (N = 1,332) in this study. Ten percent of the nursing homes that indicated willingness to participate were randomly selected by computer. The principal investigator contacted about 130 nursing homes by e-mail and telephone, and 36 nursing homes were finally enrolled as participating institutions. These included only medium- and large-sized nursing homes (30 beds or larger, as evaluated by the Korean National Health Insurance Corporation, 2013). Every 3 years, the Korean Ministry of Health Welfare is mandated to evaluate nursing homes (Korean National Health Insurance Service, 2017). On the basis of this evaluation, an evaluation grade is assigned to each nursing home. Monetary incentives are provided to the top 20% of nursing homes, and an additional inspection is conducted on nursing homes that did not pass the evaluation (Korean National Health Insurance Service, 2017).

Data Sources

Information gathered included bed size, duration of operation, ownership characteristics, chain, religious affiliation of the establishment, referral hospitals, location (metropolitan or rural), current job tenure of administrators and DONs, and numbers of administrators who, respectively, hold a nursing license, are DONs, and are RNs. All of the data were collected from primary sources because no published national data exist, and secondary data on nursing home staffing are not currently available from reliable sources (Kash, Castle, & Phillips, 2007).

Data were collected on the 15 core quality indicators related to resident outcomes that were developed by the Centers for Medicare and Medicaid in the United States and included in the 88 quality indicators of the Korean National Health Insurance Service (2017) nursing home evaluation manual (see Shin & Hyun, 2015, for details). As no official data exist on the turnover of nurse staffs, these data were collected using the American Health Care Association's (2011) Nursing Facility Staff Survey instrument.

Data Collection

A survey was used to collect the data. This survey was sent to all 1,332 nursing homes with 30 or more beds whose e-mail address was published on the long-term care insurance home page. Additional face-to-face or telephone meetings were held when requested. Approval from the institutional review board of a university in Korea was granted for this study (IRB no. 77-1).

Data Analysis

Multiple negative binomial regression was used to analyze the data. The independent variables were (a) RNs on staff/no RNs on staff, (b) DONs on staff/no DONs on staff, and (c) tenure and turnover of nursing staff. The dependent variables were the 15 quality indicators. To offset the limitations of using a cross-sectional design, we controlled heterogeneity between nursing homes as a fixed effect. Using a simple mixed-effects model for power analysis, a sample size of 36 was large enough to provide 75% power for the 15 fixed-effects dependent variables. The market characteristics of geographic location, ownership characteristics (profit vs. not for profit), market share, and size of facility were used as the control variables. The Herfindahl–Hirschman index (number of beds in an organization divided by the total number of beds in a province) was employed to control market competition characteristics (Paek et al., 2016). The long-term care insurance hierarchy (five stages) was used to adjust the case mix of residents statistically. This case mix was determined based on physical or mental competencies, cognitive status, behavior patterns, required nursing tasks, and rehabilitation (Korean National Health Insurance Service, 2017). SPSS Version 23.0 (IBM, Armonk, NY, USA) was used to identify variables with coefficients that satisfied p values below .05 and .1.

Results

Organizational Characteristics

The organizational characteristics of participating institutions are shown in Table 1. The average number of beds was 87.75 (SD = 13.24, ranging from 9 to 296 beds). Average occupancy was high (93.35%, SD = 11.43%, ranging from 50.95% to 100%), and the average stay of residents was about 8 years and 5 months (SD = 4.00, ranging from 2 to 16 years). About 86.11% were operated as nonprofit organizations. More than half were located in small cities. Most (88.9%) did not have formal referral hospitals, and 32.43% had a religious affiliation. Approximately 46.53% of residents were third-grade, long-term care beneficiaries, who are partially dependent for activities of daily living.

Staff Characteristics and Outcomes

The results indicate that neither having a nurse as the administrator nor having multiple DONs impacted resident outcomes significantly. However, significantly better resident outcomes were identified in nursing homes with RNs in terms of the following variables: fewer falls ($\beta = 0.41, p < .05$), less cognitive impairment ($\beta = 0.45, p < .01$), less incontinence

TABLE 1.

Organizational Characteristics of 36 Nursing Homes

Demographic	Mean	*SD*
Number of beds	87.75	13.24
Occupancy rate (%)	93.35	11.43
Operation duration (years)	8.42	4.00
	n	%
Ownership form		
For profit	5	13.89
Not for profit	31	86.11
Location of organizations (population)		
Large metropolitan city (≥ 1 million)	11	30.56
Local small city (50,000–500,000)	22	61.11
Rural area (≤ 50,000)	3	8.33
Long-term care insurance[†]		
First[a]		14.63
Second[b]		28.33
Third[c]		46.53
Fourth[d]		9.39
Fifth[e]		0.00
Unrated		1.12
Chain of hospitals		
Yes	4	11.10
No	32	88.90
Religious affiliation		
Yes	11	32.43
No	25	67.57

[†]percentage of total sample; [a]Older adults who are completely dependent for activities of daily living. [b]Older adults who are mostly dependent for activities of daily living. [c]Older adults who are partially dependent for activities of daily living. [d]Older adults who have limited dependence for activities of daily living. [e]Older adults with dementia.

TABLE 2.
Staff Characteristics and Outcomes

Outcome	Administrator Led by Nurse		Director of Nursing		Registered Nurse		R^2	F
	β	p	β	p	β	p		
1. Fall prevalence	−0.18	.28	0.19	.25	0.41*	.02	.22	3.00*
2. Aggressive behavior	−0.11	.56	0.14	.45	0.17	.37	.05	0.64
3. Depression	0.03	.85	0.21	.24	0.21	.26	.11	1.34
4. Cognitive impairment	−0.12	.48	0.09	.61	0.45**	< .01	.21	2.75
5. Incontinence	−0.11	.52	0.09	.60	0.41*	.03	.17	2.25
6. Urinary tract infection	−0.14	.45	−0.17	.34	0.26	.17	.07	0.18
7. Weight loss	0.08	.67	0.25	.15	0.23	.20	.16	1.99
8. Dehydration	0.04	.81	0.22	.21	0.20	.28	.11	1.33
9. Tube feeding	−0.10	.56	0.11	.50	0.47**	< .01	.23	3.11*
10. Bed rest	−0.13	.41	0.25	.10	0.52**	< .01	.35	5.66**
11. Activities of daily living	−0.59	.14	0.43	.22	−0.13	.73	.48	1.86
12. Range of motion	0.10	.59	0.05	.78	0.29	.12	.12	1.44
13. Antidepressant or sleeping pills	0.14	.40	0.14	.38	0.36*	.04	.23	3.01*
14. Physically restrained	−0.29	.12	0.02	.93	0.32	.09	.13	1.49

Note. β = standardized coefficient.
$^*p < .05$. $^{**}p < .01$.

(β = 0.41, $p < .05$), less tube feeding (β = 0.47, $p < .01$), less bed rest (β = 0.52, $p < .01$), and fewer sleeping pills or antidepressants (β = 0.36, $p < .05$; Table 2).

Staff Turnover and Resident Outcomes

The ability of staff turnover to predict resident outcomes was also examined. As shown in Table 3, RN turnover

TABLE 3.
Staff Turnover and Resident Outcomes

Outcome	Registered Nurse Turnover		Care Worker Turnover		Social Worker Turnover	
	β	p	β	p	β	p
1. Fall prevalence	1.68*	.04	0.00	.99	0.06	.75
2. Aggressive behavior	0.74	.06	−0.12	.44	0.40*	.01
3. Depression	0.46	.35	−0.22	.19	−0.31	.19
4. Cognitive impairment	1.63	.07	−0.10	.54	0.04	.85
5. Incontinence	−1.53**	< .01	0.17	.18	0.01	.94
6. Urinary tract infection	0.03	.87	−0.23	.44	−0.02	.95
7. Weight loss	0.70	.10	−0.03	.78	−0.04	.82
8. Dehydration	−0.45	.58	−0.22	.33	−0.17	.60
9. Tube feeding	1.71**	< .01	−0.01	.93	−0.21	.23
10. Bed rest	1.33	.08	−0.09	.77	−0.28	.52
11. Activities of daily living			−0.85	.10		
12. Range of motion	0.13	.66	0.02	.83	−0.09	.51
13. Antidepressant or sleeping pills	−0.18	.77	−0.33	.13	−0.02	.90
14. Physically restrained	1.31	.13	0.12	.75	−0.22	.62

Note. β = standardized coefficient.
$^*p < .05$. $^{**}p < .01$. $^{***}p < .001$.

was found to relate positively to a lower prevalence of falls (β = 1.68, $p < .05$), less tube feeding (β = 1.71, $p < .01$), and less incontinence (β = −1.53, $p < .01$); administrative staff turnover was found to relate positively to depression (β = 0.75, $p < .05$), dehydration (β = 1.02, $p < .05$), range of motion (β = 0.84, $p < .01$), and use of antidepressant or sleeping pills (β = 0.89, $p < .01$); social worker turnover was found to relate positively to aggressive behavior (β = 0.4, $p = .01$); and dietician turnover was found to relate positively to prevalence of falls (β = 1.12, $p < .001$), aggressive behaviors (β = 0.45, $p < .05$), cognitive impairment (β = 1.02, $p < .01$), incontinence (β = 0.99, $p < .001$), weight loss (β = 0.47, $p < .05$), and tube feeding (β = 1.24, $p < .001$).

Staff Tenure and Resident Outcomes

Nursing homes with RNs with tenures of more than 1 year had statistically significant reductions in the prevalence of falls (β = −0.47, $p < .05$), incontinence (β = −0.45, $p < .05$), weight loss (β = −0.53 $p < .05$), and bed rest (β = −0.54, $p < .01$) and increases in range of motion (β = 0.51, $p < .05$). Interestingly, having a DON with a tenure of over 1 year was negatively associated with the incidence of urinary tract infections among residents (β = −0.56, $p < .05$). Moreover, nursing homes with social workers and RNs with a tenure of over 1 year had significantly lower aggressive behavior (β = −0.54, $p < .05$), depression (β = −0.48, $p < .05$), and weight loss (β = −0.51, $p < .01$), as shown in Table 4.

Discussion

This article tested staff characteristics and turnover, length of tenure of employees, and resident outcomes in nursing homes. This was the first study to examine the effects of nurse-led nursing homes, staffing of nurses, staff turnover, and resident outcomes in Korea. Unexpectedly, nursing leadership of nursing homes did not significantly affect resident outcomes. Previous research indicates that the management philosophy, the awareness of importance of staffing and finance, and the experience of managers improved resident outcomes in government-funded long-term care settings (G. H. Lee & Lee, 2012). Furthermore, the general management autonomy of administrators or DONs has been deemed to guarantee the achievement of effective management with optimal quality of care (G. H. Lee & Lee, 2012). Nursing leadership plays a crucial role in advancing quality of care. The positive nursing leadership of nurse administrators favorably influences working conditions and culture and may be employed to accomplish better patient outcomes (André, Sjøvold, Rannestad, & Ringdal, 2014). Chief nurse executives promote patient safety, patient-centered care, and cost-effective systems (Adams, Erickson, Jones, & Paulo, 2009). The results of this study are inconsistent with the results of prior research in that the nursing home administrators in this study did not impact nursing home outcomes. Thus, further research is necessary to confirm the effects of staff characteristics, especially focusing on the impact of nurse-led nursing homes on resident outcomes.

Dietitian Turnover		Cook Turnover		Administrative Staff Turnover			
β	p	β	p	β	p	R^2	F
1.12***	< .001	−0.05	.75	−0.26	.21	.93	13.37**
0.45*	.040	−0.05	.79	0.35	.15	.91	9.67**
0.32	.130	0.32	.11	0.75*	.02	.90	8.56**
1.02**	.002	0.03	.87	−0.25	.33	.88	7.45*
0.99***	< .001	−0.04	.78	−0.01	.94	.94	16.56**
−0.04	.900	−0.01	.99	0.67	.16	.64	1.77
0.47*	.014	−0.04	.80	0.61*	.01	.94	16.37**
−0.22	.440	0.17	.53	1.02*	.02	.79	3.83
1.24***	< .001	0.16	.27	−0.88**	< .01	.94	16.43**
0.78	.070	−0.02	.96	0.04	.92	.64	1.76
		−0.01	.98			.64	1.97
−0.08	.600	0.15	.30	0.84**	< .01	.95	18.28***
−0.06	.840	−0.04	.88	0.89**	< .01	.83	4.80*
−0.28	.610	0.54	.26	−0.51	.38	.40	0.67

TABLE 4.
Staff Tenure and Resident Outcomes

Outcome	SEC	DON	NAD	RN	CW	SW
	β	β	β	β	β	β
1. Fall prevalence	−0.22	0.20	0.18	−0.47*	−0.01	−0.26
2. Aggressive behavior	−0.02	−0.13	0.42*	0.26	0.03	−0.54*
3. Depression	−0.20	0.01	0.34	0.17	−0.01	−0.48*
4. Cognitive impairment	−0.07	−0.07	0.21	0.39	−0.05	−0.18
5. Incontinence	−0.12	−0.02	0.23	−0.45*	0.02	−0.26
6. Urinary tract infection	−0.05	−0.56*	−0.12	−0.05	−0.01	−0.12
7. Weight loss	−0.36*	0.19	0.40*	−0.53*	−0.23	−0.51**
8. Dehydration	−0.26	0.06	0.18	0.18	0.02	−0.40
9. Tube feeding	0.21	0.06	0.25	0.44	−0.13	0.21
10. Bed rest	−0.15	0.15	0.27	−0.54**	−0.10	0.12
11. ADL						
12. Range of motion	−0.34	−0.05	0.25	0.51*	0.07	−0.28
13. Antidepressant or sleeping pills	−0.04	−0.19	0.17	0.36	−0.05	−0.34
14. Physically restrained	0.03	−0.28	0.01	−0.02	−0.02	0.34

Note. SEC = executive secretary; DON = director of nurses; NAD = administrator led by nurse; RN = registered nurse; CW = care worker; SW = social worker; AS = administrative staff; ADL = activities of daily living; β = standardized coefficient.
$^{*}p < .05$. $^{**}p < .01$.

In this study, the effects of turnover on quality outcomes are quite consistent with those identified in previous studies. High turnover of RNs aligned with the prevalence of falls, tube feeding, and incontinence, and care worker turnover impacted tube feeding. In previous studies, stability in RN staffing (i.e., lower turnover) was significantly associated with decreased falls, decreased tube feeding, and decreased incontinence; higher CNA and licensed nurse turnover (RNs and LPNs) was significantly associated with low quality of care (Lerner et al., 2014); higher CNA turnover was significantly associated with more pressure ulcers, pain, and urinary tract infections (Trinkoff et al., 2013); and a high rate of turnover of qualified care workers reduced the prevalence of residents with dehydration and bed rest (Shin & Hyun, 2015).

The turnover of administrative staffs was found to relate to resident outcomes in this study. However, Harvey (2014) found no significant relationship between administrator turnover and patient outcomes. As the turnover of administrative and other staff has yielded complex results in many studies, additional research is necessary to clarify this relationship. In this study, the high turnover of social workers caused more tube feeding and dietician turnover aligned with a prevalence of falls, aggressive behaviors, cognitive impairment, weight loss, and tube feeding. However, no researchers have investigated the relationship between the turnover rate in other occupations (social workers, dieticians, and administrative staff) and nursing home resident outcomes. More research is needed to clarify the effect of staffs other than nurses on resident outcomes in nursing homes.

In particular, nursing homes that had RNs with over 1 year of tenure had better outcomes in terms of falls, incontinence, weight loss, bed rest, and range of motion, and those that had DONs with over 1 year of tenure exhibited a lower incidence of urinary tract infection. RNs are responsible for assessing major physical or psychological changes or symptoms and for cooperating with physicians for better treatment and care plans, whereas care that is provided by assistive personnel such as CNAs is nontechnical (Konetzka, Stearns, & Park, 2008). However, some nursing homes replace RNs with CNAs to decrease staffing costs. In addition, RNs are reluctant to work in nursing homes because of deficiencies in the working environment and insufficient benefits (Konetzka et al., 2008).

In Korea, nursing homes may employ RNs or CNAs interchangeably. For example, nursing homes must have at least one RN or CNA per 25 residents for 30 or more beds and one qualified care worker per 2.5 residents (Korean National Health Insurance Corporation, 2013). However, in the United States, the federal government and each state mandate specific requirements for nurse staffing in nursing homes, specifying direct and indirect care, number of licensed versus unlicensed staff, specific nursing staff numbers during mealtimes, and size of facilities (Harrington, 2005). In 2003, the Centers for Medicare and Medicaid Services recommended that nursing homes maintain a minimum staff of one RN, with increasing staffing levels with increased resident numbers (Harrington, 2005). We studied the effects of organization and nurse staff characteristics on resident outcomes in nursing homes. Legislative regulations for long-term care facilities in Korea did not reflect differences in each staff role and responsibility, direct

Dietitian	Cook	AS				
β	β	β	R^2	*F*	*M*	*SD*
0.01	0.20	0.12	.36	1.65	12.31	25.98
−0.23	0.36	0.35	.35	1.56	7.58	9.91
0.11	0.45	0.20	.40	1.96	10.01	17.22
0.08	0.25	0.17	.31	1.29	52.94	55.34
−0.01	0.26	0.14	.31	1.30	39.75	49.06
0.25	0.10	0.55	.29	1.16	2.36	5.32
−0.16	0.47*	0.07	.56	3.69**	4.11	10.08
0.21	0.35	0.18	.37	1.63	0.97	1.90
−0.12	0.03	0.06	.32	1.28	6.86	8.94
0.02	−0.06	0.35	.56	3.50**	16.29	12.86
−0.17	0.18	0.29	.37	1.65	1.99	3.77
0.07	0.50	0.25	.42	1.99	32.51	29.68
0.26	−0.25	0.44	.28	1.10	5.20	6.41

and indirect care, licensed versus unlicensed personnel, and any specific required timing such as mealtimes (Shin & Hyun, 2015).

Unorganized staff roles and duties lead to poor practice environments and overwork problems, causing discontent and high staff turnover (Maenhout & Vanhoucke, 2013). Nurse staffing is pivotal to the delivery of high-quality care. Many studies report a relationship between higher experienced RN staffing and lower adverse outcomes. Furthermore, legislative regulations that address the issue of optimal staffing are more effective when they specify more than numbers. Well-organized direct care staffs contribute to the development of quality of care (American Nurses Association, 2017). Thus, it is necessary to introduce policies on stable nurse staffing at nursing homes to enhance residents' quality of care.

Limitations

This study had some limitations. First, the issue of how DONs control and administer their staff and resources was not examined. Further research is needed to examine how nurse administrators and DONs actually operate and the effects of this on residents' quality-of-care outcomes. Second, as participating facilities are not representative of all nursing homes in Korea, generalizations should be made cautiously. Third, the 88 quality indicators that were developed by the Korean National Health Insurance Service (2017) were not fully measured, although very important issues such as elder abuse, communication with family members, counseling with residents, quality of food, transfer, staffing benefits, and appropriate reactions to emergency situations were raised. Future research should consider a wider scope of quality measures. Last, the cross-sectional design used limits the validity of findings. Thus, more research is necessary to confirm the association between the nurse-led administration of nursing homes and resident outcomes.

Conclusions

This study examined using a cross-sectional approach the relationship between nurse-led nursing homes, staff turnover, length of tenure of employees, and resident outcomes. This was the first study to examine the relationship between nurse administrative staffing and resident outcomes in nursing homes in Korea. More research using representative sampling is required to confirm the influence of various administrative staff characteristics on resident outcomes.

Using large databases of administrative staff, future researchers may expand the current knowledge about the linkage between administrative staff characteristics and resident outcomes. In addition, accessible research materials on the effects of staff turnover and on resident outcomes are necessary for administrators or chiefs of nursing to create a more stable working environment in nursing homes (Lerner et al., 2014). Moreover, this study contributed to improving the quality of long-term care services for older adults. By assessing staff characteristics, turnover of nursing home staff, and tenure of employees, this study contributes to the more efficient management of nursing homes and to providing high-quality long-term care for older adults. Ultimately, this study contributes to enacting laws on stable staffing, especially with regard to nurse staffing in nursing homes. This study may lead to improved quality of life for older adults who need support from the government and their families and improve the quality of the work environment of employees in nursing homes.

Acknowledgments

This research was supported by Basic Science Research Program through the National Research Foundation of Korea funded by the Ministry of Science, ICT & Future Planning (2017R1A2B0032382).

References

Adams, J. M., Erickson, J. I., Jones, D. A., & Paulo, L. (2009). An evidence-based structure for transformative nurse executive practice: The model of the interrelationship of leadership, environments, and outcomes for nurse executives (MILE ONE). *Nursing Administration Quarterly, 33*(4), 280–287. https://doi.org/10.1097/NAQ.0b013e3181b9dce3

American Health Care Association. (2011). *2011 Staffing survey report.* Retrieved from http://www.ahcancal.org/research_data/staffing/Documents/2011%20Staffing%20Survey%20Report.pdf

American Nurses Association. (2017). *Safe staffing literature review.* Retrieved from http://nursingworld.org/SafeStaffing-LiteratureReview

Anderson, R. A., Issel, L. M., & McDaniel, R. R., Jr. (2003). Nursing homes as complex adaptive systems: Relationship between management practice and resident outcomes. *Nursing Research, 52*(2), 12–21. https://doi.org/10.1097/00006199-200301000-00003

André, B., Sjøvold, E., Rannestad, T., & Ringdal, G. I. (2014). The impact of work culture on quality of care in nursing homes—A review study. *Scandinavian Journal of Caring Sciences, 28*(3), 449–457. https://doi.org/10.1111/scs.12086

Blozik, E., Born, A. M., Stuck, A. E., Benninger, U., Gillmann, G., & Clough-Gorr, K. M. (2010). Reduction of inappropriate medications among older nursing-home residents: A nurse-led, pre/post-design, intervention study. *Drugs & Aging, 27*(2), 1009–1017. https://doi.org/10.2165/11584770-000000000-00000

Brannon, S. D., Kemper, P., Heier-Leitzell, B., & Stott, A. (2010). Reinventing management practices in long-term care: How cultural evolution can affect workforce recruitment and retention. *Generations, 34*(4), 68–74.

Castle, N. G., & Anderson, R. A. (2011). Caregiver staffing in nursing homes and their influence on quality of care: Using dynamic panel estimation methods. *Medical Care, 49*(6), 545–552. https://doi.org/10.1097/MLR.0b013e31820fbca9

Castle, N. G., & Engberg, J. (2007). The influence of staffing characteristics on quality of care in nursing homes. *Health Services Research, 42*(5), 1822–1847. https://doi.org/10.1111/j.1475-6773.2007.00704.x

Castle, N. G., & Lin, M. (2010). Top management turnover and quality in nursing homes. *Health Care Management Review, 35*(2), 161–174. https://doi.org/10.1097/HMR.0b013e3181c22bcb

Decker, F. H., & Castle, N. G. (2009). The relationship of education level to the job tenure of nursing home administrators and directors of nursing. *Health Care Management Review, 34*(2), 152–160. https://doi.org/10.1097/HMR.0b013e31819ea7f7

Executive Search Solutions. (2011). *Leadership turnover in long term care.* Retrieved from http://www.essusa.net/pdf/NURSINGHOMELEADERSHIPTURNOVERESSWhitePaperFinal.pdf

Harrington, C. (2005). Nurse staffing in nursing homes in the United States: Part II. *Journal of Gerontological Nursing, 31*(3), 9–15. https://doi.org/10.3928/0098-9134-20050301-05

Harvey, D. W. (2014). *Nursing home administrator turnover and quality of care: A quantitative study* (Doctoral dissertation). Retrieved from ProQuest Dissertations and Theses database. (UMI No. 3583305)

Kash, B. A., Castle, N. G., & Phillips, C. D. (2007). Nursing home spending, staffing, and turnover. *Health Care Management Review, 32*(3), 253–262. https://doi.org/10/1097/01.HMR.0000281625.20740.13

Konetzka, R. T., Stearns, S. C., & Park, J. (2008). The staffing-outcomes relationship in nursing homes. *Health Services Research, 43*(3), 1025–1042. https://doi.org/10.1111/j.1475-6773.2007.00803.x

Korean Ministry of Health and Welfare. (2013). *Medical law.* Retrieved from http://www.law.go.kr/DRF/lawService.do?OC=lrzh&target=law&MST=107499&type=HTML (Original work published in Korean)

Korean National Health Insurance Corporation. (2013). *Long term care insurance statistics* (no. 11-B550928-000038-09). Retrieved from http://khiss.go.kr/board/bbs_seq=367&bbsid=B301&tname=MINBOARD358 (Original work published in Korean)

Korean National Health Insurance Service. (2017). *Judgment rating for long-term care insurance.* Retrieved from http://www.nhis.or.kr/bbs7/boards/B0039/17025 (Original work published in Korean)

Krause, M. R. (2012). Director of nursing current job tenure and past experience and quality of care in nursing homes. *Health Care Management Review, 37*(1), 98–108. https://doi.org/10.1097/HMR.0b013e318222429a

Lee, G. H., & Lee, J. M. (2012). Impact of facility managers' characteristics on their intention to introduce a unit care system. *Health and Social Welfare Review, 32*(4), 94–122. https://doi.org/10.15709/hswr.2012.32.4.94

Lee, H. Y., Shin, J. H., & Harrington, C. (2015). Comparing the nurse staffing in Korean and U.S. nursing homes. *Nursing Outlook, 63*(2), 137–143. https://doi.org/10.1016/j.outlook.2014.08.005

Lerner, N. B., Johantgen, M., Trinkoff, A. M., Storr, C. L., & Han, K. (2014). Are nursing home survey deficiencies higher in facilities with greater staff turnover. *Journal of the American Medical Directors Association, 15*(2), 102–107. https://doi.org/10.1016/j.jamda.2013.09.003

Maenhout, B., & Vanhoucke, M. (2013). An integrated nurse staffing and scheduling analysis for longer-term nursing staff allocation problems. *Omega, 41*(2), 485–499. https://doi.org/10.1016/j.omega.2012.01.002

McGilton, K. S., Bowers, B. J., Heath, H., Shannon, K., Dellefield, M. E., Prentice, D., ... Mueller, C. A. (2016). Recommendations from the International consortium on professional nursing practice in long-term care homes. *Journal of the American Medical Directors Association, 17*(2), 99–103. https://doi.org/10.1016/j.jamda.2015.11.001

National Law Information Center. (2015). *Welfare of the Aged Act Article 22-1.* Retrieved from http://www.law.go.kr/lsInfoP.do?lsiSeq=178901&efYd=20160101#AJAX (Original work published in Korean)

Neylon, J. (2015). Nurse-led management of chronic disease in a residential care setting. *Nursing Older People, 27*(9), 22–26. https://doi.org/10.7748/nop.27.9.22.s18

Organisation for Economic Co-operation and Development. (2011). *Help wanted? Providing and paying for long-term care.* Retrieved from http://www.oecd.org/health/health-systems/help-wanted-9789264097759-en.htm

Paek, S. C., Zhang, N. J., Wan, T. T., Unruh, L. Y., & Meemon, N. (2016). The impact of state nursing home staffing standards on nurse staffing levels. *Medical Care Research and Review, 73*(1), 41–61. https://doi.org/10.1177/1077558715594733

Rantz, M. J., Hicks, L., Grando, V., Petroski, G. F., Madsen, R. W., Mehr, D. R., … Maas, M. (2004). Nursing home quality, cost, staffing, and staff mix. *The Gerontologist, 44*(1), 24–38. https://doi.org/10.1093/geront/44.1.24

Rantz, M. J., Vogelsmeier, A., Manion, P., Minner, D., Markway, B., Conn, V., … Mehr, D. R. (2003). Statewide strategy to improve quality of care in nursing facilities. *The Gerontologist, 43*(2), 248–258. https://doi.org/10.1093/geront/43.2.248

Resnick, H. E., Manard, B., Stone, R. I., & Castle, N. G. (2009). Tenure, certification, and education of nursing home administrators, medical directors, and directors of nursing in for-profit and not-for-profit nursing homes: United States 2004. *Journal of the American Medical Directors Association, 10*(6), 423–430. https://doi.org/10.1016/j.jamda.2009.03.009

Shin, J. H., & Hyun, T. K. (2015). Nurse staffing and quality of care of nursing home residents in Korea. *Journal of Nursing Scholarship, 47*(6), 555–564. https://doi.org/10.1111/jnu.12166

Siegel, E. O., Leo, M. C., Young, H. M., & Castle, N. G. (2014). Nursing home administrator self-assessed preparedness. *Health Care Management Review, 39*(3), 210–222. https://doi.org/10.1097/HMR.0b013e318294e5ce

Siegel, E. O., Young, H. M., Zysberg, L., & Santillan, V. (2015). Securing and managing nursing home resources: Director of nursing tactics. *The Gerontologist, 55*(5), 748–759. https://doi.org/10.1093/geront/gnu003

Statistics Korea. (2013). *Estimated future population.* Retrieved from http://meta.narastat.kr/metasvc/svc/SvcMetaDcDtaPopup.do?orgId=101&confmNo=10133&kosisYn=Y (Original work published in Korean)

Trinkoff, A. M., Han, K., Storr, C. L., Lerner, N., Johantgen, M., & Gartrell, K. (2013). Turnover, staffing, skill mix, and resident outcomes in a national sample of US nursing homes. *JONA: Journal of Nursing Administration, 43*(12), 630–636. https://doi.org/10.1097/NNA.0000000000000004

9

The Development of a Standardized Framework for Primary Nurse Specialists in Diabetes Care in China: A Delphi Study

Qiuling XING[1] • Mingxia ZHANG[2] • Fang ZHAO[3]* • Yingxia ZHOU[4] • Yongzhen MO[5] • Li YUAN[6]

ABSTRACT

Background: The number of patients with diabetes has been increasing rapidly according to a 2017 report by the International Diabetes Federation. Diabetes has become one of the most challenging public health problems, and there will be an estimated 143 million patients with diabetes in China by 2035. This puts considerable pressure on nurses who specialize in the care of patients with diabetes in China and increases related social and financial burdens. Clinical practice has proven that strengthening the core competencies of nurses and establishing an evaluation system of core competencies improve both healthcare quality and patient quality of life. However, no core-competence system framework currently addresses the unique characteristics of nurses in China.

Purposes: The purpose of this study was to construct a core-competence system framework for primary nurse specialists in diabetes care.

Methods: A brainstorming approach was conducted that worked to conceptualize the core competencies of nurse specialists in diabetes care in China. Next, a study group organized this information and conducted a seminar; 50 experts and patients with diabetes were invited to develop the first draft of the framework. Afterward, 50 experts were selected to participate in the Delphi survey. Most indicators were retained after a three-round Delphi process, and the superiority chart was used to determine the weights of the six dimensions.

Results: Forty-seven experts completed the consultation. The experts' rate of response ranged from 94% to 100%, the authority coefficient was .91, and the Kendall's coefficients of concordance in Grades 1–3 were .793, .418, and .542, respectively. An increasingly detailed, three-grade system framework was developed, including six first-grade indicators (diabetes professional knowledge, diabetes-related knowledge, communication skills and health education ability, specialized skills, clinical judgment, and specialty development capacity), 23 second-grade indicators, and 87 third-grade indicators. The weights of the six first-grade indicators were .221, .149, .192, .209, .160, and .069, respectively.

Conclusions: The core-competence system framework includes six core competencies, which represent the main characteristics of primary nurse specialists in diabetes care who are highly recommended by experts. It is important to keep in mind that this is only a theoretical framework and thus must be further tested in clinical practice settings in China.

Key Words:
primary nurse specialists in diabetes care, core competence, systematic framework, index weight.

Introduction

The prevalence of diabetes was estimated to be 11.6% in the Chinese adult population (Xu et al., 2013) and the patient population is increasing rapidly. It has been estimated that China will have 142.7 million patients with diabetes in 2035 (Guariguata et al., 2014). Diabetes has lifelong impacts that affect patients both physiologically and psychologically (Wang, 2017), with professional medical personnel required to manage the diabetes and improve quality of care. As nurses are the primary providers of diabetes clinical care and education, their core diabetes-related competencies have become the key factors affecting the quality of diabetes management. Clinical practice in diabetes care domestically and internationally has shown that strengthening the core competencies of nurse specialists in diabetes care, and establishing core competencies with an evaluation system, improves the quality of healthcare and of life for those living with diabetes (Chan, Bond, Adamson, & Chow, 2016; Kalb, 2008). Therefore, this study was designed to introduce international, advanced experience into current diabetes management in China, develop a core-competence system framework with China's own characteristics to meet the needs of clinical practice,

[1]*MS, RN, Professor, Department of Nursing, Tianjin Medical University Metabolic Diseases Hospital, Tianjin, China* • [2]*BSN, RN, Associate Professor of Nursing, Department of Endocrinology, Peking University People's Hospital, Beijing, China* • [3]*BSN, RN, Associate Professor, Department of Nursing, China-Japan Friendship Hospital, Beijing, China* • [4]*BSN, RN, Associate Professor of Nursing, Department of Endocrinology, Rui Jin Hospital Shanghai Jiao Tong University School of Medicine, Shanghai, China* • [5]*MS, RN, Professor, Department of Nursing, Jiangsu Province Official Hospital, Nanjing, China* • [6]*BSN, RN, Professor of Nursing, Department of Endocrinology and Metabolism, West China Hospital, Sichuan University, Chengdu, China.*

and provide guidelines for training and career development paths for nurse specialists in diabetes care. The study group focused on constructing a system framework based on the British core competence framework to ensure that the developed framework was based on evidence and applicable in terms of training and assessing nursing staff at various levels (Trend, 2011).

Background

The International Diabetes Federation estimates that 642 million people worldwide between 20 and 79 years old will have diabetes in 2040 (Ogurtsova et al., 2017). Diabetes has become one of the most challenging public health problems. With a dramatic increase in the prevalence of diabetes, China now has the largest number of people with diabetes in the world (Guariguata et al., 2014; Whiting, Guariguata, Weil, & Shaw, 2011). Because of serious dangers and complex management, diabetes places a particularly high burden on nurse specialists in diabetes care as well as on society and national finances (Bermudez-Tamayo et al., 2017). As a country with more than 90 million people with diabetes (Yang et al., 2010), China needs to do more than simply increase the numbers of nursing staff engaged in diabetes care. The clinical practice of developed countries such as the United States and United Kingdom has shown that the knowledge and skills of nurse specialists in diabetes care are key to improving the healthcare of patients and enhancing the quality of patient self-management (American Association of Diabetes Educators [AADE], 2011; Trend, 2011). Therefore, strengthening the core competencies of nurse specialists in diabetes care is the most urgent task.

The AADE (2011) established a training and evaluation system and set up the National Certification Board of Diabetes Educators. Certification is intended to improve the quality of self-management education, clinical care, and management of people with diabetes. In addition, the United Kingdom developed a career and competency framework for diabetes nursing (Douglass & Ruddle, 2009; Hicks, 2010; Trend, 2011). The British "integrated career and competency framework for diabetes nursing" model reflects this framework. There are five levels of competency for, respectively, unregistered practitioners, competent nurses, experienced or proficient nurses, senior practitioners or expert nurses, and consultant nurses. Areas of competence in the British system include prevention and early detection of Type 2 diabetes to facilitate patient self-care, care for diabetic individuals with mental illnesses, provide nutritional guidance, monitor biochemical indices, ensure the safe administration of therapies, identify and treat blood glucose, manage complications, manage gestational diabetes, support diabetic individuals who reside in prisons or young offender units, care for diabetic individuals living in residential or nursing homes, and care for patients with diabetes at the end of life.

China has the largest population of people with diabetes in the world (International Diabetes Federation, 2017). The most important difference is that patients with diabetes in China are educated and managed primarily in hospital settings, which puts considerable pressure on nurse specialists in diabetes care, especially in the areas of communication, education, and follow-up care. To date, there is no standardized framework for evaluating care implementation. Therefore, developing a comprehensive framework that provides criteria for competency evaluation, training, and guidance for the professional development of nurse specialists in diabetes care is critical. As a recently joined member of the International Council of Nurses, the Chinese Nursing Association, in establishing an effective framework, would help boost international communication and collaboration in diabetes care. Regrettably, lack of experience inhibits China from constructing a higher level, complex framework. Thus, this study aimed to construct a core-competence system framework for primary nurse specialists in diabetes care to lay the foundation for development of a multilevel framework that improves the quality of clinical nursing care.

Methods

Study Design and Sample

Theoretical basis

This study was based on the British "integrated career and competency framework for diabetes nursing" model (Trend, 2011). To address the role of nurse specialists in diabetes care in China as educators, the framework referred to some relevant studies of the AADE (2011) and the Australian Diabetes Educators Association (2008). In addition, domestic nurses in emergency care, peripherally inserted central catheter care, intensive care units, and other specialties (Fan & Xi, 2011; Yao, 2012) provided basic information for this study.

Creating the research group

This research study obtained the ethical approval of the Tianjin Medical University Metabolic Disease Hospital Ethics Committee (No. DXBYYhMEC2015-26) and guidance from the Chinese Nursing Association. The Chinese Nursing Association Diabetes Professional Committee proposed appointments to the Steering Committee and Project Execution Team.

The concept of core competencies

Twenty experts were invited by the Steering Committee to a brainstorming session to clarify the definition of core competencies of nurse specialists in diabetes care and to discuss the contents and outline of core competencies. A system framework of three grades was proposed for primary nurse specialists in diabetes care. First-grade indicators consisted of the dimensions of the core competencies. Second-grade indicators were drawn from the main competencies in the dimensions of the framework; and third-grade indicators, from the detailed content of the competencies.

Development of the first draft of the framework

After the brainstorming phase, the Project Execution Team organized the information and held a seminar to determine the first draft of the core competence framework. The 50 participants in this seminar included three diabetologists, 37 nurse specialists in diabetes care, five nursing managers, and five patients with diabetes.

Expert panel selection and recruitment

Fifty diabetes experts from 28 provinces and municipalities joined the expert panel to (a) balance the differences among regions and (b) maximize information diversity to make the framework more universal and comprehensive. The experts included clinical diabetes nurse specialists, nursing managers, and diabetologists who had 10 years or more of experience in diabetes treatment and care.

Data Collection

The Project Execution Team applied the Delphi method (Aljamal, Ashcroft, & Tully, 2016) to carry out three rounds of consultation between October 2015 and March 2016. In the first round, experts gave their advice on the first draft of the framework, with advice focused mainly on the deletion, addition, or modification of indicators. In the second round, experts continued to provide new suggestions and assigned a value to all of the indicators based on a 5-point Likert scale from 5 = *very important* to 1 = *not important.* Afterward, group members readjusted and formed new indicators based on the following screening criteria: mean > 3.5, coefficient of variation < 0.25, and expert approval rate > 70% (Guo, 2005; Wu, 2011). The third round mirrored the process in the second round and assigned weights to the first-grade indicators using the superiority chart (Cabral et al., 2005). All of the opinions were summarized to form the core competencies of primary nurse specialists in diabetes care.

Data Analysis

Microsoft Excel 2007 (Microsoft, Redmond, WA, USA) and IBM SPSS Statistics 17.0 software (SPSS, Inc., Chicago, IL, USA) were used to conduct data analysis and processing. Data were presented as means and standard deviations for continuous variables. In general, the authoritative coefficient (*Cr*) is composed on the basis of expert judgment (*Ca*) and of familiarity with the questions (*Cs*). The formula is $Cr = (Ca + Cs) / 2$. The value of *Ca* and *Cs* is obtained mainly through expert self-evaluation. The variables *Ca* and *Cs* reflect, respectively, the judgment and familiarity of the experts with regard to survey content. Kendall's coefficient of concordance (*W*) refers to the level of intraexpert agreement on all of the indicators. A nonparametric test was applied for Kendall's coefficient of concordance (*W*).

Results

Reliability of Expert Consultation

Expert information

Of the 50 consultants who participated in the Delphi survey, three did not reply and two provided incomplete information; thus, five were excluded. Demographic data on the remaining 45 included mean age, 44.69 ± 6.48 years; years of work experience in diabetes care, 15.75 ± 4.81; nursing managers, 13 (28.9%); diabetologists, 5 (11.1%); and diabetes nurse specialists, 27 (60%). In terms of education, three (6.7%) were educated to the college level, 28 (62.2%) held undergraduate degrees, 11 (24.4%) held a master's degree, and three (6.7%) held a doctoral degree.

Rate of response of experts

Fifty questionnaires were distributed, and 45 valid questionnaires were received via e-mail. The response rate for each round was 94%, 100%, and 95.7%, respectively.

Authoritative coefficient

The assignments of *Ca* and *Cs* are shown in Table 1. With the judgment coefficient of .91 and the familiarization coefficient of .90, the authority coefficient of experts was .91.

Kendall's coefficient of concordance (W)

Kendall's coefficient of concordance (*W*) values for the second and third rounds of expert consultations are shown in Table 2.

Selection of Indicators

Three rounds of Delphi consultations

In the first round of consultations, experts indicated a high level of recognition on first- and second-grade indicators. In addition, three third-grade indicators were eliminated, three third-grade indicators were added, and the descriptions of some indicators were modified based on expert opinions.

TABLE 1.
The Assignment of Expert Judgment (Ca) and Familiarity With the Questions (Cs)

Judgment Basis	Ca High	Ca Middle	Ca Low	Familiarization	Cs
Theoretical analysis (T)	.30	.20	.10	High familiarity	1.0
Experience (E)	.45	.35	.20	Familiarity	0.8
Information (I)	.20	.15	.10	Understand	0.6
Feeling (F)	.05	.05	.05	Unclear	0.4

TABLE 2.
Kendall's Coefficient of Concordance (W)

Consulting/Index	*W*	χ^2	*p*
Second round			
First grade	.892	160.56	< .001
Second grade	.378	356.96	< .001
Third grade	.485	1849.40	< .001
Third round			
First grade	.793	145.62	< .001
Second grade	.418	403.59	< .001
Third grade	.542	2021.34	< .001

In the second round, three second-grade indicators and 15 corresponding third-grade indicators were deleted on the basis of analysis methods, clinical applicability, and expert opinions.

In the third round, one second-grade indicator and five corresponding third-grade indicators were deleted. The study process is shown in Figure 1.

After three rounds of Delphi consultation, a three-grade system was constructed, consisting of six first-grade indicators, 23 second-grade indicators, and 87 third-grade indicators. The relationships among these are shown in Table 3.

Weights of the dimensions

According to the results of the consultation, the weights of the six dimensions (diabetes professional knowledge, diabetes-related knowledge, communication skills and health education ability, specialized skills, clinical judgment, and specialty development capacity) were .221, .149, .192, .209, .160, and .069, respectively.

Discussion

The Indicator Selection of the Framework

After three rounds of consultation, some indicators were deleted or added according to the analysis methods, clinical applicability, and expert opinions. Moreover, the expressions of some indicators were modified. For example, the content of "psychological knowledge" was revised from "mastering the conception of psychology," "understanding the application of psychology in nursing work," and "be able to use the psychological assessment instrument" to "learn common psychological problems in patients with diabetes" and "become familiar with the care regimen of common psychological problems" to make the framework more suitable to clinical requirements. However, the expert approval rating was only 70% for several indicators, including "ability to judge social support" and "understand the relevant laws and ethics." These indicators were retained for one or both of the following reasons: (a) These competencies facilitate the provision of individualized care and improve clinical safety, and (b) in the current healthcare environment in China, the indicator is necessary for competency among specialty nurses to meet changing healthcare demands. The final first-grade indicators represented the six dimensions of the core competencies of primary nurse specialists in diabetes care. "Diabetes professional knowledge" included five aspects (epidemiology, classification and characteristics, pathophysiology, complications, and hypoglycemia) with 16 indicators. "Diabetes-related knowledge" included three aspects (nutrition, exercise, and psychology) with 12 indicators. "Communication skills and health education ability" included four aspects (communication, assessment, organization and planning, and expression and explanation) with 17 indicators. "Specialized skills" included two aspects (specialized nursing skills and emergency response capacity) with 12 indicators. "Clinical judgment" included four aspects (clinical evaluation, judgment of social support, analysis of potential risk, and mastery of relevant laws and ethics) with 13 indicators. "Specialty development capacity" included five aspects (teaching, training, team coordination, continuous nursing, and learning) with 17 indicators.

External Validity of the Framework

This framework, which broadly reflects the professional characteristics of nurse specialists in diabetes care, was constructed

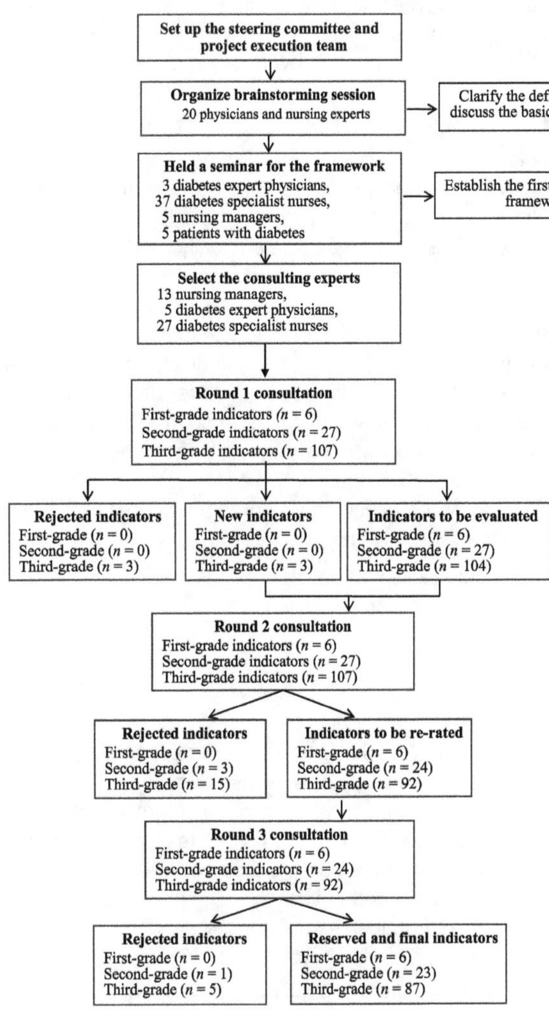

Figure 1. The study process.

TABLE 3.
Expert Opinion on First-, Second-, and Third-Grade Indicators

Indicator (First/Second/Third-Grade)	Approval Rating (%)	*M*	*SD*	Coefficient of Variation
I. Diabetes professional knowledge	100.0	5.00	0.00	0.00
1. The epidemiological trends of diabetes	81.0	4.05	0.85	0.21
(a) Know the epidemiological feature of diabetes	83.3	4.17	0.88	0.21
(b) Know the risk factors for diabetes	100.0	4.64	0.48	0.10
(c) Know the latest diabetes prevention strategies and measures	88.1	4.52	0.77	0.17
2. Classification and characteristics of diabetes	97.6	4.74	0.50	0.11
(a) Know the classification and diagnostic criteria for diabetes	100.0	4.76	0.43	0.09
(b) Know the characteristics of the different types of diabetes	100.0	4.71	0.46	0.10
(c) Identify diabetes-related metabolic parameters	100.0	4.74	0.45	0.09
3. Pathophysiology characteristics of diabetes	83.3	3.90	0.85	0.22
(a) Understand normal blood glucose metabolism	90.5	4.33	0.85	0.20
(b) Understand the causes and mechanisms of diabetes	83.3	4.19	0.77	0.18
(c) Understand the physiological role of insulin and other hormones	88.1	4.26	0.73	0.17
4. Knowledge of complications of diabetes	100.0	4.93	0.26	0.05
(a) Know diabetes acute and chronic complications	100.0	4.88	0.33	0.07
(b) Know the causes of diabetes complications	100.0	4.83	0.38	0.08
(c) Know clinical the symptoms and outcomes of various complications	95.2	4.40	0.59	0.13
(d) Master nursing key points of diabetes acute and chronic complications	100.0	4.95	0.22	0.04
5. Knowledge of hypoglycemia	100.0	4.95	0.22	0.04
(a) Know hypoglycemia prevention	100.0	5.00	0.00	0.00
(b) Know hypoglycemia cause	100.0	4.88	0.33	0.04
(c) Clear diagnosis criteria of hypoglycemia	100.0	4.95	0.22	0.04
II. Diabetes-related knowledge	97.6	4.62	0.62	0.13
1. Nutrition knowledge	100.0	4.74	0.45	0.09
(a) Clear the purpose of diabetes nutrition therapy	97.6	4.57	0.63	0.14
(b) Know the general principles of diabetes nutrition therapy very well	100.0	4.90	0.30	0.06
(c) Know the reasonable regulation of the total calories and nutrients very well	97.6	4.71	0.51	0.11
(d) Know food exchange portion and daily food glycemic index	95.2	4.43	0.59	0.13
(e) Master the principles of nutrition therapy of complications of diabetes	97.6	4.83	0.44	0.09
2. Kinematics knowledge	100.0	4.69	0.47	0.10
(a) Understand the benefits of exercise in patients with diabetes	97.6	4.71	0.51	0.11
(b) Master the indications and contraindications of exercise therapy	100.0	4.90	0.30	0.06
(c) Master the movement type suitable for patients with diabetes	100.0	4.81	0.40	0.08
(d) Master movement intensity, duration, frequency, and precautions	97.6	4.90	0.37	0.08
(e) Know the appropriate exercise tools for diabetes	90.5	4.43	0.74	0.17
3. Psychological knowledge	88.1	4.31	0.68	0.16
(a) Learn common psychological problems in patients with diabetes	92.9	4.38	0.62	0.14
(b) Become familiar with the care regimen of common psychological problems	97.6	4.55	0.55	0.12
III. Communication skills and health education ability	100.0	4.86	0.35	0.07
1. Ability to communicate with patients	100.0	4.86	0.35	0.07
(a) Evaluate effective methods of communicating with patients	100.0	4.60	0.50	0.11
(b) choose appropriate methods to communicate with diabetes	97.6	4.74	0.50	0.11
2. Ability to assess diabetes education needs	97.6	4.69	0.52	0.11
(a) Evaluate the health education needs of patients	97.6	4.76	0.48	0.10
(b) Use education methods appropriate to patient ability to comprehend	95.2	4.74	0.54	0.11
3. Ability to organize and plan diabetes education	92.8	4.38	0.70	0.16
(a) Collect and select useful educational information to make courseware	95.2	4.52	0.67	0.15
(b) Deliver specific information to patients and their families accurately	95.2	4.74	0.54	0.11
(c) Deliver educational programs together with patients	100.0	4.83	0.38	0.08
(d) Develop goals together with the patient in behavior change	97.6	4.67	0.53	0.11
(e) Evaluate educational results effectively	92.9	4.57	0.63	0.14
(f) Ability to organize different forms of educational activities	83.3	4.12	0.82	0.20

(continues)

TABLE 3.

Expert Opinion on First-, Second-, and Third-Grade Indicators, Continued

Indicator (First/Second/Third-Grade)	Approval Rating (%)	*M*	*SD*	Coefficient of Variation
4. Ability to express and explain health knowledge	100.0	4.86	0.35	0.07
(a) Make patients to master the basic knowledge of diabetes	97.6	4.83	0.44	0.09
(b) Enable patients and their families to master individualized diet regimen	97.6	4.76	0.48	0.10
(c) Enable patients and their families to master their exercise programmers	92.9	4.7	0.60	0.13
(d) Enable patients and their families to master hypoglycemic drugs including basic knowledge, intake and adverse reactions, especially their uses	97.6	4.81	0.55	0.11
(e) Enable patients to master the method of blood glucose monitoring	97.6	4.93	0.34	0.07
(f) Enable patients to master the insulin injection	100.0	4.95	0.22	0.04
(g) Enable patients to know acute and chronic complications and preventive measures	95.2	4.69	0.56	0.12
IV. Specialized skills	100.0	4.86	0.35	0.07
1. Specialized nursing skills	100.0	4.88	0.33	0.07
(a) Know the classification of oral agents, usage, and adverse reactions	97.6	4.76	0.48	0.10
(b) Know how to inject different diabetes drugs	100.0	4.98	0.15	0.03
(c) Know how to use and manage insulin pump	97.6	4.83	0.44	0.09
(d) Know how to use and manage glucose meter	100.0	4.95	0.22	0.04
(e) Know the frequency of blood glucose monitoring in a different state	100.0	4.90	0.30	0.06
(f) Know how to use continuous glucose monitoring system	88.1	4.29	0.74	0.17
(g) Know how to screen for the diabetes-related complications	71.4	4.17	0.91	0.22
(h) Master the outline of evaluation in diabetes care	90.5	4.62	0.66	0.14
2. Emergency response capacity	95.2	4.71	0.55	0.12
(a) Know how to treat hypoglycemia	100.0	5.00	0.00	0.00
(b) Know how to discern and treat acute complications of diabetes (such as ketosis)	95.2	4.86	0.47	0.10
(c) Know how to use relevant rescue equipment	95.2	4.79	0.52	0.11
(d) Ability to judge diabetes-related critical value and deal with them	95.2	4.76	0.62	0.12
V. Clinical judgment	92.6	4.50	0.63	0.14
1. Clinical evaluation capacity	92.9	4.48	0.63	0.14
(a) Ability to evaluate individual cognition levels	90.5	4.45	0.74	0.17
(b) Ability to evaluate behavioral changes in the patient	90.5	4.38	0.79	0.18
(c) Ability to evaluate compliance of the patient	92.9	4.50	0.71	0.16
(d) Ability to clearly evaluate patient condition	95.2	4.52	0.67	0.15
(e) Ability to evaluate self-care ability of the patient	95.2	4.57	0.67	0.15
(f) Ability to evaluate the psychological status of the patient	88.1	4.36	0.82	0.19
2. Ability to judge social support	70.0	3.93	0.84	0.21
(a) Ability to evaluate family support	83.3	4.21	0.84	0.20
(b) Ability to evaluate social support	78.6	4.07	0.89	0.22
(c) Ability to evaluate financial support	81.0	4.14	0.90	0.22
3. Ability to analyze potential risk	92.9	4.38	0.70	0.16
(a) Ability to evaluate diabetes complications	95.2	4.69	0.56	0.12
(b) Ability to evaluate potential adverse events (such as pressure sores, falls, and so on)	97.6	4.74	0.50	0.11
4. Understand the relevant laws and ethics	70.0	3.92	0.92	0.23
(a) Understand the relevant laws and regulations	71.4	4.02	0.90	0.22
(b) Understand the clinical ethics	70.0	3.86	0.87	0.23
VI. Specialty development capacity	88.1	4.10	0.73	0.18
1. Teaching ability	78.6	4.24	0.85	0.20
(a) Be able to use the appropriate way of teaching (such as multimedia)	95.2	4.48	0.60	0.13
(b) Be able to implement specialized teaching for students	92.9	4.38	0.70	0.16
(c) Be able to conduct case report	90.5	4.33	0.72	0.17

(continues)

TABLE 3.

Expert Opinion on First-, Second-, and Third-Grade Indicators, Continued

Indicator (First/Second/Third-Grade)	Approval Rating (%)	*M*	*SD*	Coefficient of Variation
2. Training ability	81.0	4.14	0.78	0.19
(a) Be able to offer diabetes specialized training to others	83.3	4.24	0.79	0.19
(b) Be able to supervise and guide clinical professional nurses in professional operating skills	85.4	4.24	0.79	0.19
3. Team coordination ability	92.9	4.55	0.63	0.14
(a) Ability of interpersonal communication	92.9	4.50	0.71	0.16
(b) Play a greater influence in a team	85.7	4.31	0.78	0.18
(c) Be able to communicate, coordinate, and cooperate effectively with team members	92.9	4.50	0.71	0.16
(d) Be able to adjust working pattern according to the opinions of others	88.1	4.36	0.76	0.17
(e) Ability to implement plans	92.6	4.50	0.63	0.14
4. Continuous nursing ability	92.9	4.40	0.63	0.14
(a) Be able to follow up regularly	95.2	4.50	0.67	0.15
(b) Guide patients how to check regularly	95.2	4.50	0.67	0.15
(c) Answer problems from outpatients with diabetes	95.2	4.50	0.59	0.13
(d) Develop a wellness program for patients	95.2	4.50	0.59	0.13
5. Learning ability	100.0	4.60	0.50	0.11
(a) Recognize personal learning needs	95.2	4.50	0.59	0.13
(b) Take diabetes continuing education courses	95.2	4.60	0.59	0.13
(c) Learn new knowledge and new information associated with diabetes	95.2	4.69	0.47	0.10

Note. The framework consists of six first-grade indicators, 23 second-grade indicators, and 87 third-grade indicators.

based on the British career and competency framework for diabetes nursing (Trend, 2011). The process used in this study to select experts differed from other studies in terms of number and region (Gattinger et al., 2016; Gibson & Soanes, 2000). The number of experts was relatively high (50 recruited). Moreover, clinical diabetes nurse specialists, nursing managers, and diabetologists were involved with the aim of obtaining more information from multiple perspectives. In addition, the diverse regional backgrounds of the experts (28 provinces) were expected to ensure that regional differences were considered so that the framework was universally applicable and comprehensive. Research has shown that specialty nurses have better mastery of theoretical knowledge and skills than general nurses, which certainly affects the quality of nursing care (Yao, 2012). This framework is intended to provide a reference for clinical nursing managers to cultivate and evaluate the core competencies of nurse specialists in diabetes care to help them provide more effective patient care.

Characteristics of the Indicators in the Framework

This framework was based primarily on the British career and competency framework for diabetes nursing (Trend, 2011). In addition, guidelines from the AADE (2011) and the Australian Diabetes Educators Association (2008) and domestic experience in the emergency, peripherally inserted central catheter, intensive care unit, and other settings (Fan & Xi, 2011; Yao, 2012) were incorporated. The career and competency framework for nurse specialists in diabetes care in the British model provided particularly important insights. However, the developed model differs significantly from the British model in several respects. First, the British model is a theoretical framework that emphasizes the core competencies of five different levels of nurses (unregistered practitioners, competent nurses, experienced or proficient nurses, senior practitioners or expert nurses, and consultant nurses). In contrast, the model that was developed in this study targets only nurse specialists in diabetes care. The framework contains the basic competencies that nurse specialists in diabetes care should have and provides the basis for the future establishment of a higher level framework. Because research and leadership competencies are more suited to senior nurse specialists in diabetes care, these competencies were not included in the study framework.

Second, the British framework covers competencies that focus partly on care for patients living in residential and nursing homes, confined to prisons and young offender units, and receiving end-of-life care. As patients in China are always managed in hospitals, this model did not consider patients in these categories.

Third, the two models have a number of competencies in common such as diet, exercise, blood glucose monitoring, use of antidiabetic agents, mental health, nursing for complications of the disease, and hypoglycemia prevention and treatment. However, because of differences in cultural background and health policies, certain indicators are more relevant to Chinese healthcare. These include emphasizing judgment in social support and potential risks and understanding the laws, regulations, and clinical ethics to guarantee the safety of patients and deal with medical stress. Furthermore, team coordination ability and learning ability were added to improve the quality of nursing care.

Fourth, the dimension of competencies was made more consistent with the medical background of nurses in China by classifying basic diabetes knowledge and skills into the three dimensions of diabetes professional knowledge (classification and characteristics of diabetes, knowledge of hypoglycemia, complications nursing), diabetes-related knowledge (nutrition, kinematics, psychological knowledge), and specialized skills (insulin pump management, blood glucose monitoring). Moreover, the competencies were distinguished into three grades (dimensions, competencies, and detailed indicators), which formed a detailed hierarchical system.

Finally, diabetes education is a significant component of clinical work. Thus, the model reflected the specific characteristics of diabetes educators in terms of communication skills and health education ability.

Limitations

This study showed the development process and structure of the framework for primary nurse specialists in diabetes care. Although the research design and execution were rigorous, some limitations still exist. The result of the study was the formation of a theoretical framework, which must be verified and further improved in clinical settings. The framework was constructed for primary nurse specialists in diabetes care and offers clear standards for the training of primary nurse specialists in diabetes care only. This framework is unable to meet the demands of advanced nurse specialists in diabetes care. Thus, a multilevel core-competence system framework should be developed.

Conclusions

The core-competence system framework includes six core competencies, which broadly represent the main characteristics of primary nurse specialists in diabetes care. However, as this is a theoretical framework, it must be tested in clinical practice environments in China.

Acknowledgments

The authors gratefully acknowledge the assistance of Xiuhua Li and other members of the Chinese Nursing Association diabetes professional committee. The authors acknowledge the editorial assistance of Amparo B. González and Teresa L. Pearson. Thanks to Wei Xi for assistance with statistical methods and to Zhaojun Yang, Xianghai Zhou, Yuhong Zhang, several experienced nursing staffs, and physicians with diabetes expertise for helping with the project design and implementation.

References

Aljamal, M. S., Ashcroft, D., & Tully, M. P. (2016). Development of indicators to assess the quality of medicines reconciliation at hospital admission: An e-Delphi study. *International Journal of Pharmacy Practice, 24*(3), 209–216. https://doi.org/10.1111/ijpp.12234

American Association of Diabetes Educators. (2011). *Competencies for diabetes educators: A companion document to the guidelines for the practice of diabetes education.* Chicago, IL: Author.

Australian Diabetes Educators Association. (2008). *National core competencies for credentialled diabetes educators.* Canberra, Australia: Author.

Bermudez-Tamayo, C., Besançon, S., Johri, M., Assa, S., Brown, J. B., & Ramaiya, K. (2017). Direct and indirect costs of diabetes mellitus in Mali: A case–control study. *PLoS ONE, 12*(5), e0176128. https://doi.org/10.1371/journal.pone.0176128

Cabral, D., Katz, J. N., Weinblatt, M. E., Ting, G., Avorn, J., & Solomon, D. H. (2005). Development and assessment of indicators of rheumatoid arthritis severity: Results of a Delphi panel. *Arthritis and Rheumatism, 53*(1), 61–66. https://doi.org/10.1002/art.20925

Chan, W. F., Bond, T. G., Adamson, B., & Chow, M. (2016). Identifying core competencies of infection control nurse specialists in Hong Kong. *Clinical Nurse Specialist, 30*(1), E1–E9. https://doi.org/10.1097/NUR.0000000000000174

Douglass, E., & Ruddle, G. (2009). Implementation of the NHS knowledge and skills framework. *Nursing Standard, 24*(1), 42–48. https://doi.org/10.7748/ns2009.09.24.1.42.c7260.

Fan, L., & Xi, S. H. (2011). Study on the construction of core competency evaluation index system for emergency specialized nurses. *Chinese Journal of Nursing, 46*(2), 144–146. (Original work published in Chinese)

Gattinger, H., Leino-Kilpi, H., Hantikainen, V., Köpke, S., Ott, S., & Senn, B. (2016). Assessing nursing staff's competences in mobility support in nursing-home care: Development and psychometric testing of the Kinaesthetics Competence (KC) observation instrument. *BMC Nursing, 15*(1), 65. https://doi.org/10.1186/s12912-016-0185-z

Gibson, F., & Soanes, L. (2000). The development of clinical competencies for use on a paediatric oncology nursing course using a nominal group technique. *Journal of Clinical Nursing, 9*(3), 459–469. https://doi.org/10.1046/j.1365-2702.2000.00404.x

Guariguata, L., Whiting, D. R., Hambleton, I., Beagley, J., Linnenkamp, U., & Shaw, J. E. (2014). Global estimates of diabetes prevalence for 2013 and projections for 2035. *Diabetes Research and Clinical Practice, 103*(2), 137–149. https://doi.org/10.1016/j.diabres.2013.11.002

Guo, X. H. (2005). *Practical medical investigation and analysis techniques.* Beijing, China: People's Medical Publishing House. (Original work published in Chinese)

Hicks, D. (2010). Competency in practice: Are you fit for purpose? *Journal of Diabetes Nursing, 14,* 44–46.

International Diabetes Federation. (2017). *IDF diabetes atlas—8th edition.* Brussels, Belgium: Author. Retrieved from http://www.diabetesatlas.org

Kalb, K. A. (2008). Core competencies of nurse educators: Inspiring excellence in nurse educator practice. *Nursing Education Perspectives, 29*(4), 217–219.

Ogurtsova, K., da Rocha Fernandes, J. D., Huang, Y., Linnenkamp, U., Guariguata, L., Cho, N. H., ... Makaroff, L. E. (2017). IDF diabetes atlas: Global estimates for the prevalence of diabetes for 2015 and 2040. *Diabetes Research and Clinical Practice, 128,* 40–50. https://doi.org/10.1016/j.diabres.2017.03.024

Trend, U. K. (2011). *An integrated career and competency framework for diabetes nursing* (3rd ed.). London, England: SB Communications.

Wang, R. H. (2017). Psychological care for patients with diabetes—Present and future. *The Journal of Nursing Research, 25*(2), 86–89. https://doi.org/10.1097/JNR.0000000000000207

Whiting, D. R., Guariguata, L., Weil, C., & Shaw, J. (2011). IDF diabetes atlas: Global estimates of the prevalence of diabetes for 2011 and 2030. *Diabetes Research and Clinical Practice, 94*(3), 311–321. https://doi.org/10.1016/j.diabres.2011.10.029

Wu, L. P. (2011). *Construction of a core competency evaluation index system for diabetes specialist nurse* (Master's thesis). Anhui, China: Anhui Medical University. (Original work published in Chinese)

Xu, Y., Wang, L., He, J., Bi, Y., Li, M., Wang, T., ... 2010 China Noncommunicable Disease Surveillance Group. (2013). Prevalence and control of diabetes in Chinese adults. *JAMA, 310*(9), 948–959. https://doi.org/10.1001/jama.2013.168118

Yang, W., Lu, J., Weng, J., Jia, W., Ji, L., Xiao, J., ... China National Diabetes and Metabolic Disorders Study Group. (2010). Prevalence of diabetes among men and women in China. *The New England Journal of Medicine, 362*(12), 1090–1101. https://doi.org/10.1056/NEJMoa0908292

Yao, H. (2012). *Construction of core competency evaluation indices for PICC specialized nurses and clinical investigation analysis (Master's thesis).* China: The Second Military Medical University, Shanghai City, China. (Original work published in Chinese)

10

The Smartphone Addiction Levels and the Association With Communication Skills in Nursing and Medical School Students

Ulfiye CELIKKALP[1]* • Sebnem BILGIC[2] • Munire TEMEL[3] • Gamze VAROL[4]

ABSTRACT

Background: The use of smartphones among young people is quite common. However, smartphones are associated with negative effects when used excessively. It has been reported that smartphone use may adversely affect learning in the classroom, cause safety issues, and negatively affect interpersonal communications.

Purpose: The aims of this study were to determine the level of smartphone addiction among nursing and medical school students and to examine the effect of smartphone addiction level on communication skills.

Methods: This cross-sectional study was conducted with medical school and nursing students at a public university (502 participants). Data were collected using a personal information form, the Smartphone Addiction Scale–Short Version (SAS-SV), and the Communication Skills Assessment Scale.

Results: All of the participants in the study owned smartphones. Most (70.9%) were female, and 58.2% were in the nursing program. The participants used smartphones for a mean time of 5.07 ± 3.32 hours a day, primarily for messaging. The mean total SAS-SV score for the participants was 31.89 ± 9.90, and a significant difference in SAS-SV mean scores was found with regard to the variables of department, gender, daily smartphone use duration, academic success, status regarding smartphone use in the classroom, participation in sports, easy communication with patients and relatives, preferred mode of communication, health problems tied to phone use, and injury status ($p < .05$). In addition, a positive weak-to-moderate relationship was found between SAS-SV mean scores and the variables of daily smartphone use duration and years of smartphone use, whereas a negative weak relationship was found between SAS-SV mean scores and Communication Skills Assessment Scale scores. Daily smartphone use duration was found to be the most important predictor of smartphone addiction.

Conclusions/Implications for Practice: Higher SAS-SV scores have a negative impact on interpersonal communication and social life and reduce learning efficacy in students. Therefore, students and lecturers should be better informed regarding the benefits and risks of smartphone use in education, with precautions provided against excessive and needless use.

Key Words:
academic, communication, smartphone addiction, students, university.

Introduction

Smartphones, with many applications spanning communication, information, and entertainment (Haug et al., 2015), are a ubiquitous and indispensable part of modern life (Cho & Lee, 2015). Tasks such as making phone calls, messaging, entering social networks, taking photographs and videos, sharing images and messages on social media, playing games, and surfing the Internet may be performed anywhere and anytime via smartphones (Lepp, Li, Barkley, & Salehi-Esfahani, 2015; Samaha & Hawi, 2016). In addition, smartphones have other qualities that make life easier such as making video calls and finding directions using navigation programs (Samaha & Hawi, 2016; Şata, Çelik, Ertürk, & Taş, 2016). Smartphones are very beneficial when not used excessively (Kim, Lee, Lee, Nam, & Chung, 2014). However, the recent increase in smartphone use has necessitated examinations of its negative effects (Choi et al., 2015; Mok et al., 2014; Samaha & Hawi, 2016).

A general point of concurrence in studies on smartphones is the prevalence of smartphone use among younger people and its association with addictive behavior (Davey & Davey, 2014; Kim et al., 2014; Süt, Kurt, Uzal, & Özdilek, 2016). As smartphone use is more prevalent among younger people, they are generally more exposed to the negative effects of excessive use, and smartphone addiction is seen as a particularly high risk factor for younger people (Kim et al., 2014). Smartphone addiction is defined as a condition that affects the daily life of users, inducing clinical characteristics such as loss of attention, tolerance, and control; mood disorders; and withdrawal symptoms (Lee, Chang, Lin, & Cheng, 2014). In a meta-analysis study on Indian adolescents, smartphone addiction prevalence was reported to vary between 39% and 44%, with this addiction

[1]*PhD, RN, Assistant Professor, Department of Public Health, School of Medicine, Trakya University, Edirne, Turkey* • [2]*PhD, RN, Assistant Professor, Faculty of Health Sciences, Department of Nursing, Trakya University, Edirne, Turkey* • [3]*PhD, RN, Assistant Professor, Department of Nursing, Health School Collage, Namık Kemal University, Tekirdag, Turkey* • [4]*PhD, MD, Associate Professor, Faculty of Medicine, Department of Public Health, Namık Kemal University, Tekirdağ, Turkey.*

potentially associated with psychologically negative health outcomes (Davey & Davey, 2014). Smartphone addiction has reportedly reached a prevalence of 11.4% among younger people in South Korea, with 2.2% facing smartphone-addiction-related difficulties in their daily lives (Kim et al., 2014). In a report published in the United States, 15% of 18- to 29-year-olds were identified as heavily addicted to smartphones (Smith, 2017a), with 92% of the current younger generation owning smartphones (Smith, 2017b). According to the results of the 2015 Household Information Technologies Use Survey by the Turkish Institute of Statistics, the rate of mobile phone use in Turkey is 96.9% (Turkish Statistical Institute, 2017).

In recent years, interpersonal forms of communication have been reshaped and changed because of the development and use of smartphone technologies. Time spent on social network sites and growing membership numbers on these sites are important indicators that a new form of communication has been established and that new communication habits have arisen (Aydın, 2016). A qualitative study by Çizmeci conducted on university students in Turkey found smartphones to be an essential part of relationships among today's youth, helping in both the initiation and advancement of emotional relationships. On the other hand, smartphones have been found to create trust issues in interpersonal relationships, creating behaviors related to attachment anxiety and increasing relationship fragility (Çizmeci, 2017). Similarly, a study conducted in India found that excessive telephone use has a net negative impact on the interpersonal relationships of adolescents (Davey & Davey, 2014). Using a smartphone and being online is seen as a popular activity among youth (Şata et al., 2016). However, whereas individuals "socialize" using smartphones in theory, a trend toward individualization has been noted in real (offline) life. Thus, smartphones change family and interpersonal relationships, routine daily life, habits, and even behaviors (King et al., 2013; Samaha & Hawi, 2016). This may cause problems such as loneliness, isolation, anxiety, depression, stress, sleep disorders, decreased physical activity, musculoskeletal system disorders, and academic failure (Kim, 2013; Samaha & Hawi, 2016). Concurrently, increased smartphone use by the younger generation has been shown to promote phobic behaviors such as continuously checking for messages and calls, feeling worry or anxiety in places without network coverage or with limited access, leaving the phone on constantly, and sleeping with the phone by the user's side (Bragazzi & Del Puente, 2014).

As the problems associated with smartphone and Internet addiction in current university students threaten both the present and future of society, examining the situation and determining the resultant problems are important. The smartphone addiction behaviors of students negatively affect their communication abilities, social lives, and academic performance (Cho & Lee, 2015; Davey & Davey, 2014).

In occupations such as medicine and nursing, which are concerned with human health, this type of behavioral addiction is thought to cause problems in terms of both patient safety and employee safety. Nursing and medicine students, who focus an important part of their education on clinical issues, have responsibilities regarding patient and employee safety. The excessive use of smartphones in work environments may affect the clinical performance of students. For this reason, smartphone addiction in healthcare students is an important issue to examine. Only a few studies in Turkey have examined smartphone and Internet addiction in students in healthcare-related fields (Süt et al., 2016; Yılmaz, Çınar, & Özyazıcıoğlu, 2017). Because smartphone addiction may be viewed as a new behavioral addiction, this study was conducted to determine the frequency of smartphone use among a population of students studying in medicine and nursing departments to assess their levels of addiction and examine the effect of this addiction on their communication skills.

Methods

Sample

This descriptive and cross-sectional study was conducted on a population of students studying at the medical school and nursing department of a public university between September and December 2017. Seven hundred eighty-two students were enrolled in the medical school and the nursing department of the university in the fall semester of the 2017–2018 academic year.

All of the students in the targeted medical school and nursing department were recruited as participants. Two hundred ten of the 364 students registered in the medical school and 292 of the 418 students registered in the nursing department volunteered to participate in this study, a total of 502 participants. The criteria for participation in this study included being a student in the targeted medical school or nursing department, having a smart phone, regularly attending classes, volunteering to participate, and filling in the required forms completely. The curriculum for each class was acquired from the school administration, and researchers scheduled periods when students did not have classes and were not scheduled to be in clinical practicums to conduct interviews and complete questionnaires. The researchers explained the purpose and requirements of this study to the students and obtained their verbal consent. The questionnaires were filled out by participants under direct observation and collected immediately. The completion of the data forms took approximately 10–15 minutes.

Data Collection Tools

The personal information form was prepared by the researchers based on the literature and included 20 items on age, gender, income level, academic performance, social activities, and smartphone usage characteristics.

The Smartphone Addiction Scale–Short Version (SAS-SV) is a 33-item scale designed to evaluate smartphone addiction (Kwon, Kim, Cho, & Yang, 2013). Because of the length of the scale and the lack of definitive cutoff points, 10 of the 33 items were used to create a short form that could be completed more easily and in a shorter period and that could facilitate diagnoses using cutoff points (Kwon, Lee, et al., 2013). Noyan, Darçın, Nurmedov, Yılmaz, and Dilbaz (2015) translated the 10-item SAS-SV into Turkish in 2015 and tested the validity and reliability of the translated version (Noyan et al., 2015). The scale is a 10-item, 6-point Likert-type scale with one factor and no subdimensions. The items of the scale are scored from 1 to 6, giving a possible total score range for the scale of 10–60, with higher scores indicating a higher risk of addiction. In the Korean sample, the cutoff point was determined as 31 for men and 33 for women. The internal consistency and concurrent validity Cronbach's alpha score for the original form was .91. In this study, the Cronbach's alpha value for the scale was .87. The interitem correlation matrix of SAS-SV was examined, and each item was found to correlate positively with the others. The correlation coefficient of each item was found to be medium or high. Moreover, the internal consistency coefficient did not change when the item was removed from the scale during the item analysis, and each item was in accordance with the scale.

The Communication Skills Assessment Scale (CSAS) was developed by Korkut in 1996. The CSAS was first designed to be used with high school students and later tested for validity and reliability for use with university students and adults. The CSAS is a 25-item, 5-point Likert-type scale that aims to determine how adolescents evaluate their communication skills. In the reliability study for the scale performed with university students, the reliability coefficient was found to be .78 and the internal consistency coefficient was found to be .86. Each item in the scale is scored from 1 to 5, with 1 = *never* and 5 = *always*. Because the scale includes no reverse-scored items, higher scores indicate a higher self-evaluation of personal communication skills (Korkut Owen & Bugay, 2014). In this study, the Cronbach's alpha coefficient for this scale was .93.

Data Analysis

Statistical evaluations were performed using IBM SPSS Statistics Version 21 (IBM, Armonk, NY, USA). Descriptive analyses (numbers, mean values, medians, standard deviations), the independent sample t test for the comparison of numeric variables among groups, one-way variance analysis, and correlation analysis were used to determine the relationship between students' smartphone addiction and communication skills, whereas linear regression analysis was used to determine the effect of smartphone addiction on communication skills. A p value of < .05 was considered statistically significant.

Ethical Considerations

Before the study, written permission from the institutions where the study was conducted and ethical approval from the Namık Kemal University School of Medicine Non-Invasive Clinical Studies Board of Ethics were received (2017/44/04/04). In addition, each student who stated interest to participate in the study was informed about the study, given an explanation regarding the aims and procedures, informed of their responsibilities, and asked to provide formal consent.

Results

The mean age of the participants was 21.20 ± 1.86 years. Nearly three quarters (70.9%) were female, 58.2% were studying nursing, and 41.8% were studying medicine. The participants self-reported using smartphones for a mean of 5.26 ± 2.83 years and a mean of 5.07 ± 3.32 hours a day, changing a mean of 2.58 ± 1.63 (median = 2) phones in the process. Furthermore, the participants self-reported using their smartphones mostly for messaging, followed by social media and Internet surfing, respectively.

The participants reported using smartphones in many environments and during many other activities. Phone use was especially high in classrooms and buses. More than half of the participants (55.2%) reported using smartphones during class regardless of course type, 39% reported having difficulties following courses because of smartphone use, and 13.9% had related decreases in their academic performance. A significant number (16.1%) of participants reported experiencing at least one accident or injury (falling, slipping) because of smartphone use, whereas 39.1% had at least one smartphone-related health problem (burning and dryness of eyes, sleeplessness, musculoskeletal system disorders). More than one third (39.2%) of the participants engaged regularly in sports activities (Table 1).

One quarter (27.9%) of the participants reported preferring to use their phones or social media to initiate communications. Three quarters of the participants (76.9%) stated that they communicated easily with patients and next of kin during clinical applications. The mean total CSAS score for the participants was calculated as 97.99 ± 13.17 (Table 1).

The mean total SAS-SV score of the participants was 31.89 ± 9.90. When evaluated with regard to the scores they took from each item of the Smartphone Addiction Scale, the highest mean score was for the item "I cannot stand being separated from my smartphone" (3.70 ± 1.34), whereas the lowest mean score was for the item "I feel pain in my wrist or neck because of using my smartphone" (2.78 ± 1.47; Table 2).

When the SAS-SV mean scores of the students were compared with demographic characteristics, a significant difference in SAS-SV mean score was found for the variables of department, gender, daily smartphone use duration, academic performance, smartphone use in the classroom, participation in sports, easy communication with patients and relatives, preferred mode of communication, health problems tied to phone use, and injury status ($p < .05$; Table 3).

A correlation analysis was conducted to assess whether the participants' smartphone addiction was significantly related to their communication skill level, with results showing a negative, significant, and very weak relationship ($r = -.13, p < .001$).

The results of linear regression analysis, conducted to determine the effect of participants' smartphone addiction on their communication skills, showed smartphone addiction to affect communication skills significantly ($\beta = -.130, p = .004$). Thus, smartphone addiction was found to negatively affect communication skills.

TABLE 1.
Participant Characteristics (N = 502)

Characteristic	*M*	*SD*
Age (years)	21.20	1.86
CSAS	97.99	13.17
Year of using smartphone	5.26	2.83
Smartphone usage time (hours/day)	5.07	3.32
Number of phone exchanges	2.58	1.63
Purpose and time spent using a smartphone (hours/day)		
Messaging	1.83	2.57
Social networking (Facebook, Twitter, Instagram, other)	1.81	2.38
Surfing on the Internet	1.51	0.94
	n	%
Gender		
Female	356	70.9
Male	146	29.1
Program		
Nursing department	292	58.2
Medical school	210	41.8
Smartphone use in the classroom		
Yes	277	55.2
No	225	44.8
Failure to follow course topics		
Yes	196	39.0
No	306	61.0
Situations where you use your smartphone		
While walking	34	6.8
During the conversation	10	2.0
On the bus	209	41.6
Eating	17	3.4
During sporting activities	5	1.0
Many situations	227	45.2
Injury while using the phone (falling, bumping, hanging, etc.)		
Yes	81	16.1
No	421	83.9
Health problems because of phone use (eye problems, pain, etc.)		
Yes	196	39.1
No	259	51.5
Unanswered	7	1.4
Regular sports participation		
Yes	197	39.2
No	305	60.8
Preferred communication type		
Face to face	362	72.1
Via phone or social media	140	27.9
Communicating with patients and patient relatives		
Yes	386	76.9
No	21	4.2
Some	95	18.9

Note. CSAS = Communication Skills Assessment Scale.

Discussion

In the 21st century, a large and growing number of young people and adolescents spend a significant amount of their time using and enjoying mobile phones. However, it has been highlighted in recent studies that the overuse of smartphones may result in smartphone addiction (Davey & Davey, 2014) and may already be a public health problem on par with alcohol, smoking, and drug addiction (Kuyucu, 2017).

No cutoff point was determined in the Turkish version of the SAS-SV scale used in this study. In the Korean sample, the cutoff point was determined as 31 for men and 33 for women. Overall, 26.6% of women and 16.6% of men earned scores above the cutoff point in the Korean sample (Kwon, Lee, et al., 2013). Because in large part of technological and cultural differences, the cutoff points obtained in the Korean sample may not be appropriate for Turkish settings. However, when the participants in this study were evaluated based on the cutoff points used in the Korean sample, 48.6% of women and 42.8% of men were identified as being at risk of smartphone addiction. Samaha and Hawi (2016), using the same scale in their study of 293 university students, identified a high risk of smartphone addiction in 44.6% (female: 49.1%, male: 40.7%) of students (Samaha & Hawi, 2016). These results concur with a meta-analysis study of Indian adolescents (Davey & Davey, 2014). In a study conducted in Turkey by Noyan et al. (2015), smartphone addiction was detected in 23.0% of the women and 20.5% of the men participants (Noyan et al., 2015). The difference between the studies is thought to stem from the different years in which the studies were conducted, as the prevalence of smartphone use continues to rise sharply. In Table 2, the highest mean score for the item "I cannot stand being separated from my smartphone" supports the idea of higher smartphone addiction rates. These results are important, as they show the high risk of smartphone addiction among students and the necessity of taking preventive measures to protect younger people.

In this study, the mean smartphone addiction score for the women participants was significantly higher. In the literature, gender differences have been reported in the context of smartphone addiction, usually in terms of how users of different genders use their smartphones (Choi et al., 2015; Mok et al., 2014). In a study that performed regression analysis, smartphone addiction was found to be significantly related to being female, whereas Internet addiction was found to be significantly related to being male (Choi et al., 2015). According to a study performed on South Korean adolescents, whereas women used the Internet mostly for chatting, sending messages, writing blogs, and updating their personal homepages, men used the Internet mostly for going online, searching information, and playing games (Heo, Oh, Subramanian, Kim, & Kowachi, 2014). The smartphone addiction scores for nursing students were found to be significantly higher than for medical students in this study. This difference may stem from gender as well, as most of the participants from the nursing department were women.

TABLE 2.
Smartphone Addiction Scale–Short Version Item Mean Scores (N = 502)

Item	*M*	*SD*
1. Missing planned work because of smartphone use	2.84	1.36
2. Having a hard time concentrating in class, while doing assignments, or while working because of smartphone use	3.08	1.42
3. Feeling pain in the wrists or at the back of the neck while using a smartphone	2.78	1.47
4. Won't be able to bear not having a smartphone	3.70	1.34
5. Feeling impatient and fretful when I am not holding my smartphone	3.04	1.48
6. Having my smartphone in my mind even when I am not using it	3.26	1.41
7. I will never give up using my smartphone even when my daily life is already greatly affected by it.	3.22	1.46
8. Constantly checking my smartphone so as not to miss conversations between other people on Twitter or Facebook	2.80	1.38
9. Using my smartphone longer than I had intended	3.46	1.34
10. The people around me tell me that I use my smartphone too much.	2.92	1.36

Note. Cronbach alpha = .87; scale mean = 31.89, *SD* = 9.90.

In this study, the participants were found to use smartphones mostly for messaging and connecting to social network services. These results are congruent with the motivations for smartphone use by women, as two thirds of the participants in this study were women. Choi et al. (2015) reported that smartphones were used mostly for messaging services, with the rationale behind this showing that messaging enables the use of other applications such as phone calls, blogging, and social network chatting (Choi et al., 2015). Contrary to those findings, other studies have found that smartphones are used solely as communication devices (Kwon, Kim, et al., 2013).

In this study, the result that best spotlights the excessive use of smartphones is that daily smartphone use among the participants totaled about 5 hours, which is quite high. Erdem, Kalkin, Türen, and Deniz (2016) reported daily smartphone use by students as 6.43 hours, whereas Süt et al. (2016) reported that approximately half of the students used their smartphones for over 4 hours per day on average (Süt et al., 2016). These findings concur with the findings of Haug et al.'s (2015) study of Swiss youth.

Excessive smartphone use has been associated in the literature with lower academic performance. Moreover, multiple studies have found using phones in the classroom environment to be unacceptable, distracting both to the user and to others sharing the same environment, and a cause of complaints (Choi et al., 2015; Cho & Lee, 2015; Erdem et al., 2016). This study found similar results. The SAS-SV scores, class note deficiencies, and academic scores of the participants in this study who continued to use smartphones during class were found to be significantly lowest. In Subba et al. (2013), a great majority of the Indian students reportedly used smartphones in class, laboratories, and libraries and with time limits. In Cho and Lee (2015), smartphone use was shown to affect classroom learning negatively and it was recommended that rules and policies to control smartphone use in clinical applications be developed. Furthermore, another study identified smartphone use as affecting classroom performance, obstructing studies, and causing psychological problems (Davey & Davey, 2014). Yıldırım, Yaşar, and Duru (2016) examined smartphone use in educational environments under a different light, concluding that the educational functions of smartphones were being ignored and that smartphones could support teaching and learning if an appropriate technical and contextual substructure were developed (Yıldırım et al., 2016).

In the literature, the effects of smartphones on daily life, habits, and behaviors have been emphasized (Samaha & Hawi, 2016). Of special interest is the consistent controlling behavior of constantly using and checking smartphone applications. This causes problems in users such as anxiety, stress, sleep disorders, decreased physical activity, decreased academic performance, and disrupted well-being (Haug et al., 2015; Samaha & Hawi, 2016). In this study, dovetailing with the literature, the SAS-SV scores of those who reported health problems related to smartphone use faced a significantly higher risk of experiencing falling and slipping accidents during smartphone use and participated in sports less than their non-smartphone-using peers (Haug et al., 2015). These results are important in terms of showing the effects on behavior, especially among those addicted to smartphone use.

In this study, participants were shown to have good communication skills. Although several studies have reported student communication skills similar to this study (Abdrbo, 2017; Cerit, Çıtak Bilgin, & Ak, 2018), other studies have found that students had an unacceptably low level of communication skills (Acar & Buldukoglu, 2016). Communication skills facilitate interpersonal relationships in all areas of life, especially in the professional field. Communication is a high-priority competency for healthcare professionals who work in human-centered environments. Communication is a basic tool that is necessary to determine the needs of healthy individuals as well as patients and to plan the provision of appropriate care. Thus, it is important to establish effective

TABLE 3.

Comparison of Smartphone Addiction Scale–Short Version Mean Scores by Characteristics of Students (N = 502)

	Smartphone Addiction Scale–Short Version			
Characteristic	*M*	*SD*	*t*/*F*	*p*
Program			3.864	< .001
Medical school	29.32	9.93		
Nursing department	33.32	9.54		
Gender			3.033	.002
Female	32.74	9.89		
Male	29.81	9.66		
Daily use (hours/day)			*F* = 41.284	< .001
0–2	26.07	8.66		
3–5	30.38	8.86		
6–8	36.91	9.94		
Smartphone use in the classroom			3.826	< .001
Yes	33.39	9.78		
No	30.04	9.77		
Failure to follow course topics			6.070	< .001
Yes	35.13	10.13		
No	29.81	9.19		
Course performance			*F* = 28.310	< .001
Successful	30.84	1.02		
Partially successful	32.27	9.36		
Unsuccessful	35.26	1.09		
Regular sports participation			4.677	< .001
Yes	29.37	9.67		
No	33.52	9.73		
Health problems because of phone use (eye problems, pain, etc.)			4.276	.001
Yes	34.11	9.69		
No	30.12	9.98		
Injury when using the phone (falling, bumping, hanging, etc.)			3.021	.003
Yes	34.91	11.16		
No	31.31	9.55		
Preferred communication type			−2.857	.004
Face to face	31.06	9.14		
Via phone or social media	33.79	11.28		
Communicating with patients and patient relatives			−1.798	.043
Yes	31.44	9.65		
No/some	33.30	10.59		

communication to understand the patient, build mutual trust, and improve quality of care and thus improve the condition of patients. Therefore, good communication skills may be considered a positive outcome.

Because smartphones enable people to communicate at any place and time, they are a highly favored tool for communication (Davey & Davey, 2014). However, studies indicate that excessive use of smartphones affects social relations negatively (Choi et al., 2015; Samaha & Hawi, 2016; Süt et al., 2016). Choi et al. (2015) reported that smartphone addiction affected interpersonal relationships and mental health negatively. Smartphones, which have an important place in the lives of university students, also affect their ability to communicate. In this study, approximately one third of the participants preferred communicating via smartphones or social media in the communication initiation process, with the SAS-SV scores of these students significantly higher. Moreover, a negative relationship was found between the SAS-SV mean scores of the participants and CSAS mean scores. Thus, the communication skill scores of the participants decreased as their addiction scores increased. Moreover, the result of the regression analysis revealed that smartphone addiction negatively and significantly predicted the communication skills of the participants.

Another important result supporting this finding was the higher SAS-SV scores of the students who stated that they could not communicate comfortably with patients and next of kin. Other studies indicate that the young generation and the medical and nursing students who are part of this generation are at risk of smartphone addiction. One of the most important consequences of this risk is the negative effects on interpersonal communication. The few previous studies of students enrolled in health programs yielded results that are similar to this study, finding that increased levels of smartphone addiction reduced communication skills (Cerit et al., 2018; Cho & Kim, 2014; Süt et al., 2016). These skills play a key role in the ability of students to express their emotions and thoughts and to use listening and body language skills effectively. Students are required to be able to show appropriate skills to communicate effectively with their peers, educators, families, healthcare professionals, and the group that they are serving. One of the most important skills of health workers, whose job is centered on the care of humans, is effective and therapeutic communication skills. It should not be forgotten that effective communication is a key element in correct treatment and good care. Thus, addictions such as smartphone addiction are thought to cause problems in professional life. According to the results of this study, regulating the smartphone usage and reducing the smartphone addiction levels of students are critical to improving their communication skills.

Limitations

The results of this study may not represent all nursing and medical students because the study was conducted at a single center in Turkey. In addition, the results presume that participants self-reported in an honest manner on the questionnaire. Finally, as the cutoff point of the Turkish version of the SAS-SV scale was not previously determined, the researchers in this study were unable to determine the addiction status of the students in this study group.

Conclusions

The participants in this study self-reported spending a significant amount of time using smartphones, indicating a high level of smartphone addiction. The increase in the SAS-SV scores of the participants negatively affected communication skills, academic performance, and social life. The interest of younger people in novel technologies is important for Turkey, which is evolving into an information-based society. However, it should not be ignored that excessive smartphone use forms a basis for the development of various health, education, and social problems. Thus, it is necessary to control the smartphone usage behavior of students to avoid negatively affecting communication skills to ensure better service to patients and a better understanding of the language of care.

It has been reported in the literature that the clinical learning, problem-solving skills, and skill development of students may be made easier by incorporating technology into the learning environment (Doyle, Garret, & Currie, 2014; Strandell-Laine, Stolt, Leino-Kilpi, & Saarikoski, 2015). Thus, student and lecturer awareness of the benefits of smartphones to education should be increased, while balanced by precautions against excessive and needless use. These precautions could include increasing sporting and artistic activities on campus, referring students with a high addiction risk to counseling services, and promoting awareness of the potential harms of inappropriate smartphone use.

Acknowledgment

Special thanks to the students who participated in this study and donated their time.

Author Contributions

Study conception and design: All authors
Data collection: All authors
Data analysis and interpretation: UC, MT, GV
Drafting of the article: UC, SB, MT
Critical revision of the article: UC, SB, MT

References

Abdrbo, A. (2017). Assessment of nursing students' communication skills. *Nursing Education Perspectives, 38*(3), 149–151. https://doi.org/10.1097/01.NEP.0000000000000126

Acar, G., & Buldukoglu, K. (2016). Difficulties of students' in communication with patients and their perception of difficult patient. *Journal of Psychiatric Nursing, 7*(1), 7–12. https://doi.org/10.5505/phd.2016.20592

Aydın, İ. E. (2016). A study on usage of social media among university students: Anadolu University case. *Selçuk University Journal of Social Sciences Institute, 35*, 373–386. Retrieved from http://dergisosyalbil.selcuk.edu.tr/susbed/article/download/1256/1073 (Original work published in Turkish)

Bragazzi, N. L., & Del Puente, G. (2014). A proposal for including nomophobia in the new DSM-V. *Psychology Research and Behavior Management, 7*, 155–160. https://doi.org/10.2147/PRBM.S41386

Cerit, B., Çıtak Bilgin, N., & Ak, B. (2018). Relationship between smartphone addiction of nursing department students and their communication skills. *Contemporary Nurse, 54*(4–5), 532–542. https://doi.org/10.1080/10376178.2018.1448291

Cho, G. Y., & Kim, Y. H. (2014). Factors affecting smartphone addiction among university students. *Journal of the Korean Academia-Industrial Cooperation Society, 15*(3), 1632–1640. https://doi.org/10.5762/KAIS.2014.15.3.1632

Cho, S., & Lee, E. (2015). Development of a brief instrument to measure smartphone addiction among nursing students. *Computers, Informatics, Nursing, 33*(5), 216–224. https://doi.org/10.1097/CIN.0000000000000132

Choi, S. W., Kım, D. J., Choi, J. S., Ahn, H., Choi, E. J., Song, W. Y., ... Youn, H. (2015). Comparison of risk and protective factors associated with smartphone addiction and Internet addiction. *Journal of Behavioral Addictions, 4*(4), 308–314. https://doi.org/10.1556/2006.4.2015.043

Çizmeci, E. (2017). Both sides of the coin: Smartphones in romantic relationships of youth. *Electronic Journal of Social Sciences, 16*(63), 1400–1415. Retrieved from https://dergipark.gov.tr/download/article-file/346329 (Original work published in Turkish)

Davey, S., & Davey, A. (2014). Assessment of smartphone addiction in Indian adolescents: A mixed method study by systematic-review and meta-analysis approach. *International Journal of Preventive Medicine, 5*(12), 1500–1511.

Doyle, G. J., Garrett, B., & Currie, L. M. (2014). Integrating mobile devices into nursing curricula: Opportunities for implementation using Rogers' diffusion of innovation model. *Nurse Education Today, 34*(5), 775–782. https://doi.org/10.1016/j.nedt.2013.10.021

Erdem, H., Kalkin, G., Türen, U., & Deniz, M. (2016). The effects of no mobile phone phobia (nomofobi) on academic performance among undergraduate students. *The Journal of Faculty of Economics and Administrative Sciences, 21*(3), 923–936. Retrieved from https://www.researchgate.net/publication/305851086

Haug, S., Castro, P. R., Kwon, M., Filler, A., Kowatsch, T., & Schaub, M. P. (2015). Smartphone use and smartphone addiction among young people in Switzerland. *Journal of Behavioral Addictions, 4*(4), 299–307. https://doi.org/10.1556/2006.4.2015.037

Heo, J., Oh, J., Subramanian, S. V., Kim, Y., & Kawachi, I. (2014). Addictive internet use among Korean adolescents: A national survey. *PLOS ONE, 9*(2), e87819. https://doi.org/10.1371/journal.pone.0087819

Kim, D., Lee, Y., Lee, J., Nam, J. K., & Chung, Y. (2014). Development of Korean smartphone addiction proneness scale for youth. *PLOS ONE, 9*(5), e97920. https://doi.org/10.1371/journal.pone.0097920

Kim, H. (2013). Exercise rehabilitation for smartphone addiction. *Journal of Exercise Rehabilitation, 9*(6), 500–505. https://doi.org/10.12965/jer.130080

King, A. L. S., Valença, A. M., Silva, A. C. O., Baczynski, T., Carvalho, M. R., & Nardi, A. E. (2013). Nomophobia: Dependency on virtual environments or social phobia? *Computers in Human Behavior, 29*(1), 140–144. https://doi.org/10.1016/j.chb.2012.07.025

Korkut, F. (1996). Developing the communication skills scale: Reliability and validity studies. *Turkish Psychological Counseling and Guidance Journal, 2*(7), 18–23. Retrieved from http://turkpdrdergisi.com/index.php/pdr/article/view/401/342 (Original work published in Turkish)

Korkut Owen, F., & Bugay, A. (2014). Developing a communication skills scale: Validity and reliability studies. *Mersin University Journal of the Faculty of Education, 10*(2), 51–64. Retrieved from http://dergipark.gov.tr/mersinefd/issue/17394/181805 (Original work published in Turkish)

Kuyucu, M. (2017). Use of smart phone and problematic of smart phone addiction in young people: "Smartphone (colic)" university youth. *Global Media Journal TR Edition, 7*(14), 328–359. Retrieved from http://globalmediajournaltr.yeditepe.edu.tr/bahar-2017-sayisi-spring-2017-issue (Original work published in Turkish)

Kwon, M., Kim, D. J., Cho, H., & Yang, S. (2013). The Smartphone Addiction Scale: Development and validation of a short version for adolescents. *PLOS ONE, 8*(12), e83558. https://doi.org/10.1371/journal.pone.0083558

Kwon, M., Lee, J. Y., Won, W. Y., Park, J. W., Min, J. A., Hahn, C., ... Kim, D. J. (2013). Development and validation of a Smartphone Addiction Scale (SAS). *PLOS ONE, 8*(2), e56936. https://doi.org/10.1371/journal.pone.0056936

Lee, Y. K., Chang, C. T., Lin, Y., & Cheng, Z. H. (2014). The dark side of smartphone usage: Psychological traits, compulsive behavior and technostress. *Computers in Human Behavior, 31*, 373–383. https://doi.org/10.1016/j.chb.2013.10.047

Lepp, A., Li, J., Barkley, J. E., & Salehi-Esfahani, S. (2015). Exploring the relationships between college students' cell phone use, personality and leisure. *Computers in Human Behavior, 43*, 210–219. https://doi.org/10.1016/j.chb.2014.11.006

Mok, Y. J., Choi, S. W., Kim, D. J., Choi, J. S., Lee, J., Ahn, H., ... Song, W. Y. (2014). Latent class analysis on internet and smartphone addiction in college students. *Neuropsychiatric Disease and Treatment, 10*, 817–828. https://doi.org/10.2147/NDT.S59293

Noyan, C. O., Darçın, A. E., Nurmedov, S., Yılmaz, O., & Dilbaz, N. (2015). Validity and reliability of the Turkish version of the Smartphone Addiction Scale–Short Version among university students. *Anatolian Journal of Psychiatry, 16*(1), 73–81. https://doi.org/10.5455/apd.176101 (Original work published in Turkish)

Samaha, M., & Hawi, N. S. (2016). Relationships among smartphone addiction, stress, academic performance, and satisfaction with life. *Computers in Human Behavior, 57*, 321–325. https://doi.org/10.1016/j.chb.2015.12.045

Şata, M., Çelik, İ., Ertürk, Z., & Taş, U. E. (2016). The study of adapting Smartphone Addiction Scale for Turkish high school students. *Journal of Measurement and Evaluation in Education and Psychology, 7*(1), 156–169. https://doi.org/10.21031/epod.95432 (Original work published in Turkish)

Smith, A. (2017a). *Record shares of Americans now own smartphones, have home broadband.* Retrieved from http://www.pewresearch.org/fact-tank/2017/01/12/evolution-of-technology/

Smith, A. (2017b). *US smartphone use in 2017.* Retrieved from http://www.pewinternet.org/2015/04/01/us-smartphone-use-in-2015/

Strandell-Laine, C., Stolt, M., Leino-Kilpi, H., & Saarikoski, M. (2015). Use of mobile devices in nursing student–nurse teacher cooperation during the clinical practicum: An integrative review. *Nurse Education Today, 35*(3), 493–499. https://doi.org/10.1016/j.nedt.2014.10.007

Subba, S. H., Mandelia, C., Pathak, V., Reddy, D., Goel, A., Tayal, A., ... Nagaraj, K. (2013). Ringxiety and the mobile phone usage pattern among the students of a medical college in South India. *Journal of Clinical and Diagnostic Research, 7*(2), 205–209. https://doi.org/10.7860/JCDR/2013/4652.2729

Süt, H. K., Kurt, S., Uzal, Ö., & Özdilek, S. (2016). Effects of smartphone addiction level on social and educational life in health sciences students. *Eurasian Journal of Family Medicine, 5*(1), 13–19. Retrieved from http://ejfm.trakya.edu.tr/userfiles/2016/April/3-hatice-sut.pdf

Turkish Statistical Institute. (2017). *Household information technology use survey 2017. Number: 24862.* Retrieved from http://afyonluoglu.org/PublicWebFiles/stats/hbtk/2017-HBTK.pdf (Original work published in Turkish)

Yıldırım, K., Yaşar, Ö., & Duru, M. (2016). Based on the views of teachers and students analysing the usage of smartphones in teaching and learning environments and effects. *International Journal of Education, Science and Technology, 2*(2), 72–84. Retrieved from http://dergipark.gov.tr/download/article-file/227994 (Original work published in Turkish)

Yılmaz, D., Çinar, H. G., & Özyazıcıoğlu, N. (2017). The examination of relationship between smart phone, internet addiction and upper extremity functional activity levels among nursing students. *Journal of Health Science, 8*(3), 34–39. https://doi.org/10.22312/sdusbed.311497 (Original work published in Turkish)

The Lived Experiences of Indonesian Nurses Who Worked as Care Workers in Taiwan

Nursalam NURSALAM[1]* • Ching-Min CHEN[2] • Ferry EFENDI[3] • Eka Misbahatul Mar'ah HAS[4] • Laily HIDAYATI[5] • Setho HADISUYATMANA[6]

ABSTRACT

Background: Despite the large number of Indonesian nurses currently working as migrant care workers in Taiwan, no studies in the literature have been found that explore this phenomenon or assess the working situation of Indonesian nurses working in care facilities in Taiwan.

Purpose: This study aimed to elicit and describe the lived experiences of Indonesian nurses serving as care workers in Taiwan.

Methods: Phenomenological research was used to explore the experiences of Indonesian nurses working in long-term care facilities. The participants were recruited from care facilities in Taiwan. This study utilized semistructured interviews conducted with 16 Indonesian nurses in a suitable setting. All of the interviews were transcribed, and the work of Van Manen was used to analyze the data.

Results: Four main themes were identified, including motives for working abroad, feelings of being trapped, experiencing a difficult journey, and the feeling of being supported. These themes reflect the lived experiences of Indonesian nurses who work in Taiwan's long-term care industry.

Conclusions: Nurses from Indonesia choose to who work as nurses in Taiwan because of poor financial background and the chance of gaining a better life. However, the participants in this study felt stressed, challenged, and disappointed when faced with the unmet expectations of being employed as care workers without a clear career path. Furthermore, the need to communicate in an unfamiliar language was mentioned as a significant barrier to fulfilling their role. Better policies should be put in place to achieve improved outcomes for both countries.

KEY WORDS:
lived experience, Indonesian nurses, foreign care workers, Taiwan.

Introduction

A critical shortage of nurses in developed countries contributed to the active recruitment of nurses from other, particularly developing, countries such as Indonesia (Efendi, Chen, Nursalam, Indarwati, & Ulfiana, 2016; Efendi, Mackey, Huang, & Chen, 2017). Using migrant nurses is used by receiving countries as a quick remedy to meet the growing needs of aging populations and to achieve adequate staffing levels (Buchan, 2006). Indonesia is a major provider of care workers to meet the global demand (Efendi, Nursalam, Kurniati, & Gunawan, 2018; National Board for the Placement and Protection of Indonesian Overseas Workers [NBPPIOW], 2014). In the last decade, Indonesia has encouraged nurse migration based on economic benefit (Efendi, Nursalam, Dang, & Arief, 2015).

Responding to the international recruitment of health personnel, the World Health Organization (WHO) began regulating this movement by issuing the WHO Global Code of Practice (WHO, 2010). This code emphasizes and promotes the ethical recruitment of health personnel to minimize brain drain and brain waste, specifically from developing countries. This code is intended as a guide for receiving countries to promote and respect fair labor practices for all health personnel (WHO, 2010, 2011).

Recent data show that Taiwan is the most common destination for migrant nurses from Indonesia, with a total placement of 597 nurses as of the end of 2013 (NBPPIOW, 2014). It is surprising to know that Taiwan is the top destination for Indonesian nurses, as 75% (178,205) of the migrant workers in Taiwan are employed in the informal employment sectors (Economic and Trade Office of Indonesia, 2015). However, little is known regarding the level of education, placement channels, type of employment, or background of the Indonesians who work as migrant nurses in Taiwan. Moreover, there are incomplete and inconsistent data on migration in the literature (Clemens & Pettersson, 2008).

[1]PhD, RN, Professor, Faculty of Nursing, Universitas Airlangga, Surabaya, Indonesia • [2]DNS, RN, Professor, Research Center for Humanities and Social Sciences, Department of Nursing, College of Medicine, National Cheng Kung University, Taiwan, ROC • [3]PhD, RN, Assistant Professor, Faculty of Nursing, Department of Community and Mental Health, Universitas Airlangga, Surabaya, Indonesia • [4]MS, RN, Assistant Professor, Faculty of Nursing, Department of Community and Mental Health, Universitas Airlangga, Surabaya, Indonesia • [5]MS, RN, Lecturer, Faculty of Nursing, Department of Basic, Medical-Surgical and Critical Care, Universitas Airlangga, Surabaya, Indonesia • [6]MSN, RN, Lecturer, Faculty of Nursing, Department of Community and Mental Health, Universitas Airlangga, Surabaya, Indonesia.

Taiwan, as a developed and wealthy country, has attracted foreign workers from many countries, including Indonesia. The Council of Labour Affairs first opened Taiwan to foreign workers in 1989, and migrant care workers were first hired in 1992 to meet the rising care needs of Taiwan's aging population (Kung, 2002). Recently, the number of foreign labor workers in Taiwan has increased significantly, to over 600,000, with most originating from the Philippines, Thailand, Indonesia, Malaysia, Mongolia, and Vietnam (Department of Statistics, Ministry of Interior, 2019). The Economic and Trade Office of Indonesia reported that 245,180 Indonesians worked as registered care workers in Taiwan in 2015. Although this number was slightly less in 2017 (190,587), Indonesia remains the largest source of migrant care workers in Taiwan (Ministry of Labor, Taiwan, ROC, 2017).

Despite the movement of Indonesian nurses to Taiwan, few studies have explored their experiences or examined their motivations in pursuing work as care workers in Taiwan. Foreign care workers have become an important part of care provision in Taiwan's long-term care (LTC) industry despite the paucity of information about their lived experience. This study was designed to explore the lived experiences of Indonesian migrant care workers in Taiwan. The insights gathered from their perspectives may be used to improve future placements and maximize the mutual benefits to both countries.

Methods

Research Design

A qualitative study using a phenomenological approach was used to reveal the nature of being a care worker in Taiwanese LTC institutions. The interpretive phenomenology employed both interpretive and descriptive elements to better understand the nature of the essence of the daily lived experiences of the participants (Van Manen, 1997). To conduct precise analysis and interpretation, participant-friendly settings were prearranged to allow their provision of rich and deep information.

Participants

Indonesian nurses who have worked as care workers in Taiwan's LTC institutions were recruited purposively as participants in this study. The inclusion criteria were that they were Indonesian nurses who (a) have lived and worked as a care workers in Taiwan for a minimum of 6 months and (b) are an enrolled nurse in Indonesia. Although the size of the research participant population was predetermined, once data saturation was reached, no additional interviews were held. The study was advertised to three potential participants, and afterward, further recruitment proceeded using a snowballing technique, which was selected because of the dispersed locations of the nurses and the limited access that researchers had to databases of Indonesian nurses working in Taiwan. The potential participants were contacted by phone and asked to provide verbal consent to participate. Twenty-four care workers from different locations of Taiwan (Taipei, Tainan, and Kaohsiung) were contacted as potential participants.

Data Collection

Data collection was carried out between August and September 2017. The participants were contacted, provided information on the study, and informed that their participation would be voluntary and that they could withdraw at any time. All communications with participants were conducted in their mother tongue, Bahasa Indonesia. The participants were interviewed for 45–90 minutes each using a semi-structured questionnaire. The questionnaire was designed to assess (a) the reason for migration, (b) their lived experiences while working as care workers, (c) perceived barriers in addition to cultural differences, (d) unwanted events, (e) experiences that they have lived, and (f) recommendations for nurses who want to come to work in Taiwan. We collected the data using interviews and gathered in-depth information that reflected the perceptions and experiences of the participants. The interviews were audio-recorded and transcribed verbatim. Transcribed data were then cleaned, de-identified, and translated into English, and the transcriptions of both the original version and the English-translated version were reviewed for authenticity. No additional themes emerged after 16 interviews.

Ethical Considerations

Approval to conduct the study was granted by the ethical committee of Universitas Airlangga, Surabaya, Indonesia (513/KEPK). Written consent from the participants was obtained before conducting the interviews. The participants were assured that their data would be kept confidential and used for research purposes only. Access to the data was limited to members of the research study only.

Data Analysis

The data were carefully analyzed after transcription following the six steps of van Manen's (1997) phenomenological approach, which include (a) emphasizing the phenomenon by developing the research question around the experience of becoming a care worker in Taiwan, (b) selecting the participants and undertaking face-to-face interviews to explore the experience, (c) recognizing and reflecting on the important themes, (d) writing and rewriting to describe the phenomenon, (e) preserving the focus through in-depth exploration, and (f) considering both the parts and the whole to balance out the research context. We analyzed both versions of the transcripts using NVivo 11 (QSR International, Burlington, USA). Four themes emerged, which were subsequently used to describe the participants' lived experiences accompanied by one verbatim excerpt each.

Rigor and Trustworthiness

The rigor and trustworthiness of this study were examined in accordance with Lincoln and Guba (1985) to maintain the concepts of credibility, dependability, confirmability, and transferability. Three ways were used to improve the credibility of the data. First, the researchers were trained by an expert investigator in the qualitative method of data collection. Second, the researchers asked for feedback from an experienced researcher in hermeneutic phenomenology regarding the data quality and subsequent interpretations. Third, the participants were invited to provide suggestions and to comment on the data.

A professional transcriber was hired to transcribe the data for each interview session verbatim. The transcribed data were then reviewed by all of the team members in this study and an external expert to address the issue of dependability. The confirmability of this study was maintained by showing the results to the participants. Finally, the transferability of this study was evaluated by providing a thick description of the study that fits with other contexts.

Results

Participants' Description

Sixteen Indonesian nurses who have worked as care workers were enrolled as participants and interviewed individually. The settings for interview were selected by the nurses as places where the participants would feel comfortable to communicate their story. Most of the participants were women (n = 11). Their ages ranged from 22 to 41 years, most were single (n = 11), and most held a diploma in nursing (n = 12) or a BSN (n = 4) as their highest level of education. The nurses were mostly from the province of Jawa Tengah (n = 9) and were currently working and living in Taipei City (n = 8). Most of the participants had lived in Taiwan for more than 2 years (n = 11). The net monthly salary of the participants ranged from 15,000 to 30,000 Taiwan dollars (see Table 1).

TABLE 1.

Demographic Distribution of the Participants (N = 16)

Characteristic	Migrant Caregiver	
	n	%
Age (years; *M* and *SD*)	27.6	5.3
Gender		
Female	11	68
Male	5	32
Marital status		
Single	11	68
In a relationship	5	32
Children in household		
One or more	5	32
None	11	68
Province of origin		
East Java	5	32
West Java	2	12
Central Java	9	56
Current area		
Taipei	8	50
Tainan	3	19
Kaohsiung	5	31
Highest education		
Diploma 3 in nursing	12	75
Having work experience before emigrating		
Yes	16	100
Years of residence in Taiwan		
≥ 2	11	68
< 2	5	32
Salary while abroad (TWD; mean and *SD*)	20,271	4,063

Note. Age range is 22–41 years; salary range is TWD 10,000–30,000.

Findings

Following the work of van Manen's phenomenology, this study revealed four themes and eight subthemes, including (a) "motives for working abroad: financial motives and seeking different life experiences"; (b) "feelings of being trapped: victimized by fraud, losing professional identity, and losing professional skills"; (c) "difficult journey: communication inadequacy and limited career pathway"; and (d) "feelings of being supported: support from their employer and support from their recruiting agent."

Theme 1: Motives for Working Abroad

Coming from a poor financial background drove most of the participants to seek migrant work in Taiwan, with most expecting to have a better future as a result. Nevertheless, some of the participants stated that gaining the experience of working abroad was their primary reason for seeking migrant work in Taiwan. All of these responses refer to the first theme in this study, which reflects on the meaning behind deciding to move to Taiwan to live and work. Nearly every participant initially believed Taiwan to be a place where they could earn money and gain more experience. Most of the respondents identified financial gain as a motivation to work in Taiwan.

Financial motives

Most of the participants had sought migrant work in Taiwan because of the poor economic situation of their families. They expected that working in Taiwan would improve their financial situation and, thus, support their family needs. As Participant 5 described: "...my family needs my support to live a decent life."

Several participants were attracted by the higher salary offered by the recruiting agents in their home country. As Participants 3 and 5 noted:

"...Second, was the economic (motive).... I know that the salary was low. It was far under my expectations. Here, good-Lord, it is far better than in Indonesia."

"I am here because the salary offered is much higher than in Indonesia. By doing a similar job, I can earn five times more...."

In search of a different life experience

Some of the participants stated that money was secondary for them in taking migrant work in Taiwan. More important, they said, was acquiring experience working outside their country of birth. Participants 11 and 1, respectively, recalled:

"I really want to go abroad to acquire new experience. Working in foreign countries has been a personal challenge. Frankly speaking, I was hoping to go to Japan, but I failed, and, so, came here."

"I was just, like...I wanted to know better the differences between the medical and nursing instruments used in caring for patients here and in Indonesia...yeah, especially about the instruments they (Taiwanese nurses) use..."

However, still other participants said that the life experience of working abroad had been their priority in seeking overseas employment. Participant 4 shared that:

"...My most important reason (for working abroad) was just wanting to go abroad to look for new life experiences."

Theme 2: Feelings of Being Trapped

The participants revealed that they faced unexpected experiences while working and living in Taiwan. They expressed feeling trapped by the different nursing qualification system in Taiwan, which prevented their working as professional nurses while here.

Victimized by fraud

Some of the participants shared that they did not initially realize that they would be required to do work that is typically done by people holding lower qualifications. They said that they had been persuaded to come to Taiwan by the offer of a higher salary and promises of easy work. Participant 10 recalled:

"I was lulled by the (recruiting agency's) sweet offer... a high salary and a load (workload) that wouldn't be heavy. Only five days of work per week, eight hours per day. But it didn't work out that way. I have to work 12 hours a day, and the five-day work week was just an empty promise...."

Losing their professional identity

Almost all of the participants soon realized that it would not be possible to transfer their qualifications and work in Taiwan, as the system in Taiwan does not permit foreign nurses to work as professional nurses. Participant 8 stressed that:

"...we felt very sad. Our status is not clear here. We have a high degree in nursing from our country, but here we are nothing. Maybe there is another way to solve this problem."

Participant 10 stated that obtaining work that was in line with their professional background was a promise without truth.

"...To be honest, it was not like what I expected. When I first arrived, I didn't see it (as part of my job) .... I was given the dirty parts to clean, told to tidy up the mess...or just (to help) old people do they want to do."

Losing their professional skills

The participants also discussed how they felt losing their skills while working in nursing homes and LTC facilities, where they were not permitted to continue practicing their professional skills. They felt that they were being forced to stop using these skills and saw no future for their career. As Participant 15 stated:

"...I am not allowed to practice some of the skills that I know I can do. Like suction, for example. As long as you were qualified, you are allowed to do that back home. I think that only Taiwanese nurses are allowed to perform this procedure."

Some of the participants began to perceive the restrictions on what they were allowed to do. As Participant 10 recalled:

"...We don't have the right to give an injection or to do other things that nurses in Indonesia may do in their job...."

Theme 3: Difficult Journey

There was no consensus regarding the challenges that Indonesian nurses experience in Taiwan. However, communicating with older adult care recipients and their local counterparts was generally viewed as another significant hurdle at work. Other participants identified that this situation inhibited their career development.

Communication inadequacy

Failure to understand the local language hindered the participants from fully understanding conversations and instructions. The participants agreed that this contributed to their hardship and significantly exacerbated their stress. As one participant noted:

"Taiwanese speak in a different intonation and so quickly. As you can guess, it causes a lot of stress when I cannot understand anything about my patients."

For the younger participants, the language barrier made them bear others' problems as their own and take on all of the consequences, as they were unable to voice their thoughts and opinions. Participant 9 related:

> *"...as a first-timer, I didn't fully understand the language. If other care workers made a mistake, all of them were older than me and put the guilt on me. I couldn't speak for myself...so silence was my only option."*

Limited career pathway

Their limited career opportunities in Taiwan were another significant issue for the participants. They reported that this significantly impacted their future plans. Participant 11 stated:

> *"Here, it is impossible to advance my career. It is only about settling myself, and just a matter of moving to another country."*

Participant 4 agreed, stating that:

> *"There is no such a thing as a career. We're not Taiwanese. Otherwise (if we wanted to develop a career in Taiwan), we would have to take another test and attend school again...."*

Finding the situation difficult, the participants even suggested that the younger generation of nurses should think twice before deciding to work as care workers in Taiwan. Participant 1 stressed:

> *"If they are able to put Taiwan as the last option, they should. If they can, they should think of Japan or the Middle East. Indonesian nurses would have a brighter future in those places...."*

Theme 4: Feeling of Being Supported

Nevertheless, the participants felt that their management was supportive at work, although, for others, their agents in Taiwan always offered help whenever the nurses needed help to cope with their current situation.

Support from the employer

The participants agreed that support from their employer and nursing home/LTC institution was critical to creating a supportive workplace environment. Participant 7 suggested:

> *"My nursing home is doing its best to help me adjust and adapt to the new environment. They are motivating us to learn and study Mandarin in every situation. So far, we seldom have problems with our employer."*

Participant 6 added:

> *"They told me to keep smiling while working...."*

Support from the recruiting agent

The participants voiced that the placement agencies played a nurturing role, particularly when dealing with problems in the workplace. Participant 9 said:

> *"I was prepared because the agency that helped us gave us a few suggestions for when we are dealing with any problems in our life. They will come when I complain about almost anything."*

Participant 3 highlighted the support received from her recruiting agent, recalling that:

> *"...My agent came to handle just about all of my problems. If I have any problems with my employer, they send someone. They are very helpful."*

Discussion

This study explored the lived experiences of migrant nurses working as care workers in Taiwan. This study revealed the motivations for participants choosing to work abroad and their personal experiences while working as care workers, including the situations that they were required to face and their learning from these experiences. The current trends suggest the popularity of working abroad, as informed by the NBPPIOW (2014), which narrows the gap in understanding by unveiling the learned experience from the firsthand perspective of the participants.

The latest data from NBPPIOW (2019) show that Taiwan was the second largest recipient of Indonesians as migrant labor, after Malaysia. The nurses who participated in this study highlighted the desire to improve their poor financial situation as the most important reason for applying to work in Taiwan. This finding echoed previous studies that identified economic motive as a primary factor attracting migrant workers to a destination country (Aiken, Buchan, Sochalski, Nichols, & Powell, 2004; Buchan, 2015). All of the participants agreed that Taiwan was one of the most popular destination countries for Indonesian nurses to live and work in. The participants noted that they were attracted by the ease of access when applying to work as care workers in Taiwan. Furthermore, the opportunity to have a better life was underscored by the nurses, as the currency conversion between the two countries gave them a higher income when compared with working as a nurse in Indonesia. They expected that being a care worker in Taiwan would allow them to help their families improve their economic situation. Nevertheless, other participants asserted that gaining experience working abroad was a factor that encouraged them to seek work in Taiwan (Aiken et al., 2004; Buchan, 2015; Kingma, 2007). However, they ultimately felt neglected in their current position because of their inability to continue performing in the professional capacity they were accustomed to in Indonesia.

The expectation of being employed in an advanced technological and sophisticated health system was emphasized by the participants. However, some revealed dissatisfaction with their identity and their skills going unused abroad. Before coming to Taiwan, the nurses perceived that being a care worker would allow them to hold a role equivalent to their professional nursing role in Indonesia. This misunderstanding was a cause for dissatisfaction. The term "care worker" is widely associated in Indonesia with geriatric nursing. Therefore, many Indonesian migrant nurses expect that they will be able to work as professional nurses in Taiwan. This situation is similar to that of Indonesian nurses working as care workers in Japan under the bilateral scheme (Kurniati, Chen, Efendi, & Ogawa, 2017).

A clear career path for foreign care workers should be addressed as an important component in sustaining the migration cycle within the nursing sector (Buchan, 2015). Nevertheless, the different approach between Taiwan and Indonesia has failed to address this issue. The Government of the Republic of Indonesia recognizes nursing as a profession with a set of responsibilities to be carried out by the certificate holder (Law on Health Workers, 2014). On the other hand, the health system in Taiwan does not allow foreign nurses to work at their certified level of qualification. This finding urges the need for a clear, informed, and well-explained contract for Indonesian nurses interested in working as care workers in Taiwan. The term "care worker" should be clarified, as it confuses nurses who sign up to work in Taiwan's LTC facilities.

Thorsteinsson (2002) reasoned that more effective communication is necessary to encourage nurses to involve feeling, trust, and empathy in care delivery. In addition, the findings of this study highlighted the importance of effective communication at work. The participants argued that it signified the accuracy of the transfer of information among the nurses, care workers, residents, and their manager. They indicated that language difficulties posed a significant challenge in delivering care and coordinating work. Language differences were perceived by the participants as requiring specific sets of skills, techniques, and processes. Therefore, the different languages used in their work became an inevitable barrier against the participants conducting their role as care workers.

The uniqueness of the migration scheme is related to the support of the care facilities and the healthcare agencies of Taiwan. The participants noted that support from Taiwan LTC institutions was critical in their initial adjustment to working and living in Taiwan. Furthermore, they stressed that the private recruitment agencies in Taiwan and in the sending countries should provide services for both employers and foreign care workers. Cooperation with recruiting agencies in the sending countries should help ensure that information on foreign care workers is provided to prospective employers. Once a foreign care worker is selected by an employer, the agency in the sending country will assist the foreign care worker to complete the requisite procedures before entering Taiwan (Chen, 2013). As most of Indonesian nurses do not speak Mandarin fluently, the services of these agencies should be given a greater emphasis in the future.

Limitations

Given the nature of qualitative research, the findings in this study may only be transferred to gain an understanding of the phenomenon within similar contexts and settings. Moreover, the lack of the Indonesian Nurses' Association as a potential source of information in Taiwan may have limited diversity among the participants.

Conclusions

Most nurses who participated in this study were prompted to work in Taiwan by poor financial background and the expectations of a better life. They expected to be able to help improve the economic situation of their families and to upgrade their skills in their destination country. The participants expressed feelings of being stressed, challenged, and disappointed. Their unmet expectations of being employed as nurses increased because of their relegation to relatively menial tasks that did not reflect their professional nursing backgrounds. This situation highlights the need for a clear definition of work responsibilities for those who sign up to work in Taiwan's LTC facilities. Language problems were raised as a barrier for nurses migrating from Indonesia to Taiwan. Fortunately, the participants felt somewhat supported by the LTC management and recruiting agencies. It is hoped that structured policies related to strengthening the support provided by LTCs to Indonesian care workers are standardized in Taiwan.

Implications for Practice

Some findings of this study reveal the challenges encountered by Indonesian nurses working in Taiwan's LTC industry. The results of this study highlight the need for better predeparture preparation and better recruitment processes. Nurses who intend to work abroad must be made aware in their native language of the details of what they are applying for. This study is expected to contribute to the formulation of appropriate future-migration policies based on the contexts that are specific to Taiwan. This study recommends that policies be changed to facilitate professional nursing career development, particularly for overseas nurses who work in Taiwan. Putting the experiences of Indonesian care worker nurses into the context of the global market reveals a cycle of brain gain, brain drain, and brain waste that hinders the career path of Indonesian nurses. Taiwan, as a receiving country, should play a more positive role in promoting and encouraging good practices by recruitment agencies in compliance with the WHO global code.

Acknowledgment

Special thanks to Universitas Airlangga, Surabaya, Indonesia, for funding this study.

Author Contributions

Study conception and design: All authors
Data collection: FE, SH
Data analysis and interpretation: FE, EM, LH, SH
Drafting of the article: All authors
Critical revision of the article: All authors

References

Aiken, L. H., Buchan, J., Sochalski, J., Nichols, B., & Powell, M. (2004). Trends in international nurse migration: The world's wealthy countries must be aware of how the "pull" of nurses from developing countries affects global health. *Health Affairs, 23*(3), 69–77. https://doi.org/10.1377/hlthaff.23.3.69

Buchan, J. (2006). The impact of global nursing migration on health services delivery. *Policy, Politics, & Nursing Practice, 7* (3, Suppl.), 16S–25S. https://doi.org/10.1177/1527154406291520

Buchan, J. (2015). *Nursing workforce sustainability: The international connection.* Philadelphia, PA: International Centre on Nurse Migration.

Chen, Y. (2013). *(Re)-regulating care: Employing foreign carers for older persons in Taiwan.* Queensland University of Technology, Australia.

Clemens, M. A., & Pettersson, G. (2008). New data on African health professionals abroad. *Human Resources for Health, 6*(1), 1–11. https://doi.org/10.1186/1478-4491-6-1

Department of Statistics, Ministry of Interior, Taiwan, ROC. (2019). *Annual statistics report of Ministry of Interior, 2017.* Retrieved from https://www.moi.gov.tw/stat/node.aspx?cate_sn=&belong_sn=6463&sn=6465 (Original work published in Chinese)

Economic and Trade Office of Indonesia. (2015). *Distribution of Indonesian workers in Taiwan.* Retrieved from http://simpati.kdei-taipei.org/v2/index.php/peta_p (Original work published in Bahasa Indonesia)

Efendi, F., Chen, C. M., Nursalam, N., Indarwati, R., & Ulfiana, E. (2016). Lived experience of Indonesian nurses in Japan: A phenomenological study. *Japan Journal of Nursing Science, 13*(2), 284–293. https://doi.org/10.1111/jjns.12108

Efendi, F., Mackey, T. K., Huang, M. C., & Chen, C. M. (2017). IJEPA: Gray area for health policy and international nurse migration. *Nursing Ethics, 24*(3), 313–328. https://doi.org/10.1177/0969733015602052

Efendi, F., Nursalam, Dang, L. T. N., & Arief, Y. S. (2015). *Nursing education in Indonesia: Today's and future trends.* Paper presented at the Shanghai International Nursing Conference, Shanghai, China. https://doi.org/10.13140/RG.2.1.3270.2562

Efendi, F., Nursalam, N., Kurniati, A., & Gunawan, J. (2018). Nursing qualification and workforce for the Association of Southeast Asian Nations Economic Community. *Nursing Forum, 52*(2), 197–203. https://doi.org/10.1111/nuf.12243

Kingma, M. (2007). Nurses on the move: A global overview. *Health Services Research, 42*(3p2), 1281–1298. https://doi.org/10.1111/j.1475-6773.2007.00711.x

Kung, L. (2002). Migrant workers in Taipei: Biased central state policy and alternative administration strategy of local state. *Taiwan: A Radical Quarterly in Social Studies, 48,* 235–286.

Kurniati, A., Chen, C. M., Efendi, F., & Ogawa, R. (2017). A deskilling and challenging journey: The lived experience of Indonesian nurse returnees. *International Nursing Review, 64*(4), 494–501. https://doi.org/10.1111/inr.12352

Law on Health Workers (Law No. 36 of 2014), Government of the Republic Indonesia/36 (October 17, 2014).

Lincoln, Y. S., & Guba, E. G. (1985). *Naturalistic inquiry* (1st ed.). Newbury Park, CA: Sage Publications.

Ministry of Labor, Taiwan, ROC. (April, 2017). *Foreign workers in productive industries and social welfare by industry and nationality.* Retrieved from http://statdb.mol.gov.tw/html/mon/212040.htm

National Board for the Placement and Protection of Indonesian Overseas Workers. (2014). *Data on placement and protection of Indonesian workers in 2015.* Retrieved from http://goo.gl/8u9xSH (Original work published in Bahasa Indonesia)

National Board for the Placement and Protection of Indonesian Overseas Workers. (2019). *Data collection placement and protection of Indonesian overseas worker.* Retrieved from https://www.unescap.org/sites/default/files/3%20Session%207%20Country%20presentation%20Indonesia.pdf (Original work published in Bahasa Indonesia)

Thorsteinsson, L. S. (2002). The quality of nursing care as perceived by individuals with chronic illnesses: The magical touch of nursing. *Journal of Clinical Nursing, 11*(1), 32–40. Retrieved from http://www.ncbi.nlm.nih.gov/pubmed/11845753

van Manen, M. (1997). From meaning to method. *Qualitative Health Research, 7*(3), 345–369. https://doi.org/10.1177/104973239700700303

World Health Organization. (2010). *WHO global code of practice on the international recruitment of health personnel.* Retrieved from http://www.who.int/hrh/migration/code/WHO_global_code_of_practice_EN.pdf

World Health Organization. (2011). *Health workforce: User's guide to the WHO global code of practice on the international recruitment of health personnel.* Retrieved from http://www.who.int/hrh/resources/guide/en/index.html

12

Effects of an Education Intervention on Nursing Students' Knowledge and Attitudes Regarding Skin Self-Examination and Skin Cancer Risks

Özüm ERKİN[1] • Özcan AYGÜN[2]*

ABSTRACT

Background: The incidence of skin cancers is increasing in Turkey as well as worldwide. Nurses have a potentially influential role to play in educating the public about skin cancer prevention.

Purpose: The purpose of this study was to teach nursing students the risks of skin cancer and the steps involved in conducting related skin self-examinations to encourage positive attitudes toward skin cancer protection and early detection.

Methods: This research used a quasi-experimental, single-group, pretest–posttest design. The study population was composed of all the nursing students who were currently enrolled in a university in Muğla, a city in southern Turkey ($n = 900$). The study analysis included the 332 nursing students who had completed both the pretest and posttest assessments. An intervention to raise awareness about skin cancer risks and skin self-examination was carried out using educational materials that included posters/pictures, brochures, a PowerPoint slideshow, and a video. The posttest assessment was done 6 weeks after the pretest.

Results: The participants were 18–23 years old, and 67.5% were female. Furthermore, 3.6% had undergone a routine (external) screening for skin cancer, and 14.5% believed that they were at risk for skin cancer. The mean score for knowledge of skin cancer risks for those participants who had completed the program was 5.75 ± 1.20 in the pretest and 6.84 ± 1.17 in the posttest (minimum: 0, maximum: 8). The mean posttest score was higher than the pretest score in this group, $F(1, 329) = 6.49$, $p = .011$, and a significant difference was found between the mean pretest and posttest score for knowledge of the ABCDE rule ($p < .05$).

Conclusions: Educating nursing students about skin self-examination increased their level of knowledge about both skin cancer risks and the ABCDE rule. We believe that this and similar educational programs are an effective way to increase the knowledge and awareness of nurses regarding skin cancer and to improve their attitudes toward performing skin self-examination.

KEY WORDS:
early detection, education, nurse, skin self-examination, student.

Introduction

The incidence of skin cancer in predominantly fair-skinned populations has risen steadily over the last 50 years. Recent reports indicate that this increase has leveled off in North America, Australia, New Zealand, and various European countries (Erdmann et al., 2013). In 2014, skin cancers were the third most common cancer in Turkey, with an incidence of 29.2 per 100,000 in men and 19.1 per 100,000 in women (Gültekin & Boztaş, 2014).

Certain types of skin cancer have been associated with skin, hair, and eye color; familial history; the presence of numerous moles; sensitivity to sunlight; and long-term exposure to ultraviolet radiation (Etzkorn et al., 2013). The best way to diagnose skin cancer early is to recognize new skin growths or changes in the skin, especially those that look different from existing moles. Although most nonmelanoma skin cancers develop on sun-exposed parts of the body, many melanomas appear on parts of the body that are normally covered by clothing. Therefore, skin should be examined at regular intervals, and any changes should be evaluated by a physician (Nikolaou & Stratigos, 2014). Because of the increased incidence of melanoma worldwide, adherence to preventive measures such as skin self-examination (SSE) must be improved (Secker, Bergman, & Kukutsch, 2016). Anyone aged 20 years or older should be able to perform SSE easily at home (Arnold & DeJong, 2005). The steps involved in SSE include examination of the front upper body, especially the face and neck, as well as the arms, shoulders, chest, and stomach; the front lower body (the groin/genital region, legs, and feet); and the back of the body, including the back of the neck, upper back, lower back, and legs (Arnold & DeJong, 2005). One study suggested that SSE could reduce melanoma mortality by 63% (Berwick, Oliveria, Luo, Headley, & Bolognia, 2000). Any moles or pigmented spots detected in SSE should be evaluated according to the ABCDE rule,

[1]*PhD, RN, Associate Professor, Faculty of Health Sciences, Department of Nursing, İzmir Democracy University, Turkey;* [2]*PhD, RN, Assistant Professor, Fethiye Faculty of Health Sciences, Department of Nursing, Mugla Sitki Kocman University, Turkey.*

which includes the following criteria: Asymmetry, Border, Color, Diameter, and Evolving (American Society for Dermatologic Surgery, 2010).

Community educational campaigns aimed at reducing melanoma mortality rates in North America, Australia, and Europe have had positive impacts on SSE performance (Arnold & DeJong, 2005). Moreover, several studies have revealed that campaigns to raise awareness and encourage SSE facilitate earlier skin cancer detection, which may improve prognosis (Etzkorn et al., 2013; Gordon, 2014; Yagerman & Marghoob, 2013). The goal of primary prevention is to educate the public and healthcare providers to increase skin cancer awareness and reduce risky behaviors (Göl & Erkin, 2018). Secondary prevention promotes early diagnosis using strategies such as SSE and skin screening to reduce mortality and morbidity (Erkin, Ardahan, Temel, & Temel, 2018; Roman, Lugo-Somolinos, & Thomas, 2013).

The role of health professionals in prevention has been highlighted in various studies and guidelines. Educational campaigns conducted by nurses in the community have successfully raised awareness of the risks and early warning signs of skin cancer and of how to perform SSE (Oliveria et al., 2004). Nurses are accepted as more influential sources of information in the community than many other healthcare professionals. Thus, nurses should play a key role in community-based interventions that promote both primary and secondary skin cancer prevention. To this end, nurses should be provided specific education and training on skin cancer prevention to bring this crucial information to the public (Mahon & Yackzan, 2011). In one study, a nurse-led education program on SSE was shown to increase the rate of SSE performance (Berwick et al., 2000). However, nurses have expressed a belief that they do not have sufficient training to enable them to integrate skin cancer detection activities into their practice and stated that they desire more training on this topic (Christos, Oliveria, Mâsse, McCormick, & Halpern, 2004).

Nurses contribute to individual, family, and societal health by serving as role models (Özçam et al., 2014; Siegel, 2010). Thus, it is important that nursing students are equipped with adequate knowledge of SSE so that they are prepared to fulfill their roles as public educators and advisers (Erkin et al., 2018).

The purpose of this study was to teach nursing students the risks of skin cancer and the steps involved in SSE to encourage positive attitudes toward skin cancer protection and early detection. In line with this aim, the subaims of this study were to (a) determine the participants' knowledge and attitudes regarding skin cancer risks and the steps involved in SSE, (b) evaluate their changes in knowledge regarding the risks of skin cancer after training, and (c) determine what percentage of the participants were able to perform SSE effectively and accurately.

Methods

Design and Sample

The study used a quasi-experimental, single-group, pretest/posttest design and was carried out between March and April 2016 in the Faculty of Health Sciences at Mugla Sitki Kocman University in southern Turkey. The study population was composed of all the nursing students at this school (n = 900). To determine the sample size required for covariance analysis, selecting the effect size as 0.25 and the sampling error as 0.05 within a 95% confidence interval, it was calculated that 323 persons would be required to obtain a power of 95%. The G*power 3.1 software program was used to perform all of the related calculations (Faul, Erdfelder, Buchner, & Lang, 2009). The data of all the 332 students who attended the training program, participated in both the pretest and posttest evaluations, and volunteered to participate were used in the analysis (Figure 1).

Measures

Data were collected using a questionnaire developed by the researchers based on previous studies (Balyacı, Koştu, & Temel, 2012; Erkin et al., 2018; Koştu, Erkin, & Bayık Temel, 2014). The questionnaire consisted of two sections: The first section (descriptive characteristics) included 13 questions about age, gender, natural hair color, eye color, complexion, number of freckles and moles, skin reaction to ultraviolet radiation, use of tanning beds/solariums, family history of skin cancer, self-perceived skin cancer risk, and whether or not the participant was currently seeing a dermatologist for skin cancer screening. The second section contained another 17 items assessing knowledge of skin cancer risk (eight questions) and knowledge and practice of SSE (nine questions). Knowledge of skin cancer risk was assessed based on their ability to correctly identify the following as risk factors: light skin; light-colored eyes; a blood relative diagnosed with skin cancer; large, brown moles on the body; birthmarks; history of blistering sunburn (even once); using a tanning bed/solarium; and lifetime sun exposure experience. Correct answers received 1 point, and wrong answers received no points, resulting in a possible total score of 0–8, with higher scores indicating better knowledge of skin cancer risks (Balyacı et al., 2012). Knowledge of the SSE ABCDE rule was evaluated using the following questions and expected (correct) answers: "Who should perform a skin self-exam?" ("everyone"), "How frequently should a skin self-exam be performed?" ("once a month"), "Should a full-length mirror be used in skin self-exams?" ("yes, always"), "Should a hand mirror be used in SSE?" ("yes, always"), and "Which parts of the body should be examined in a skin self-exam?" ("every part of the body"). Furthermore, each participant was asked if they had performed SSE and to explain why not if they answered no. These questions were not scored. Content validity (.81) and the Kuder–Richardson value (.85) were calculated for the questionnaire.

Intervention

The intervention that was implemented in this study was designed to raise awareness of skin cancer risks and SSE using educational materials including posters and pictures, brochures, a PowerPoint slideshow, and a video (Figure 1).

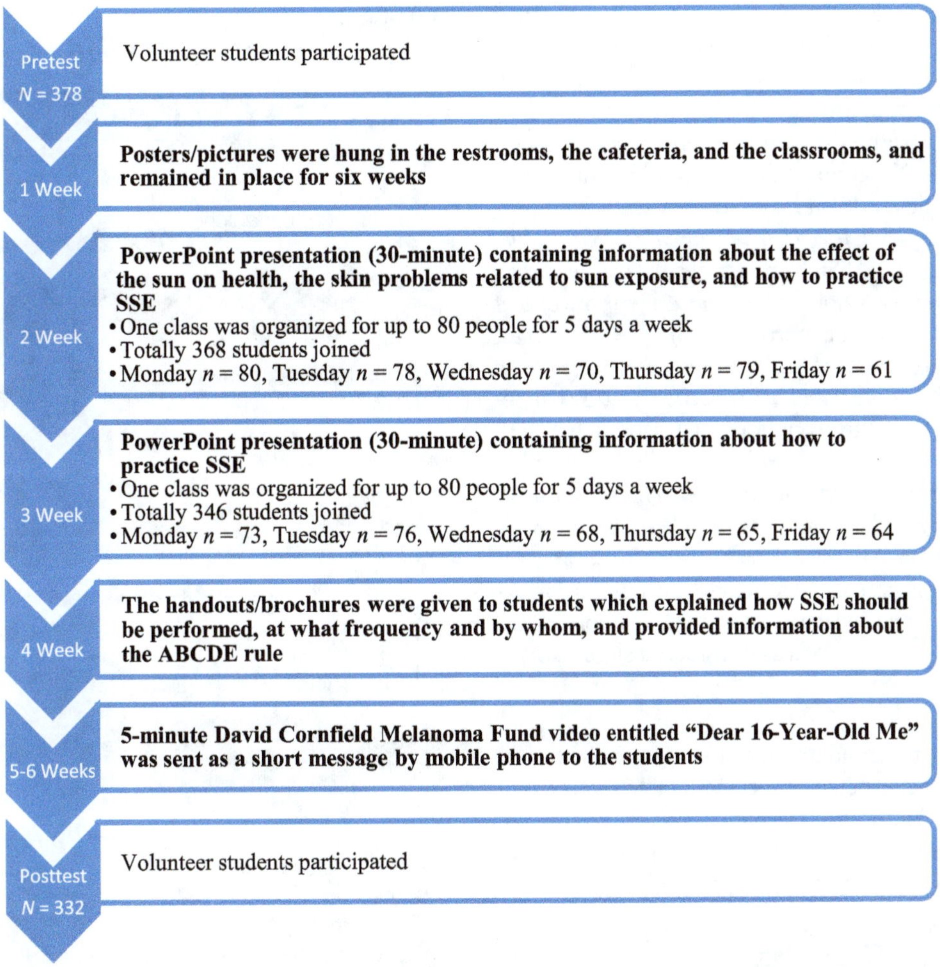

Figure 1. Data collection and intervention flow of the study. SSE = skin self-examination; ABCDE = asymmetry, border, color, diameter, and evolving.

The posters and pictures contained information about the steps required to perform SSE, skin cancer risks, and early detection. The materials were created based on a guide developed by Friedman, Rigel, and Kopf (1985). The eight-step SSE guide from the Skin Cancer Foundation and pictures illustrating the steps were translated into Turkish and adapted for Turkish cultural settings (Koştu et al., 2014). The guide was pilot tested on 30 students, and its content validity was found to be .98 based on the opinions of nine experts (Koştu et al., 2014) who had backgrounds in medical nursing, public health nursing, fundamentals of nursing, and dermatology (Balyacı et al., 2012).

The handouts used in the program were prepared in line with the literature and distributed to all of the students. This brochure explained how, at what frequency, and by whom SSE should be performed and provided information about the ABCDE rule. The students were then shown an hour-long PowerPoint presentation (in two, 30-minute parts) containing information about the effects of the sun on health, skin problems related to sun exposure, and how to practice SSE. Finally, the 5-minute David Cornfield Melanoma Fund video entitled *Dear 16-Year-Old Me* with Turkish subtitles was shown to all of the participants and sent with a short message to their mobile phones. In addition, related educational materials were displayed in restrooms, the cafeteria, and classrooms for 6 weeks. These materials were removed before administering the posttest assessment (Figure 1).

Data Collection

Data collection was carried out in two stages: pretest and posttest. The students were asked about their descriptive characteristics, self-perceived risk of skin cancer, and knowledge about skin cancer risk and SSE before and after the education intervention. The posttest was conducted 6 weeks after the pretest. Codes assigned to each student at the beginning of the study were used to pair the pretest and posttest questionnaires (Figure 1).

Data Analysis

The data were analyzed using the SPSS 20.0 (IBM, Armonk, NY, USA) program and descriptive statistics, Wilcoxon signed rank test, and covariance analysis. Skewness and kurtosis values showed that the data had a normal distribution, and parametric tests were utilized in their analysis. Asymmetry and kurtosis values between −2 and +2 are considered acceptable to prove normal univariate distribution (Gravetter

& Wallnau, 2014). A McNemar test was used in pretest comparison of binary variables such as yes–no and true–false. Wilcoxon signed rank test was used to examine the change in knowledge and attitudes in the posttest according to the pretest. The variables in Table 4 were reclassified and then subjected to the Wilcoxon signed rank test. These classifications are as follows: "Who should perform SSE? "(1 = *women*, 2 = *men*, 3 = *young people*, 4 = *children*, 5 = *old people*, 6 = *all*), "How often should SSE be performed?" (1 = *every day*, 2 = *once a week*, 3 = *every 6 months 1*, 4 = *once a year*, 5 = *once a month*), "Using a wall and hand mirror" (1 = *no*, 2 = *sometimes*, 3 = *yes, always*), "Body parts in SSE?" (1 = *only the mole regions of the body*, 2 = *only sun-exposed areas of the body*, 3 = *all regions of the body*), and "Reasons for not performing SSE?" (1 = *I do not know*, 2 = *I'm busy and forget*, 3 = *I'm afraid of finding something*, 4 = *I do not believe it is effective*, 5 = *I do*).

In covariance analysis, the pretest was considered as the covariate and seeing the educational material, participating in the program in full (all 6 weeks) or in part, and discussing the educational material with others were considered the main factors. The confidence interval was 95%, and $p < .05$ was considered significant.

Ethics

Written permission for conducting the study was obtained from the scientific ethics committee (Mugla Sitki Kocman University Ethics Committee Decision No. 159) and the Nursing Department. The participants were informed about the study, and their consent was obtained.

Results

The participants were 18–23 years old; 67.5% were female (n = 224), and 32.5% were male (n = 108). In terms of descriptive characteristics, 15.7% had sandy red/blond hair; 10.2% had blue, gray, or light-colored eyes; 36.7% had fair skin; and 42.2% had 1–10 moles. Responses regarding skin cancer family history, screening, and perceived risk indicated that 0.6% of the participants had a blood relative who had been diagnosed with skin cancer, 3.6% of the participants had received physical checkups for skin cancer screening, and 14.5% of the participants believed that they were at risk for skin cancer. Furthermore, 25.0%, 66.7%, and 8.3% of the participants were at low, medium, and high risk, respectively. The descriptive characteristics of the participants are presented in Table 1. The skewness and kurtosis values, which indicate the normal distribution suitability of the data, were between ± 2 and symmetry.

A comparison of the numbers of respondents who responded correctly to the pretest and posttest for their skin cancer risk information and for their protection against skin cancer is presented in Table 2. When skin cancer risk information was examined, the number of participants who gave a correct response of light skin was 278 in the pretest and 298 in the posttest (χ^2 = 5.30, p = .021), the number of correct responders to light eye color was 116 in the pretest and 140 in the posttest (χ^2 = 5.08, p = .024), the number of those who correctly responded to the number of freckles/moles on their body was 304 in the pretest and 326 in the posttest (χ^2 = 14.70, p < .001), the number of participants who gave a correct response for birthmarks was 114 in the pretest and

TABLE 1.
Characteristics of Participants (N = 332)

Characteristic	*n*	%
Natural hair color		
Sandy red, blond	52	15.7
Chestnut or dark blond	68	20.5
Brown	118	35.5
Black	94	28.3
Eye color		
Light	10	3.0
Blue, gray, or green	24	7.2
Dark	130	39.2
Brown	116	34.9
Black	52	15.7
Skin color		
Reddish	122	36.7
Pale	56	16.9
Beige or olive	60	18.1
Brown	30	9.0
Dark brown	64	19.3
Freckles, moles		
≥ 31	13	3.9
11–30	139	41.9
1–10	140	42.2
None	40	12.0
Skin is sensitive		
Very sensitive, easily reacts	68	20.5
Sensitive	36	10.8
Sometimes	118	35.5
Reacts normal	62	18.7
Very resistive, hardly reacts	48	14.5
Skin turns brown		
Never	24	7.2
Rarely	76	22.9
Sometimes	122	36.8
Frequently	82	24.7
Always	28	8.4
A blood relative diagnosed with skin cancer		
Yes	2	0.6
No	330	99.4
Self-perceived skin cancer risk		
Yes	48	14.5
No	284	85.5
Level of risk (*n* = 48)[a]		
Low	12	25.0
Medium	32	66.7
High	4	8.3
Skin cancer screening: seeing a dermatologist		
Yes	12	3.6
No	320	96.4

[a]Participants believed they were at risk for skin cancer.

TABLE 2.

Changes in Participant Responses Regarding Skin Cancer Risks, Knowledge, and Practices of Skin Self-Examination (SSE) Between Pretest and Posttest

	Pretest (n = 332)		Posttest (n = 332)			
Skin Cancer Risk	n	%	n	%	χ^2	p
Light skin					5.30	.021
True	278	83.7	298	89.8		
False	54	16.3	34	10.2		
Light eye color					5.08	.024
True	116	34.9	140	42.2		
False	216	65.1	192	57.8		
Family history of skin cancer					0.04	.845
True	312	94.0	314	94.6		
False	20	6.0	18	5.4		
Many freckles/moles					14.70	< .001
True	304	91.6	326	98.2		
False	28	8.4	6	1.8		
Birthmarks					40.17	< .001
True	114	34.3	190	57.2		
False	218	65.7	142	42.8		
Blistering sunburns					35.80	< .001
True	208	62.7	274	82.5		
False	124	37.3	58	17.5		
Tanning bed/solariums					0.12	.286
True	316	95.2	322	97.0		
False	16	4.8	10	3.0		
Sun exposure/ultraviolet radiation					4.32	.038
True	312	94.0	324	97.6		
False	20	6.0	8	2.4		
Knowledge of ABCDE criteria					65.87	< .001
True	12	3.6	90	27.1		
False	320	96.4	242	72.9		
Performing SSE					22.08	< .001
Yes	58	17.5	96	28.9		
No	274	82.5	236	71.1		

190 in the posttest (χ^2 = 40.17, p < .001), the number who gave a correct response for blistering sunburn experience was 208 in the pretest and 274 in the posttest (χ^2 = 35.80, p < .001), and the number who gave a correct response to the sun exposure/ultraviolet radiation question was 312 in the pretest and 324 in the posttest (χ^2 = 4.32, p = .038), which all represented statistically significant changes. However, no statistically significant pretest–posttest change was noted for either the number of respondents providing a correct family history of skin cancer (312 vs. 314; χ^2 = 0.04, p = .845) or the number of correct responses to tanning bed/solariums (316 vs. 322; χ^2 = 0.12, p = .286). When the participants were assessed for protection from skin cancer, the number of respondents who correctly answered the knowledge of ABCDE question was only 12 in the pretest and 90 in the posttest (χ^2 = 65.87, p < .001). Furthermore, the number of participants performing SSE significantly increased from 58 in the pretest to 96 in the posttest (χ^2 = 22.08, p < .001; Table 2).

The mean score for recognition of skin cancer risks among the participants with complete program participation was 5.75 ± 1.20 in the pretest and 6.84 ± 1.17 in the posttest (minimum: 0, maximum: 8). In the covariance analysis, the mean pretest scores were used as a covariate and seeing the educational materials, attending the entire program, and discussing the program with friends were accepted as the main factors affecting scores for recognition of skin cancer risks. Posttest scores increased significantly compared with pretest with complete program participation, F(1, 329) = 6.49, p = .011 (Table 3). However, seeing the educational materials or discussing them with friends was not associated with significant differences in mean scores for recognition of skin cancer risks, F(1, 329) = 3.61, p = .058, and F(1, 329) = 2.48, p = .116, respectively (Table 3).

Table 4 shows the distribution of pretest and posttest responses related to knowledge and practices of SSE. The differences in pretest and posttest scores of those participants who reported knowing who should perform SSE (Negative

TABLE 3.

Pretest–Posttest Comparison of Mean Scores on Knowledge of Skin Cancer Risks (N = 332)

Main Effect	*n*	Pretest *M*	Pretest *SD*	Posttest *M*	Posttest *SD*	*df*	Mean Square	*F*	*p*
Seeing the educational materials	142	5.81	1.21	6.72	1.19	1	5.66	3.61	.058
Not seeing the aleducation materials	190	5.97	1.21	6.41	1.40				
Complete program participation	136	5.75	1.20	6.84	1.17	1	10.09	6.49	.001*
Partial program participation	196	6.09	1.21	6.40	1.36				
Discussing about the education	46	5.80	1.42	6.50	1.30	1	3.90	2.48	.116
Not discussing about the education	286	6.50	1.15	6.60	1.30				

Note. The sample size with complete data at baseline and the posttest scores were included in analyses. *F* = analysis of covariance.
$^*p < .05$.

Ranks = 22.79, $p = .432$) and the body parts involved in SSE (Negative Ranks = 17.50, $p = .066$) were not significant. However, significant differences were found between the pretest and posttest scores of participants who reported knowing how often SSE should be performed (Positive Ranks = 101.81, $p < .001$) and knowing to use a wall mirror (Positive Ranks = 48.93, $p < .001$) and a hand mirror (Positive Ranks = 63.52, $p < .001$) in SSE as well as those who reported a reason for not performing SSE (Positive Ranks = 67.90, $p = .019$; Table 4).

Discussion

In this study, providing SSE education resulted in positive changes in the participants in terms of knowledge of the risks of skin cancer. There were also significant changes between

TABLE 4.

Pretest–Posttest Change in Knowledge and Practices of Skin Self-Examination (SSE; N = 332)

Variable/Ranks	*n*	Pretest–Posttest Median	Mean Rank	Sum of Ranks	*Z*	*p*
Who should perform SSE?		5.75–5.81			−0.78	.432
Negative Ranks	14		22.79	319.00		
Positive Ranks	24		17.58	422.00		
Ties	294					
How often should SSE be performed?		3.71–4.13			−4.61	< .001
Negative Ranks	68		76.62	5,210.00		
Positive Ranks	116		101.81	11,810.00		
Ties	148					
Using a wall mirror		2.56–2.77			−5.58	< .001
Negative Ranks	20		42.20	844.00		
Positive Ranks	74		48.93	3,621.00		
Ties	238					
Using a hand mirror		2.42–2.59			−4.19	< .001
Negative Ranks	38		63.45	2,411.00		
Positive Ranks	88		63.52	5,590.00		
Ties	206					
Body parts in SSE		2.77–2.92			−1.84	.066
Negative Ranks	16		17.50	280.00		
Positive Ranks	12		10.50	126.00		
Ties	304					
Reasons for not performing SSE		1.84–2.54			−7.24	< .001
Negative Ranks	20		65.20	1,304.00		
Positive Ranks	114		67.90	7,741.00		
Ties	198					

pretest and posttest in level of knowledge of the ABCDE rule, performance of SSE, accurate knowledge of body parts to be examined in SSE, and awareness of the necessity to use both a full-length mirror and a hand mirror during SSE. These findings indicate that the students learned about skin cancer risk and prevention through the intervention.

At present, nurses play an increasingly significant role in the detection of early-stage skin cancer and in advocating primary and secondary prevention (Lucas, Chung, Marchetti, & Marghoob, 2016; Siegel, 2010). Nurses should be aware of the risk factors and early signs of skin cancer to provide the best patient care (Erkin et al., 2018; Koştu et al., 2014; Lucas et al., 2016; Özçam et al., 2014). More than half of the participants in this study reported that they did not consider themselves at risk for skin cancer. Close to half of the participants said that they had fewer than 10 moles on their bodies. Perceived risk of future skin cancer and awareness of early symptoms of skin cancer have been associated in the literature with willingness to perform SSE (Janda et al., 2004). In this study, more than half of the participants displayed low-to-moderate perceived skin cancer risk, suggesting that they were aware of skin types and skin cancer risks. Furthermore, nurses must be aware of the necessity of taking a detailed patient history to identify those patients who are at a higher risk of developing skin cancer (Gordon, 2014).

The pretest assessment of our study showed that using tanning beds/solariums was the most known skin cancer risk for a large majority of the students, whereas birthmarks were the least known risk. In the posttest assessment, however, the students showed significantly more knowledge of skin cancer risks and were able to recognize more of the risks. A previous study reported a significant and positive relationship between the presence of four or more risk factors and SSE (Arnold & DeJong, 2005). Similarly, another study stated that a personal risk for skin cancer is the strongest determinant of SSE performance (Saitta, Cohen, Rigel, Grekin, & Brancaccio, 2011). In this study, the intervention caused a significant increase in the mean score for knowledge of skin cancer risks ($p = .011$). Education interventions such as these may be used as active learning tools to increase awareness of skin cancer risks. Specifically, the participants who participated in the entire educational program showed significantly increased scores for knowledge of skin cancer risks ($p < .05$). The intervention also had a significant and positive effect on the SSE performance of participants in the posttest.

Atlases, photographs, and pictures are tools that have gained acceptance in promoting SSE in the general population (Loescher, Janda, Soyer, Shea, & Curiel-Lewandrowski, 2013). Previous studies have drawn attention to the relationship between SSE performance and increased knowledge of skin cancer and its risks (Gordon, 2014; Roebuck, Moran, MacDonald, Shumer, & McCune, 2015; Roman et al., 2013). Similarly, this study shows that an intervention may effectively promote knowledge and awareness of the risks of skin cancer as well as the rate of SSE performance.

It was striking that, although the participants in this study were nursing students, very few had received education about SSE and skin cancer risks before the intervention. On the basis of the change in pretest–posttest scores, the intervention changed participants positively toward SSE. Increased recognition of skin cancer risks in the posttest may be associated with reading the provided SSE educational materials. This underscores the impact of education on the early detection of skin cancer.

All adults should perform SSE monthly starting at the age of 20 years (American Society for Dermatologic Surgery, 2010). Efforts to encourage screening are hindered by the lack of standardized guidelines regarding who should be screened and when screenings should be performed (Oliveria, Heneghan, Cushman, Ughetta, & Halpern, 2011). Most of the participants in this study gave the correct answer in the posttest that everyone should perform SSE, and there was a positive change between pretest and posttest in the number of participants who knew that SSE should be performed monthly. Another study on SSE reported that 77.1% of high-risk individuals had performed SSE at least once during the previous 1-year period and that 14.5% of these individuals did so regularly every month (Secker et al., 2016). In this study, the intervention was found to be effective in teaching the participants how, when, and what to look for during SSE.

There is currently no screening test for detecting skin cancer other than the direct examination of an individual's skin by a trained professional (Loescher et al., 2013). Both healthcare professionals and laymen have utilized the ABCDE rule widely during the past 30 years (Lucas et al., 2016). This study increased the awareness among participants of the ABCDE rule between pretest and posttest. A previous Turkish study similarly reported that education tools such as posters and photographs helped reduce the proportion of nursing students who did not know the ABCDE rule from 94.5% to 20.9% (Erkin et al., 2018). Approximately 75% of melanomas are either self-detected by patients or detected by a spouse orfriend (Berwick et al., 2000; Körner, Coroiu, Martins, & Wang, 2013). Therefore, it is important that individuals know what to look for and what warning signs and skin changes occur so that patients may detect skin cancers themselves. Before healthcare professionals teach the community about the ABCDE criteria for skin cancer protection, they must be thoroughly knowledgeable about these criteria themselves.

In this study, awareness that a full-length mirror should be used when performing SSE increased between pretest and posttest. Previous studies have found associations between using a mirror, having a partner, and personal risk perceptions and the frequency of performing SSE (Oliveria et al., 2011; Secker et al., 2016). A mirror is important in SSE to check the entire body, especially high-risk areas. It has been reported that the back is the least examined area, despite being the most common location of melanomas (Arnold & DeJong, 2005). Most of the participants in this study knew that the entire body must be examined during an SSE. A study conducted in the United States found that only 35.3% of students who reported performing SSE checked their entire body (Arnold & DeJong, 2005). The comparatively higher proportion of participants in this study who knew that all areas of the body must be checked may be related to the fact that the participants were nursing students.

In this study, a relatively high proportion of participants already performed SSE. Moreover, this proportion increased further after the intervention. A previous study reported that 33.2% of university students performed SSE (Arnold & DeJong, 2005). A French study determined that approximately 60% of university students performed SSE at least once a year (Isvy, Beauchet, Saiag, & Mahé, 2013). Another study stated that 22% of Hispanic people performed SSE (Roman et al., 2013). A different Turkish study revealed that, of a group of Turkish university students who knew about SSE (n = 40), only 18 students actually practiced it (Uğrlu et al., 2016). The prevalence of SSE among general and high-risk populations is influenced by healthcare-provider-related factors such as physician and nurse recommendations (Loescher et al., 2013). Of particular note, previous studies have shown the positive effects of nursing interventions on SSE performance (Erkin et al., 2018; Oliveria et al., 2004). In a different study of Turkish nursing students, 6.0% performed SSE in the pretest and 42.3% did so in the posttest (Erkin et al., 2018). Another study reported an increase in the rate of SSE performance from 10% to 61% after an intervention (Oliveria et al., 2004). Consistent with the literature, this study further showed the positive effects of an intervention on SSE performance.

The number of participants who cited "not knowing what to look for" as their reason for not performing SSE declined between pretest and posttest. In another study, of the 78% of the participants who stated that they did not perform SSE, 49% stated that it was because they were not told to do so and 29% stated that it was because they did not know what to look for (Roman et al., 2013). Another study of young adults revealed that more than half of the participants did not know what to look for or never thought about performing SSE (Arnold & DeJong, 2005). In this study, the participants being healthcare providers may have made it easier for the intervention to raise awareness about skin cancer and SSE. In addition, encouraging active learning through posters and brochures may have had a positive effect on SSE performance. When health professionals know about self-examinations and practice it themselves, they will be better equipped to advocate for and support positive health-promoting behaviors.

Nurses are not currently considered successful agents in skin cancer prevention (Roebuck et al., 2015). Therefore, nurses should become more familiar with the warning signs and risk factors of skin cancer as well as with SSE to enable them to design and implement public education campaigns (Lucas et al., 2016). This study shows that awareness of skin cancer and SSE skills may be raised easily through nursing education.

Limitations

This study had several limitations. One was that the research was conducted at only one institution, which precludes the generalization of the findings. Furthermore, the design and sample selection also represent study limitations. Matching numbers of participants were necessary to compare pretest and posttest results. Therefore, data obtained from those participants who were unable to take either the pretest or the posttest were not included in the analysis. A further limitation is that the results of this study were based on individual self-reporting. Nevertheless, the authors believe that the data collection tool that was used was useful in evaluating SSE education in the context of skin cancer detection. Finally, another limitation was that the SSE education intervention was restricted to the use of posters and images.

Conclusions

This study showed that SSE education for the early detection of skin cancer had a positive influence on the knowledge and practices of SSE in the sample of nursing students. Moreover, the education intervention increased knowledge or awareness of the ABCDE rule and of skin cancer risks. Nurses should educate the community regarding skin cancer prevention and early detection and act as role models. If nurses are able to further raise awareness about skin cancer and SSE, they will make a substantial additional contribution to public health. One strategy that may be used to improve skin cancer and SSE counseling among nurses is to use the screening guidelines for skin cancer SSE in primary care settings. Furthermore, nurses should play a more active role in the primary care setting for screening patients and detecting skin cancer at early stages. In addition, nurses should increase their skin-cancer-related knowledge and skills and should specialize in continuing education and dermatology nursing.

Acknowledgments

Portions of this article were presented in an oral presentation given at the II. International Graduate Education Congress in Manisa, Turkey, on May 12–14, 2017. The authors acknowledge the cooperation of the university management, teaching staff, and students who participated in this study.

References

American Society for Dermatologic Surgery. (2010). *Skin cancer self-exam kit.* Retrieved from https://www.asds.net/Skin_Cancer_Self_Exam_Kit/

Arnold, M. R., & DeJong, W. (2005). Skin self-examination practices in a convenience sample of US university students. *Preventive Medicine, 40*(3), 268–273. https://doi.org/10.1016/j.ypmed.2004.05.031

Balyacı, O. E., Koştu, N., & Temel, A. B. (2012). Training program to raise consciousness among adolescents for protection against skin cancer through performance of skin self examination. *Asian Pacific Journal of Cancer Prevention, 13*(10), 5011–5017. https://doi.org/10.7314/APJCP.2012.13.10.5011

Berwick, M., Oliveria, S., Luo, S. T., Headley, A., & Bolognia, J. L. (2000). A pilot study using nurse education as an intervention to increase skin self-examination for melanoma. *Journal of Cancer Education, 15*(1), 38–40.

Christos, P. J., Oliveria, S. A., Mâsse, L. C., McCormick, L. K., & Halpern, A. C. (2004). Skin cancer prevention and detection by nurses: Attitudes, perceptions, and barriers. *Journal of Cancer Education, 19*(1), 50–57.

Erdmann, F., Lortet Tieulent, J., Schüz, J., Zeeb, H., Greinert, R., Breitbart, E. W., & Bray, F. (2013). International trends in the incidence of malignant melanoma 1953–2008—Are recent generations at higher or lower risk? *International Journal of Cancer, 132*(2), 385–400. https://doi.org/10.7314/APJCP.2012.13.10.5011

Erkin, Ö., Ardahan, M., Temel, A. B., & Temel, A. B. (2018). Effects of creating awareness through photographs and posters on skin self-examination in nursing students. *Journal of Cancer Education, 33*(1), 52–58. https://doi.org/10.1007/s13187-016-1037-y

Etzkorn, J. R., Parikh, R. P., Marzban, S. S., Law, K., Davis, A. H., Rawal, B., ... Lien, M. H. (2013). Identifying risk factors using a skin cancer screening program. *Cancer Control, 20*(4), 248–254.

Faul, F., Erdfelder, E., Buchner, A., & Lang, A. G. (2009). Statistical power analyses using G* Power 3.1: Tests for correlation and regression analyses. *Behavior Research Methods, 41*(4), 1149–1160. https://doi.org/10.3758/BRM.41.4.1149

Friedman, R. J., Rigel, D. S., & Kopf, A. W. (1985). Early detection of malignant-melanoma: The role of physician examination and self-examination of the skin. *CA: A Cancer Journal for Clinicians, 35*(3), 130–151. https://doi.org/10.3322/canjclin.35.3.130

Göl, İ., & Erkin, Ö. (2018). Knowledge and practices of primary care providers on skin cancer and skin self-examination. *Revista da Escola de Enfermagem da USP, 52*, e03359. http://dx.doi.org/10.1590/s1980-220x2017039703359

Gordon, R. (2014). Skin cancer: Increasing awareness and screening in primary care. *The Nurse Practitioner, 39*(5), 48–54. https://doi.org/10.1097/01.NPR.0000446024.75947.16

Gravetter, F., & Wallnau, L. (2014). *Essentials of statistics for the behavioral sciences* (8th ed.). Belmont, CA: Wadsworth.

Gültekin, M., & Boztaş, G. (2014). *Cancer statistics of Turkey* (p. 43). Ankara, Turkey: Ministry of Health, Public Health Institution of Turkey. (Original work published in Turkish).

Isvy, A., Beauchet, A., Saiag, P., & Mahé, E. (2013). Medical students and sun prevention: Knowledge and behaviours in France. *Journal of the European Academy of Dermatology and Venereology, 27*(2), e247–e251. https://doi.org/10.1111/j.1468-3083.2012.04621.x

Janda, M., Youl, P. H., Lowe, J. B., Elwood, M., Ring, I. T., & Aitken, J. F. (2004). Attitudes and intentions in relation to skin checks for early signs of skin cancer. *Preventive Medicine, 39*(1), 11–18. https://doi.org/10.1016/j.ypmed.2004.02.019

Körner, A., Coroiu, A., Martins, C., & Wang, B. (2013). Predictors of skin self-examination before and after a melanoma diagnosis: The role of medical advice and patient's level of education. *International Archives of Medicine, 6*(1), 8. https://doi.org/10.1186/1755-7682-6-8

Koştu, N., Erkin, Ö., & Bayık Temel, A. (2014). Turkish validity study of skin self examination. *Dokuz Eylül Nursing Faculty E-Journal, 7*(1), 7–11. Retrieved from http://www.deuhyoedergi.org/index.php/DEUHYOED/article/view/38/273 (Original work published in Turkish)

Loescher, L. J., Janda, M., Soyer, H. P., Shea, K., & Curiel-Lewandrowski, C. (2013). Advances in skin cancer early detection and diagnosis. *Seminars in Oncology Nursing, 29*(3), 170–181. https://doi.org/10.1016/j.soncn.2013.06.003

Lucas, A. S., Chung, E., Marchetti, M. A., & Marghoob, A. A. (2016). A guide for dermatology nurses to assist in the early detection of skin cancer. *Journal of Nursing Education and Practice, 6*(10), 71–79. https://doi.org/10.5430/jnep.v6n10p71

Mahon, S. M., & Yackzan, S. G. (2011). Skin cancer. In C. H. Yarbro, D. Wujcik, & B. H. Gobel (Eds.), *Cancer nursing: Principles and practice* (7th ed., pp. 1650–1682). Sudbury, MA: Jones & Bartlett.

Nikolaou, V., & Stratigos, A. J. (2014). Emerging trends in the epidemiology of melanoma. *British Journal of Dermatology, 170*(1), 11–19. https://doi.org/10.1111/bjd.12492

Oliveria, S. A., Dusza, S. W., Phelan, D. L., Ostroff, J. S., Berwick, M., & Halpern, A. C. (2004). Patient adherence to skin self-examination. effect of nurse intervention with photographs. *American Journal of Preventive Medicine, 26*(2), 152–155. https://doi.org/10.1016/j.amepre.2003.10.006

Oliveria, S. A., Heneghan, M. K., Cushman, L. F., Ughetta, E. A., & Halpern, A. C. (2011). Skin cancer screening by dermatologists, family practitioners, and internists: Barriers and facilitating factors. *Archives of Dermatology, 147*(1), 39–44. https://doi.org/10.1001/archdermatol.2010.414

Özçam, H., Çimen, G., Uzunçakmak, C., Aydın, S., Özcan, T., & Boran, B. (2014). Evaluation of the knowledge, attitude, and behavior of female health workers about breast cancer, cervical cancer, and routine screening test. *Istanbul Medical Journal, 15*(3), 154–160. (Original work published in Turkish).

Roebuck, H., Moran, K., MacDonald, D. A., Shumer, S., & McCune, R. L. (2015). Assessing skin cancer prevention and detection educational needs: An andragogical approach. *The Journal for Nurse Practitioners, 11*(4), 409–416. https://doi.org/10.1016/j.nurpra.2015.01.036

Roman, C., Lugo-Somolinos, A., & Thomas, N. (2013). Skin cancer knowledge and skin self-examinations in the Hispanic population of North Carolina: The patient's perspective. *JAMA Dermatology, 149*(1), 103–104. https://doi.org/10.1001/2013.jamadermatol.263

Saitta, P., Cohen, D. E., Rigel, D., Grekin, S. K., & Brancaccio, R. (2011). The frequency of self-skin examination and full body skin examination in dermatologists. *The Journal of Clinical and Aesthetic Dermatology, 4*(6), 20–24.

Secker, L. J., Bergman, W., & Kukutsch, N. A. (2016). Total body photography as an aid to skin self-examination: A patient's perspective. *Acta Dermato-Venereologica, 96*(2), 186–190. https://doi.org/10.2340/00015555-2228

Siegel, V. (2010). The role of the nurse in skin cancer prevention, screening, and early detection. *Dermatology Nursing, 22*(6), 18–22.

Uğurlu, Z., Işık, S. A., Balanuye, B., Budak, E., Elbaş, N. Ö., & Kav, S. (2016). Awareness of skin cancer, prevention, and early detection among Turkish university students. *Asia-Pacific Journal of Oncology Nursing, 3*(1), 93–97. https://doi.org/10.4103/2347-5625.170969

Yagerman, S., & Marghoob, A. (2013). Melanoma patient self-detection: A review of efficacy of the skin self-examination and patient-directed educational efforts. *Expert Review of Anticancer Therapy, 13*(12), 1423–1431. https://doi.org/10.1586/14737140.2013.856272

13

The Professional Identity of Nursing Students and Their Intention to Leave the Nursing Profession During the Coronavirus Disease (COVID-19) Pandemic

Shengxiao NIE[1]* • Chao SUN[2] • Lei WANG[3] • Xia WANG[3]

ABSTRACT

Background: The COVID-19 pandemic has affected China and other countries since December 2019. The effects of this pandemic on nursing students in terms of their professional identity, intention to leave the nursing profession, and perception of clinical nursing work remain unclear.

Purpose: The aims of this study were, first, to investigate nursing students' professional identity, intention to leave the nursing profession, and perception of clinical nursing work during the COVID-19 pandemic and, second, to explore factors influencing professional identity to help develop effective strategies to enrich and strengthen this factor in the future.

Methods: This cross-sectional, descriptive survey study was conducted on 150 nursing students in China in February 2020.

Results: The 14 (9.3%) participants who reported intending to leave the nursing profession earned lower scores for professional identity than their peers who reported intending to remain. The participants who believed that the COVID-19 pandemic had made them "more passionate about clinical nursing work" earned the highest scores, followed by those who believed the pandemic had "no effect." The lowest scores were earned by those who believed clinical nursing work to be "too dangerous to engage in." COVID-19 knowledge scores, the perceived effectiveness of preventive and control measures, the number of cases seen on the day the study survey was taken, and time spent daily on COVID-19 events were the variables found to influence professional identity.

Conclusions: COVID-19 outbreak is not merely a time of crisis but also an opportunity to reconstruct the professional identity of nursing students.

Key Words:
COVID-19, professional identity, retention, nursing student, cross-sectional study.

Introduction

The new coronavirus pneumonia (COVID-19) pandemic has affected China and other countries since December 2019. The number of COVID-19 cases worldwide surpassed 1,600,000 on April 11, 2020 (World Health Organization, 2020a). COVID-19 is highly contagious and generally susceptible and directly threatens the health and life of the public. However, no medicine is currently recommended for the prevention or treatment of COVID-19 (World Health Organization, 2020b), which has caused widespread panic among the public. In China, by February 24, 2020, more than 3,300 healthcare workers had contracted COVID-19 and several nurses had died of the disease.

Nursing students in China during this critical period were removed from all clinical placements in training hospitals. The main reason was safety, and the other reasons were that they were neither covered by health insurance for this type of epidemic disease nor seen as sufficiently competent to help. In this regard, they may have experienced a feeling of own inadequacy as well as unachieved professionalism. As nursing jobs certainly present elements of risk when caring for patients with COVID-19, especially undetected cases, nursing students at this moment were likely to be motivated to clarify their devotion to and reaffirm the meaning of nursing from a personal perspective.

The worldwide nursing shortage, high rates of attrition for both nursing students and new nurses, and workforce aging highlight the importance of recruiting and retaining suitable candidates (McCallum et al., 2006). Nursing students are the future of the nursing workforce. Thus, their retention within the nursing profession has been the focus of a considerable amount of research worldwide (Glew et al., 2019; Ten Hoeve et al., 2017; Powers et al., 2018). Individual factors

[1]*MSN, RN, Department of Nursing, Beijing Hospital, National Center of Gerontology; Institute of Geriatric Medicine, Chinese Academy of Medical Sciences, People's Republic of China* • [2]*MSc, RN, Director, Department of Nursing, Beijing Hospital, National Center of Gerontology; Institute of Geriatric Medicine, Chinese Academy of Medical Sciences, People's Republic of China* • [3]*BSN, RN, Deputy Director, Department of Nursing, Beijing Hospital, National Center of Gerontology; Institute of Geriatric Medicine, Chinese Academy of Medical Sciences, People's Republic of China.*

that have been reported to contribute to attrition rates include common reasons such as academic failure, personal/family difficulties, nursing as a wrong career choice, and financial difficulties (Urwin et al., 2010). Other reasons also contributing to attrition rates include, among others, disappointed dreams and lack of academic support (Glew et al., 2019; Ten Hoeve et al., 2017). Although there are many reasons why nursing students may choose to leave the nursing profession, the focus of this study is on the relationship that professional identity has on nursing student retention during the current COVID-19 pandemic.

Professional identity, defined as the attitudes, values, knowledge, beliefs, and skills that are shared with others within a professional group, may affect how people interact with, compare themselves with, and differentiate themselves from other professional groups in the workplace (Worthington et al., 2013). Professional identity has direct relationships with student retention in nursing programs and intention to leave the nursing profession (Worthington et al., 2013; Yang & Yin, 2019). The clinical internship is a transitional stage for nursing students from being a student to being a nurse. This stage is a critical period for the formation of nursing students' professional identity, as clinical placements help student nurses experience their future professional reality and compare this reality with what they had been taught in theoretical and academic classes (Arreciado Marañón & Isla Pera, 2015).

During the outbreak of severe acute respiratory syndrome (SARS) in early 2003, a study conducted in China found that some students reported that the SARS incident had made them better understand the dangers they may face in nursing work and made them concerned regarding their future work safety, fostering thoughts of leaving nursing work in the future (Sun et al., 2004). Although there are risks involved in caring for infected patients, there were also many moving stories of nurses in connection with this event. Nurses have been portrayed by the media as heroic, self-sacrificing, and having a strong sense of morality. Both the negative and positive information of the COVID-19 pandemic may impact the professional identity of nursing students, which may affect their retention in the nursing profession. Thus, this study was designed to explore how the COVID-19 pandemic has affected the professional identity, intention to leave the nursing profession, and clinical nursing work perceptions of nursing students. Therefore, the aims of this study were to (a) investigate nursing students' professional identity, intention to leave the nursing profession, and perception of clinical nursing work during the COVID-19 pandemic and (b) explore factors influencing professional identity to help develop effective strategies to enrich and strengthen this factor in the future.

Methods

Design and Sample

A cross-sectional study was conducted in seven medical schools with 150 participants. All of the participants were nursing students who had completed an 8-month internship in a general hospital and were currently enrolled in either a junior college or a bachelor's degree study program. The internship for nursing students in China is scheduled during the final year of the nursing educational program, starting in late summer and finishing in late spring. Over these 8 months, nursing students should take a rotation in a general hospital in the surgical, medical, gynecological, or pediatric wards; emergency room; or operating room.

Instruments

Four instruments and a demographic survey comprised the 55-item survey questionnaire that was provided to participants.

Professional identity

This variable was assessed using the 17-item Professional Identity Questionnaire for Nurse Students (PIQNS) developed by Hao Yu-fang. This questionnaire includes the five dimensions of professional self-image, benefit of retention and risk of turnover, social comparison and self-reflection, independence of career choice, and social modeling. The PIQNS items are scored using a 5-point Likert-type scale, ranging from 1 (*strongly disagree*) to 5 (*strongly agree*), with higher scores correlated with increasingly positive professional identity. The test–retest reliability, Cronbach's alpha, and split-half reliability of the scale were .74, .83, and .84, respectively, indicating good reliability and validity (Hao et al., 2014).

Intention to leave the nursing profession and the impact of the COVID-19 pandemic on perceptions of clinical nursing work

Nursing students' intention to leave the nursing profession was assessed using the question: "Would you like to be a nurse in the future?" (yes/no). The impact of the COVID-19 pandemic on perceptions of clinical nursing work was assessed using the question: "What do you think the impacts of COVID-19 pandemic on your perception of clinical nursing work?" (no impact/clinical frontline work was too dangerous to engage in/more passionate about clinical nursing work).

Fear of COVID-19

This variable was assessed using a one-item numeric rating scale, ranging from 0 (*no fear at all*) to 10 (*very scared*), with higher scores correlated with greater fear of COVID-19.

Knowledge, Attitude, and Practice of COVID-19

These variables were assessed using a self-designed, three-part questionnaire. The knowledge part includes nine items scored using a 5-point Likert-type scale, ranging from 1 (*very strange*) to 5 (*very familiar*), with higher scores correlated with greater knowledge of COVID-19. The attitude part includes six dimensions and 10 items. Each item is scored using a 5-point Likert-type scale, ranging from 1 (*strongly disagree*) to 5 (*strongly agree*). The practice part includes nine items scored using a 5-point Likert-type scale, with 1 = *never*, 2 = *rarely*, 3 = *sometimes*, 4 = *usually*, and 5 = *always*. Items 6 and 7 in the practice part employ reverse scoring. The average score for each item was calculated, with higher scores correlated with better practice of COVID-19. Five clinical experts were invited to evaluate the validity of this questionnaire. The average content validity index of all items was 1.0. In this study, the Cronbach's α of the knowledge part was .90, that of the attitude part was .72, and that of the practice part was .65.

Demographic survey

This survey included seven items, including gender; educational level; place of residence; number of confirmed cases; current cases in their city of residence; whether nurses in the internship hospital were participating in the anti-COVID-19 pandemic medical team in Wuhan, China; and time spent on COVID-19 events daily.

Data Collection and Management

A link to the questionnaire was sent to the participants through WeChat workgroups in February 2020. Concurrently, the internship leader at each school was invited to send the link to her classmates who were interns in other hospitals. Any invited nursing students could fill in the questionnaire. To ensure the quality of completed questionnaires, all of the items were flagged as "required questions." In addition, each device was limited to one questionnaire submission to avoid repeated submissions. Finally, the collected questionnaires were checked individually, and the questionnaires with all of the same options were deleted.

Data Analysis

All of the items were transferred into an SPSS database from the electronic survey site. SPSS 16.0 statistical software (SPSS, Inc., Chicago, IL, USA) was used for data analysis. All of the demographic questions and the nursing students' professional identity, fear, knowledge, attitude, and practice scores were described in terms of mean and standard deviation (*SD*) values. To analyze the influence of professional identity on intention to leave the nursing profession and perception of clinical nursing work, we used *t* test, one-way analysis of variance, Pearson correlation, and Spearman correlation to identify if significant differences in professional identity existed between different demographic characteristics, fear scores, knowledge scores, attitude scores, or practice scores. Finally, after setting the professional identity of nursing students as the dependent variable and the statistically significant factors as the independent variables, a stepwise multiple linear regression was conducted. The alpha was set at $p < .05$.

Results

Characteristics of the Participants

One hundred sixty-two questionnaires and 150 valid questionnaires were collected in this study (validity rate: 92.6%). The characteristics of the participants are shown in Table 1.

Professional Identity, Intention to Leave the Nursing Profession, the Impacts of COVID-19 Pandemic on Their Perception of Clinical Nursing Work, and Fear of COVID, Knowledge, Attitude, and Practice Scores of COVID-19

The mean overall and dimension scores for the PIQNS, fear of COVID, knowledge, attitude, and practice scores of COVID-19; distribution of intention to leave the nursing profession; and the impacts of COVID-19 pandemic on nursing students' perception of clinical nursing work are shown in Table 2. The mean PIQNS score was 3.95 (*SD* = 0.61), with participants earning the highest mean score on social modeling (mean = 4.29, *SD* = 0.78) and the lowest score on independence of career choice (mean = 3.75, *SD* = 0.69). Of the 150 participants, 14 (9.3%) affirmed their intention to leave the nursing profession, 100 (66.7%) answered that the COVID-19 pandemic had no impact on their perception of clinical nursing work, 46 (30.7%) answered that the COVID-19 pandemic had made them "more passionate about clinical nursing work," and four (2.7%) expressed the opinion that "clinical frontline work was too dangerous to engage in." The mean scores for fear of COVID-19, knowledge, and practice of COVID-19 were 5.11 (*SD* = 2.04), 3.84 (*SD* = 0.59), and 4.24 (*SD* = 0.46), respectively.

Influences of the Professional Identity on Intention to Leave the Nursing Profession and Perceptions of Clinical Nursing Work

The results with regard to the influence of professional identity on intention to leave the nursing profession and the perception of clinical nursing work are shown in Table 3. The participants who expressed an intention to leave the nursing profession had lower professional identity scores than those who expressed an intention to remain. Professional identity has been positively associated with perception of clinical nursing work. On the basis of the least significant difference one-way analysis of variance, the participants who expressed the opinion that the COVID-19 pandemic had made them "more passionate about clinical nursing work" had the highest professional identity scores, followed by those reporting

Table 1

Characteristics of Participants and Factors Influencing Professional Identity in Nursing Students

Variable	*n*	%	*M*	*SD*	*t*/*F*/*r*	*p*
Gender					$t = 2.88$	.005
Male	9	6.0	4.50	0.36		
Female	141	94.0	3.91	0.61		
Educational level					$t = -1.41$	.162
Bachelor degree	107	71.3	3.90	0.56		
College degree	43	28.7	4.07	0.73		
Area of residence					$F = 0.72$	.488
City	70	46.7	3.97	0.62		
Town	37	24.7	3.84	0.68		
Village	43	28.7	4.00	0.54		
Number of cases on the survey day, [a] P_{50} and (P_{25}, P_{75})	146		(6, 157)		$r = .29$	< .001
Confirmed cases on the survey day, [b] P_{50} and (P_{25}, P_{75})	410		(32, 410)		$r = .23$	.005
Participating in the anti-COVID-19 pandemic medical team in the internship hospital [c]					$F = 1.80$	.169
Yes	138	92.0	3.97	0.62		
No	4	2.7	3.59	0.49		
Do not know	8	5.3	3.72	0.13		
Time spent on COVID-19 cases daily					$F = 3.95$	.021
> 2 hours	24	16.0	4.19	0.62		
1–2 hours	60	40.0	4.00	0.53		
< 1 hour	66	44.0	3.81	0.65		

Variable	*r*	*p*
Fear score	.06	.441
Knowledge score	.48	< .001
Worrying about infection	.03	.745
Attitude score		
High possibility of being infected	−.19	.019
Perceptions of the consequences of infection	.06	.468
Feeling calm in the COVID-19 pandemic	.02	.786
Perceived importance of prevention and control measures	.34	< .001
Perceived effectiveness of preventive and control measures	.45	< .001
Practice scores	.38	< .001

Note. P_{25} = 25th percentiles; P50 = 50th percentiles; P75 = 75th percentiles.
[a] Minimum is 0, and maximum is 198. [b] Minimum is 2, and maximum is 576. [c] Whether there were nurses in the internship hospital participating in the anti-COVID-19 pandemic medical team in Wuhan, China.

"no effect" and, finally, by those reporting "clinical nursing work is too dangerous to engage in" ($F = 6.98$, $p < .05$).

Factors Influencing Professional Identity

The factors influencing professional identity are shown in Table 1. Men earned a higher mean score for professional identity than women ($t = 2.88$, $p = .005$). Those spending over 2 hours on COVID-19 daily earned higher scores for professional identity than those who spent less than 1 hour daily. Moderate but statistically significant and positive relationships were identified between number of confirmed cases, number of existing cases, COVID-19 knowledge scores, perceived importance of prevention and control measures, perceived effectiveness of preventive and control measures, practice scores, and professional identity ($r = .23$–$.48$). Moreover, a negative relationship was found between having a high possibility of being infected and professional identity ($r = -.19$). However, educational level ($t = -1.41$, $p = .162$); place of residence ($F = 0.72$, $p = .488$); whether there were nurses in the internship hospital participating in the anti-COVID-19 pandemic medical team in Wuhan, China ($F = 1.80$, $p = .169$); fear scores ($r = .06$, $p = .441$); worrying about infection ($r = .03$, $p = .745$); perceptions of the consequences of infection ($r = .06$, $p = .468$); and feeling calm in the COVID-19 pandemic ($r = .02$, $p = .786$) were not found to influence professional identity.

The results of stepwise multiple linear regression analysis of professional identity and influencing factors are shown in

Table 2

Mean Scores for PIQNS, Fear and KAP Scores of COVID, Distribution of Intention to Leave the Nursing Profession, and the Impacts of COVID-19 Pandemic on Nursing Students' Perception of Clinical Nursing Work

Scale	Mean	*SD*	Min	Max
PIQNS				
Overall professional identity	3.95	0.61	2.12	5
Professional self-image	4.01	0.74	1.17	5
Benefit of retention and risk of turnover	3.77	0.75	1.00	5
Social comparison and self-reflection	3.98	0.64	2.00	5
Independence of career choice	3.75	0.69	2.50	5
Social modeling	4.29	0.78	1.50	5
Fear of COVID-19	5.11	2.04	0.00	10
KAP of COVID-19				
Knowledge	3.84	0.59	3.00	5
Attitude				
Worrying about infection	3.18	1.00	1.00	5
High possibility of being infected	2.25	1.00	1.00	5
Perceptions of the consequences of infection	3.46	0.93	1.00	5
Perceived importance of prevention and control measures	4.50	0.70	2.00	5
Feeling calm in the COVID-19 event	3.22	0.83	1.00	5
Perceived effectiveness of preventive and control measures	4.45	0.67	2.00	5
Practice	4.24	0.46	2.78	5
Variable	***n***	**%**		
Intention to leave the nursing profession				
Yes	14	9.3		
No	136	90.7		
Impact of COVID-19 pandemic on perception of clinical nursing work				
No impact	100	66.7		
More passionate about clinical nursing work	46	30.7		
Clinical frontline work is too dangerous to engage in	4	2.7		

Note. PIQNS = Professional Identity Questionnaire for Nurse Students; KAP = knowledge, attitude, and practice.

Table 4. The final model included four independent variables that together accounted for 33.8% of the variation in professional identity. Higher COVID-19 knowledge scores, perceived effectiveness of preventive and control measures, and more cases on the day of the survey were shown to correlate significantly and positively with stronger professional identity, whereas less time spent on COVID-19 events daily was found to correlate with weaker professional identity.

Discussion

In this study, the mean score for professional identity was found to be higher than in other studies (Chen & Zhang,

Table 3

Influences of the Professional Identity of Nursing Students on Intention to Leave the Nursing Profession and Perception of Clinical Nursing Work

Variable	*M*	*SD*	*t/F*	*p*
Intention to leave the nursing profession			*t* = −4.50	< .001
Yes	3.29	0.67		
No	4.01	0.57		
Perception of clinical nursing work			*F* = 6.98	.001
No effect	3.88	0.63		
More passionate about clinical nursing work	4.16	0.51		
Clinical nursing work is too dangerous to engage in	3.21	0.45		

Table 4

Stepwise Multiple Linear Regression Analysis of Predictors of Professional Identity (N = 150)

Variable	β	*SE*	β'	*t*	*p*
Constant	1.04	0.38	—	2.77	.006
Knowledge score	0.41	0.09	0.34	4.67	< .001
Perception of the effectiveness of preventive and control measures	0.27	0.07	0.27	3.79	< .001
The number of cases on the survey day	0.00	0.00	0.21	3.10	.002
Time spent on COVID-19 cases is < 1 hour	−0.20	0.08	−0.16	−2.42	.017

Note. R^2 = .355, adjusted R^2 = .338, F = 19.978, and $p < .001$.

2015; T. T. Wang & Luo, 2018; C. Wu et al., 2020). The reason for this may be differences in the surveyed populations. Chen and Zhang's study included students of all grades, and Wu et al.'s study enrolled first-year, post-associate-degree baccalaureate nursing students. However, only students in the final year of their nursing programs were included in this study. Furthermore, nursing students at different grade levels have been shown to differ in terms of professional identity (Chen & Zhang, 2015). Moreover, the COVID-19 outbreak is a unique and unanticipated event that provided a stage for nurses to establish a good professional image. Nursing work has been universally respected and recognized by society, and the positive attitude of society toward nursing is likely to enhance the positive, professional attitude of nursing students. It may also be that, similar to during the previous SARS outbreak, nursing during the COVID-19 pandemic has helped nursing students recognize the value of nursing as a profession that focuses on the lives of others and on being altruistic, moral, and concerned with understanding more about those around them, providing a unique opportunity to mature and grow into their profession, thereby profoundly enhancing their professional identity (Heung et al., 2005). The dimension of "social modeling" earned the highest score in this study, which differs from other studies (Chen & Zhang, 2015; Q. R. Wang, 2018), indicating that the public's positive attitude toward nursing work has improved the professional identity of nursing students. The dimension of "independence of career choice" earned the lowest score. There are currently limited career choices for nursing graduates, and most will become a nurse, with only a very few with the best academic records continuing to study for a master's degree. In addition, nursing students' choice of career is influenced by other factors such as family members and the general employment situation (L. T. Wu et al., 2015), which limits career choice autonomy.

Significant differences were found in terms of professional identity, with different intentions to leave the nursing profession and perceptions of clinical nursing work, which is consistent with the findings of other research (Chênevert et al., 2016). Of the 150 participants in this study, 46 (30.7%) expressed that the COVID-19 event had made them "more passionate about clinical nursing work" and earned the highest scores for professional identity. However, four (2.7%) of the participants in this study expressed the opinion that "clinical nursing work is too dangerous to engage in," supporting job security as an important factor affecting career choice (L. T. Wu et al., 2015) in light of the large overall population of nursing students in China.

The COVID-19 knowledge score was found to play an important role in enhancing professional identity, with higher knowledge scores correlating with stronger professional identity, indicating that improving the awareness of nursing students regarding COVID-19 will help improve their professional identity. This may be because nursing students with higher professional identity hold deeper understandings, convictions, and emotions toward the nursing profession and therefore pay more attention to knowledge related to the COVID-19 pandemic. Another possible reason for this phenomenon is that information on the COVID-19 pandemic help nursing students more deeply perceive the important role played by nurses in controlling this pandemic and the resultant high level of professional prestige, inspiring feelings of social responsibility and love for the nursing profession. Desire to help others, personal interest in healthcare, and professional prestige are important factors that influence the career choices of nursing students (L. T. Wu et al., 2015) and that thus enhance their professional identity.

The self-perceived effectiveness of preventive and control measures was shown to influence professional identity in this study, with higher "perception of the effectiveness of preventive and control measures" scores associated with stronger professional identity scores. The participants with higher scores of "perception of the effectiveness of preventive and control measures" were shown to be more likely to take good protective behaviors to ensure their own safety and thus to have a more reasonable understanding of the safety of nursing work, which also increased their perceived professional identity.

Number of confirmed cases was also found to be a factor that influences professional identity, although these did not necessarily share a positive relationship. A large number of current confirmed cases means that the COVID-19 pandemic situation is more serious, which also encourages nursing students to pay close attention to the pandemic situation, thereby improving their awareness of this situation, enhancing their self-perceived value of nursing work, and improving their professional identity.

In this study, those participants who paid attention to COVID-19 less than 1 hour every day had the lowest professional identity scores. Nursing students who pay less attention to the COVID-19 pandemic likely have a lower understanding of the value of nursing work, which, in turn, affects their professional identity. Nursing students with poor professional identity may not pay sufficient attention to the most currently important nursing-work-related events such as the COVID-19 pandemic.

Conclusions

The professional identity of nursing students and its influences on intention to leave the nursing profession and perception of clinical nursing work were explored in this study. The factors that significantly influence professional identity were also explored. We found the professional identity of the participants to be at the upper middle level and that significant differences exist among perceived professional identity, with different intentions to leave the nursing profession and different perceptions of clinical nursing work. COVID-19 knowledge, the perceived effectiveness of preventive and control measures, the number of confirmed cases, and the time spent on COVID-19 events daily were identified as factors that significantly influence professional identity in nursing students. The COVID-19 outbreak is a time of crisis and an opportunity to reconstruct the professional identity of nurses. The pandemic has an affirming effect on the professional identity of nursing students. Making sense of this pandemic and incorporating related findings into educational activities have the potential to promote professional identity in nursing students and increase their commitment to remaining in the nursing profession.

Author Contributions

Study conception and design: SN
Data collection: All authors
Data analysis and interpretation: SN
Drafting of the article: SN
Critical revision of the article: SN

References

Arreciado Marañón, A., & Isla Pera, M. P. (2015). Theory and practice in the construction of professional identity in nursing students: A qualitative study. *Nurse Education Today, 35*(7), 859–863. https://doi.org/10.1016/j.nedt.2015.03.014

Chen, H. Z., & Zhang, C. Y. (2015). Investigation of the undergraduate nursing students' professional identity: A case study of the nursing school of Lanzhou University. *Chinese Clinical Nursing, 7*(6), 537–541. https://doi.org/10.3969/j.issn.1674-3768.2015.06.029 (Original work published in Chinese)

Chênevert, D., Jourdain, G., & Vandenberghe, C. (2016). The role of high-involvement work practices and professional self-image in nursing recruits' turnover: A three-year prospective study. *International Journal of Nursing Studies, 53*, 73–84. https://doi.org/10.1016/j.ijnurstu.2015.09.005

Glew, P. J., Ramjan, L. M., Salas, M., Raper, K., Creed, H., & Salamonson, Y. (2019). Relationships between academic literacy support, student retention and academic performance. *Nurse Education Practice, 39*, 61–65. https://doi.org/10.1016/j.nepr.2019.07.011

Hao, Y.-F., Niu, H.-J., Li, L.-P., Yue, S.-J., & Liu, X.-H. (2014). Measurement of professional identity in Chinese nursing students. *International Journal of Nursing Sciences, 1*(2), 137–144. https://doi.org/10.1016/j.ijnss.2014.05.002

Heung, Y. Y., Wrong, K. Y., Kwong, W. Y., To, S. S., & Wong, H. C. (2005). Severe acute respiratory syndrome outbreak promotes a strong sense of professional identity among nursing students. *Nurse Education Today, 25*(2), 112–118. https://doi.org/10.1016/j.nedt.2004.11.003

McCallum, J., Donaldson, J. H., & Lafferty, P. (2006). Can an interview score sheet assist with student selection onto the bachelor of science/diploma of higher education (adult) nursing programme? Findings from a pilot study. *Nurse Education Today, 26*(7), 586–592. https://doi.org/10.1016/j.nedt.2006.01.015

Powers, K., Herron, E. K., Sheeler, C., & Sain, A. (2018). The lived experience of being a male nursing student: Implications for student retention and success. *Journal of Professional Nursing, 34*(6), 475–482. https://doi.org/10.1016/j.profnurs.2018.04.002

Sun, Y. M., Guo, J. M., Guan, M. Y., & Li, X. P. (2004). Study of the relations between SARS and the professional attitude of nursing students. *Chinese Journal of Nursing, 39*(4), 278–280. (Original work published in Chinese)

Ten Hoeve, Y., Castelein, S., Jansen, G., & Roodbol, P. (2017). Dreams and disappointments regarding nursing: Student nurses' reasons for attrition and retention. A qualitative study design. *Nurse Education Today, 54*, 28–36. https://doi.org/10.1016/j.nedt.2017.04.013

Urwin, S., Stanley, R., Jones, M., Gallagher, A., Wainwright, P., & Perkins, A. (2010). Understanding student nurse attrition: Learning from the literature. *Nurse Education Today, 30*(2), 202–207. https://doi.org/10.1016/j.nedt.2009.07.014

Wang, Q. R. (2018). The relevance research of hardy personality and professional identification for undergraduate nursing students. *Tianjin Journal of Nursing, 26*(3), 287–290. https://doi.org/10.3969/j.issn.1006-9143.2018.03.011 (Original work published in Chinese)

Wang, T.-T., & Luo, Y. (2018). Correlation between care atmosphere perception in hospital and professional identity of nursing students in clinical training. *Chinese Nursing Research, 32*(5), 825–828. https://doi.org/10.3969/j.issn.1009-6493.2018.05.041 (Original work published in Chinese)

World Health Organization. (2020a). *Coronavirus disease 2019 (COVID-19) situation report-82*. https://www.who.int/docs/default-source/coronaviruse/situation-reports/20200411-sitrep-82-covid-19.pdf?sfvrsn=74a5d15_2

World Health Organization. (2020b). *Coronavirus disease (COVID-19)*. https://www.who.int/news-room/q-a-detail/q-a-coronaviruses

Worthington, M., Salamonson, Y., Weaver, R., & Cleary, M. (2013). Predictive validity of the Macleod Clark professional identity scale for undergraduate nursing students. *Nurse Education Today, 33*(3), 187–191. https://doi.org/10.1016/j.nedt.2012.01.012

Wu, C., Palmer, M. H., & Sha, K. (2020). Professional identity and its influencing factors of first-year post-associate degree baccalaureate nursing students: A cross-sectional study. *Nurse Education Today, 84,* Article 104227. https://doi.org/10.1016/j.nedt.2019.104227

Wu, L. T., Low, M. M., Tan, K. K., Lopez, V., & Liaw, S. Y. (2015). Why not nursing? A systematic review of factors influencing career choice among healthcare students. *International Nursing Review, 62*(4), 547–562. https://doi.org/10.1111/inr.12220

Yang, H., & Yin, Y. L. (2019). A qualitative research on professional identification of male nursing postgraduate students. *Chinese Journal of Modern Nursing, 25*(22), 2892–2895. https://doi.org/10.3760/cma.j.issn.1674-2907.2019.22.029 (Original work published in Chinese)

14

Effect of Scenario-Based Simulation Training on the Obstetrics and Gynecology Nursing Clinical Practicum

Ayten ŞENTÜRK ERENEL[1] • Şengül YAMAN SÖZBİR[2] • Mehtap UZUN AKSOY[3*] • Esra ARSLAN GÜRCÜOĞLU[4] • Sıdıka PELİT AKSU[5] • Filiz ÜNAL TOPRAK[6] • Canan UÇAKCI ASALIOĞLU[5]

ABSTRACT

Background: Simulation practices in obstetrics and gynecology (OB-GYN) nursing are used in education, practice, assessment, and the investigation of interventional and behavioral skills related to both routine and emergency conditions.

Purpose: This study was conducted in an OB-GYN nursing course to determine the effect of simulation practices on clinical practice satisfaction, clinical stress, and self-confidence in nursing students.

Methods: A cluster randomized controlled experimental trial was conducted on 122 students (experimental group, n = 58; control group, n = 64). After theoretical training, all of the students applied six scenarios in the OB-GYN nursing simulation laboratory. The students in the experimental group began clinical practice after simulation training, whereas their peers in the control group began clinical practice without prior simulation training. Data in this study were collected using a personal information form, the Pagana Clinical Stress Questionnaire, a self-confidence scale, and a satisfaction subscale from the Clinical Learning Environment Scale on, respectively, the first day and final day of clinical practice.

Results: At the end of the clinical practice, average clinical stress in the control group was higher than that in the experimental group (p = .001). No intergroup difference was found in self-confidence levels (p > .05). For the control group, at posttest, the average satisfaction with the clinical learning environment was higher (p = .046) and the average satisfaction with the clinical learning environment was lower (p = .05). In contrast, no mean pretest–posttest differences were found in clinical stress and self-confidence levels in the experimental group (p > .05). In the control group, no mean pretest–posttest difference was found for the clinical learning environment (p > .05), whereas mean clinical stress (p < .001) and self-confidence (p = .012) levels were higher at posttest (p < .05).

Conclusions/Implications for Practice: The findings of this study indicate that simulation training interventions reduce clinical satisfaction and stress in students but do not influence self-confidence. Nursing educators may provide scenario-based simulation training to students taking OB-GYN courses to enhance their preparedness for clinical practice.

Key Words:
nursing, students, simulation, self-confidence, clinical stress.

Introduction

Nursing education consists of theoretical and clinical applications. In nursing education, students are expected to acquire basic competencies in patient-centered care, teamwork, and collaboration; evidence-based practices; quality improvement; safety; and informatics (Cronenwett et al., 2007). Nevertheless, in most vocational courses, nursing students currently gain a theoretical understanding of these topics in their syllabus and begin clinical training after limited classroom practice. However, this approach does not provide adequate opportunities for practice, causing students to experience anxiety and a lack of self-confidence (Woda et al., 2017). The World Health Organization has identified technological and innovative methods as the gold standard in nursing and midwifery education (World Health Organization, 2013), which suggests that students should practice all key skills/practices in simulated laboratory settings (Maas & Flood, 2011; Skrable & Fitzsimons, 2014; Yuan et al., 2012). In prior studies, simulation training has been reported to increase clinical satisfaction, the benefits perceived by patients, acceptance from working nurses, self-confidence, and performance in nursing students while reducing their anxiety (Labrague et al., 2019; Oh et al., 2015; Smith et al., 2012). In addition, simulation training has been identified as an effective method for improving psychomotor and problem-solving skills and rates of accurate

[1]*PhD, Professor, Faculty of Health Sciences, Nursing Department, Gazi University, Ankara, Turkey* • [2]*PhD, Associate Professor, Faculty of Health Sciences, Nursing Department, Gazi University, Ankara, Turkey* • [3]*PhD, RN, Lecturer, Faculty of Health Sciences, Nursing Department, Gazi University, Ankara, Turkey* • [4]*PhD, RN, Research Assistant, Faculty of Health Sciences, Nursing Department, Çankırı Karatekin University, Çankırı, Turkey* • [5]*MSN, RN, Research Assistant, Faculty of Health Sciences, Nursing Department, Gazi University, Ankara, Turkey* • [6]*PhD, RN, Assistant Professor, Faculty of Health Sciences, Nursing Department, Abant Izzet Baysal University, Bolu, Turkey.*

application of these skills among students (Eyikara & Baykara, 2018; Işık & Kaya, 2014; Mete et al., 2017).

One of the areas in which simulation is needed in nursing education is obstetrics and gynecology (OB-GYN). Simulation practices in OB-GYN nursing include education, practice, assessment, and the investigation of interventional and behavioral skills related to routine or emergency obstetric-gynecological conditions (Şendir, 2013). Thus, when applied before the start of clinical practice, OB-GYN nursing-related simulation programs allow students to gain hands-on skills, become familiar with situations that they may encounter in clinical settings, develop clinical decision-making skills, hone their abilities to choose appropriate interventions, and experience teamwork (Gardner & Raemer, 2008; Şendir, 2013). In the literature, it has been reported that conducting simulation training in OB-GYN nursing courses achieves certain positive results. Pınar and Doğan (2013) found simulation-based education in OB-GYN nursing to be effective in improving students' technical skills in the area of perinatal patient management. In another study, it was found that a simulation activity held in OB-GYN nursing course improved students' perceptions of learning (Pınar et al., 2015). Moreover, scenario-based simulation practice in OB-GYN nursing courses was found to improve students' clinical knowledge and skill performance (Pınar et al., 2016). In addition, use of different types of simulators to improve students' psychomotor and communication skills was found to be effective in preparing students for clinical practice and increasing their competences in clinical practice (Terzioğlu et al., 2016). Furthermore, it was found that postpartum care simulation increases the confidence of nursing students to perform patient assessments (Germain et al., 2018).

Although most nursing education departments in Turkey have a general skills laboratory, none currently operates simulation laboratories equipped with simulators for OB-GYN nursing courses. Therefore, the use of simulation in OB-GYN nursing is not very common domestically, and exclusively theory-based nursing education remains prevalent throughout Turkey. Thus, students encounter patients in real hospital environments without the opportunity to apply the information they have learned in theoretical lectures. In this study, increasing the care and communication skills of students using preclinical simulations was presumed to decrease the clinical stress of these students by increasing their self-confidence, decreasing their stress, and, subsequently, increasing their clinical satisfaction. Therefore, this study was designed to determine the effects of a pre-clinical-practice simulation practice program on satisfaction related to clinical practice, clinical stress, and self-confidence in OB-GYN nursing students.

Hypotheses

The following are the hypotheses used for this study:

H_1 = Preclinical simulation training increases students' clinical practice satisfaction.

H_2 = Preclinical simulation training reduces students' clinical stress level.

H_3 = Preclinical simulation training increases students' self-confidence.

Methods

Setting

This cluster-randomized controlled experimental trial study was carried out in the nursing department of a state university. Simulation practices were conducted in the Application Laboratory of Obstetrics and Gynecology Nursing, which was established within the university's Faculty of Health Sciences. The research team consisted of two faculty members (an associate professor and a lecturer doctor) and five research assistants (all were doctoral students) in the Department of Obstetrics and Gynecology Nursing.

Participants

The study population consisted of 136 third-year students in the Nursing-301: Obstetrics and Gynecology Nursing course in the Faculty of Health Sciences in the 2016–2017 academic year. This course was convened in both fall and spring semesters. Using lots, the researchers randomly assigned spring semester participants to the experimental group and fall semester participants to the control group. Using power analysis (GPower 3.1 program), 128 students (64 in each group) was deemed necessary to achieve a Type 1 error value of 5%, a power level of 80%, and a medium effect size of .50. One hundred thirty-six students were enrolled. However, 13 of the students in the experimental group were unable to participate in all of the scenarios and were thus excluded from the sample. One student in the control group was excluded from the sample because of unwillingness to participate. Thus, the study was conducted on 122 students, with 58 in the experimental group and 64 in the control group.

Study Procedures

Before the students in both groups started clinical practice in the hospital, they were given theoretical courses specific to each target skill. The theoretical courses in OB-GYN nursing were performed in the first 7 weeks (84 hours) for both groups for 6 hours a day on Monday and Tuesday of each week. Theoretical courses and clinical practice were administered to both groups by the same instructors. Theoretical lectures' content, lecture period, services that were used for the clinical practice, and clinical practice period (7 weeks, 2 days a week for a total of 112 hours) were the same for both groups.

Experimental Group

For the experimental group, after the theoretical courses, the students practiced (16 hours) on simulation scenarios in the OB-GYN nursing simulation laboratory. Simulation practices were conducted in the simulation laboratory (using three birth simulators, three newborn simulators, and three breast models) using real-life OB-GYN scenarios that were developed by the researchers. The National League for Nursing Jeffries simulation theory was used as a framework to design and implement the simulation session (Jeffries et al., 2015). Six scenarios were created by the research team for the simulation. Each scenario was developed to provide the basic information and skills typically targeted in women's health nursing courses (Table 1). The first scenario trained participants on pregnancy monitoring, risky situation handling skills, and family planning counseling. The second scenario trained participants on providing care during vaginal birth, providing mother–infant care during the postpartum period, and breastfeeding training skills. The third scenario trained participants on treating gestational diabetes mellitus and providing counseling and caring in situations such as polyhydramnios and Rh mismatch. The fourth scenario trained participants on conducting gynecological

Table 1

Scenarios and Skills Expected to be Developed

Scenario	Skill Expected to be Developed
Pregnancy scenario • Monitoring pregnancy • Family planning counseling	✓ Pregnancy follow-up ✓ Gathering information about obstetric and gynecological history ✓ Routine examinations during pregnancy ✓ A scenario involving risky situations during pregnancy ✓ Complications during pregnancy ✓ Family planning counseling
Childbirth scenario • Vaginal childbirth • Mother and infant care postpartum period • Breastfeeding counseling	✓ Admission of the pregnant woman to the delivery room ✓ Labor follow-up ✓ Application of Leopold maneuvers ✓ Evaluation of risky situations at birth ✓ Emotional support for the mother at birth ✓ First examination and care of the newborn ✓ First breastfeeding, initiating the mother–infant relationship ✓ Postpartum mother care
Gestational diabetes scenario • Gestational diabetes mellitus • Polyhydramnios • Rh mismatch	✓ Physiopathology, symptoms, and findings of gestational diabetes ✓ Complications of gestational diabetes ✓ Insulin administration, exercise, and diet ✓ Problems that may occur in the mother and the infant during postpartum period
Sexual violence scenario • Gynecological examination • Sexual violence • Sexually transmitted diseases	✓ Nursing approaches during gynecological examination ✓ Sexual violence symptoms ✓ Sexually transmitted diseases ✓ Conditions needing caution and procedures to be followed when sexual violence is determined
Infertility scenario • Definition of infertility and defining the factors that affect • The diagnosis and treatment methods used in infertility • Ovarian hyperstimulation syndrome • Termination of pregnancy or loss	✓ Risk factors for female–male infertility ✓ Signs and symptoms ✓ Diagnostic tests ✓ Treatments and nursing care ✓ Psychosocial problems in infertility ✓ Assisted reproduction techniques
Endometrial cancer scenario • Endometrial cancer • Total abdominal hysterectomy, bilateral salpingo-oophorectomy surgery • Postoperative nursing care • Discharge training (menopause, sexuality, postoperative risk factors, dangerous situations, etc.)	✓ Endometrial cancer risk factors ✓ Endometrial cancer signs and symptoms ✓ Endometrial cancer treatments ✓ Surgical treatment of gynecologic cancers ✓ Preoperative nursing care ✓ Postoperative nursing care

examinations, providing care for victims of sexual violence, and recognizing and treating sexually transmitted diseases. The fifth scenario provided skills necessary to identify infertility and related factors, understand how to diagnose and treat infertility, and provide care in situations such as ovarian hyperstimulation syndrome and termination of pregnancy or loss. The sixth scenario helped participants improve skills related to endometrium cancer, total abdominal hysterectomy, bilateral salpingo-oophorectomy surgery, postoperative nursing care, and discharge training (e.g., menopause, sexuality, postoperative risk factors, dangerous situations). Each scenario consists of the scenario, objectives, actors, scenario cases, discussion questions, and evaluation form (Table 1). The students were given a week to prepare the scenarios after receipt. The scenarios were performed simultaneously in three different stations in groups of five people. Each student was present in each scenario. The scenarios were performed under the supervision of the researchers. Each scenario lasted for 1–1.5 hours. Researchers observed the scenario practice sessions, asked the discussion questions at the end of the scenario, and filled out the evaluation forms for the students. In addition, the simulation laboratory was open weekdays during normal work hours to enable students to repeat the same scenarios. The experimental group students started their clinical practice in the hospital after having practiced all of the scenarios in the laboratory. On the first day of clinical practice (pretest), the students completed the personal information form (PIF), the Pagana Clinical Stress Questionnaire (PCSQ), the Self-Confidence Scale (SS), and the satisfaction subscale of the Clinical Learning Environment Scale (CLES). On the last day of the clinical practice (posttest), students completed the latter three measures again (Figure 1).

Control Group

The parameters examined in our research may also be affected by the content of theoretical coursework. The control group was used to control for this potential effect. For the control group, clinical practice started in the hospital without simulation practice after they had completed their theoretical courses. On the first day of clinical practice (pretest), students completed the PIF, PCSQ, SS, and the satisfaction subscale of the CLES. On the last day of the clinical practice (posttest), students completed the latter three measures again (Figure 1).

Instruments

The data for this study were collected using a PIF, the satisfaction subscale of the CLES, PCSQ, and SS.

Personal information form

This form consisted of two items: age and grade point average (GPA).

Clinical learning environment scale

This scale was developed by Dunn and Burnett (1995) to identify factors that characterize the clinical learning environment. The CLES is a 5-point Likert-type scale (Dunn & Burnett, 1995). A Turkish validity and reliability study of this scale was done by Sarı (2001). The Turkish version of the CLES consists of 22 items and five subscales, including staff–student relationships (six items), responsibilities of the instructor (four items), patient relationships (four items), student satisfaction (four items), and hierarchy and routines (four items). The Cronbach's alpha value of the Turkish version of the CLES was determined to be .81, with item–total correlations ranging from .21 to .55. On the basis of the results of content validity analysis, the Kendall coefficient of concordance of this scale is 0.20 ($\chi^2 = 33.61$, $p = .03$). As this study was designed to evaluate the satisfaction of the participants, only the student satisfaction subscale of this scale was used. The Cronbach's alpha value of the student satisfaction subscale in the Turkish version was determined to be .81. In this study, the Cronbach's alpha value of this subscale was found to be .67 at pretest and .79 at posttest. The highest possible score for the subscale is 20, and the lowest is 4. Lower scores correlate with a lower level of satisfaction, whereas higher scores correlate with higher levels of satisfaction (Sarı, 2001).

Pagana clinical stress questionnaire

This questionnaire was developed by Pagana (1989) to evaluate the stress experienced by nursing students during clinical practice. On the basis of Kaiser's criterion (eigenvalues of 1 or greater), four factors were extracted, accounting for 58% of the variance. Factor loadings ranged from .31 to .81 in the original scale, and Cronbach's alpha values ranged between .85 and .84 for the factors (Pagana, 1989). In a validity and reliability study of the PCSQ conducted by Şendir and Acaroğlu (2008) in Turkey, the Cronbach's alpha was value determined as .70 (Pagana, 1989; Şendir & Acaroğlu, 2008). The PCSQ consists of four factors that explain 58.6% of the variance. Factor loadings were found to range between .52 and .83 in the Turkish version (Şendir & Acaroğlu, 2008). The PCSQ is a 5-point Likert-type scale, with 20 items classified into four subscales of emotional expression, including threat, challenge, harm, and benefit. The "threat" scale includes six statements, the "challenge" scale includes seven statements, the "harm" scale includes five statements, and the "benefit" scale includes two statements. Total possible PCSQ scores range between 0 and 80, with low scores correlated with lower levels of stress and higher scores correlated with higher levels of stress (Pagana, 1989). In this study, the Cronbach's alpha value of the PCSQ was found to be .81 for pretest and .84 for posttest.

Self-confidence scale

This scale was designed by Akın (2007) to assess self-confidence in university students in Turkey. This 5-point Likert-type scale consists of 33 items, with a possible score range of 33–165. Higher scores correlate with higher levels of self-confidence. Dividing the total score by the number of items (33) gives an estimate of self-confidence, with scores of < 2.5 indicating low self-confidence, 2.5–3.5 indicating

Figure 1

Flowchart of study

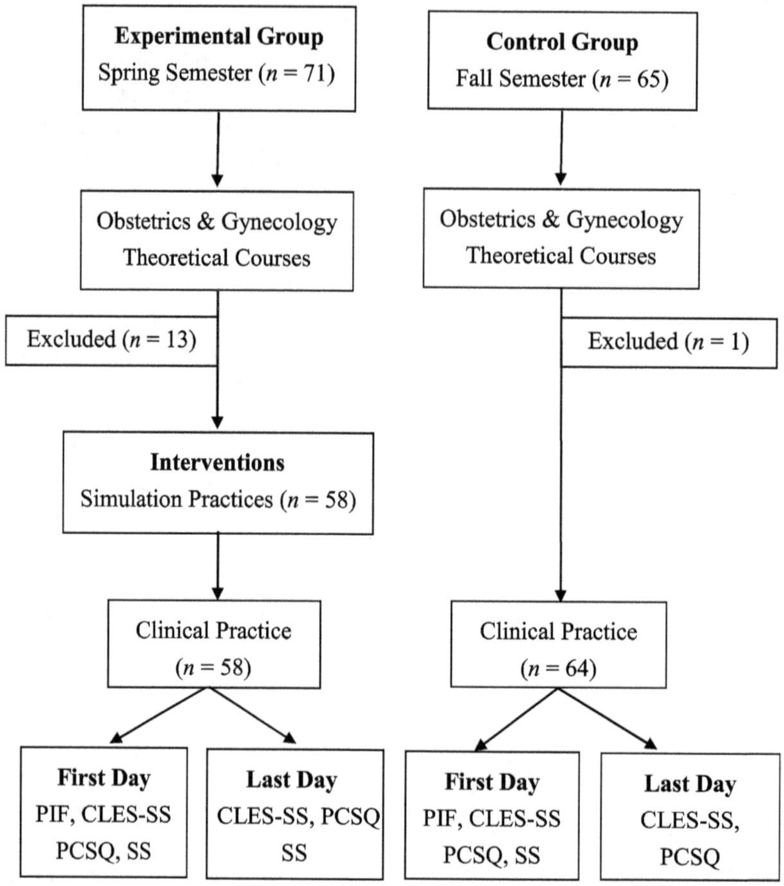

Note. PIF = personal information form; CLES-SS= satisfaction subscale of the clinical learning environment scale; PCSQ = Pagana clinical stress questionnaire; SS = self-confidence scale.

moderate self-confidence, and > 3.5 indicating higher self-confidence. The internal consistency coefficient for the SS is .83, and the test–retest reliability coefficient is .94 (Akın, 2007). Factor loadings ranged from .31 to .74, and according to confirmatory factor analysis, fit index values are as follows: root mean square error of approximation = .044, normed fit index = .90, comparative fit index = .96, incremental fit index = .96, relative fit index = .89, goodness of fit index = .94, adjusted goodness of fit index = .91, and standardized root mean square residual = .058 (χ^2 = 700.41, df = 488, p < .001; Akın, 2007). In this study, the Cronbach's alpha was found to be .94 for both pretest and posttest.

Ethical Considerations

Written permission from the university and approval from the university's ethics committee were obtained before launching the program (date: March 31, 2015; No. 77082166-604.01.02-39505).

At the outset, all of the students were informed of the purpose and procedures of the study. Students were ensured that their participation would not affect their formal education scores. The 14 students who were excluded from this study took the normal, theoretical courses before starting clinical practice in the hospital and did not complete any of the scales or the questionnaire during clinical practice. All students were anonymized using codes during and after distribution of the measures. Thus, the researchers did not know which students chose not to participate in the study. All of the simulation training after the clinical practice and the application of the study was implemented in the laboratory setting with the same instructors in the control group.

Data Analysis

The data obtained from this study were analyzed using SPSS Version 20.0 (IBM, Inc., Armonk, NY, USA). Mean and standard deviation were used to evaluate the quantitative variables, and frequency and percentage values were used to evaluate the qualitative variables. Mann–Whitney U and independent sample t test statistics were used to analyze the difference between the experimental and control groups. Paired-sample t test and

Table 2

Participant Sociodemographic Characteristics (N = 112)

Characteristic	Experimental Group (*n* = 58)		Control Group (*n* = 64)		Statistical Value	*p*
	M	*SD*	*M*	*SD*		
Age	20.50	0.68	20.39	0.93	*U* = 1613.50	.21[a]
GPA	2.88	0.32	2.87	0.34	*t* = 0.125	.90[b]

Note. GPA = grade point average (indicator of academic achievement).
[a] Mann–Whitney *U* test. [b] Independent sample *t* test.

Wilcoxon signed-rank test statistics were used to analyze the difference between pretest and posttest scores. Level of significance was defined as $p \leq .05$ in this study.

Results

The mean age of the participants in the experimental and control groups was 20.50 ± 0.68 and 20.39 ± 0.93 years, respectively ($p = .21$). Mean GPA was 2.88 ± 0.32 in the experimental group and 2.87 ± 0.34 in the control group ($p = .90$; Table 2). To confirm that the groups were homogeneous, it was shown that there was no difference between groups in terms of age or GPA ($p > .05$; Table 2).

No differences were found in terms of pretest mean/median scores ($p > .05$) between the groups. However, intergroup differences were significant at posttest in terms of mean PCSQ score ($p < .001$) and median score for the satisfaction subscale of CLES ($p = .046$), with the posttest scores for the control group found to be higher (Table 2). PCSQ threat ($p = .019$), challenge ($p = .048$), and harm ($p = .005$) subscale posttest scores in the control group were found to be significantly higher than those in the experimental group. No significant difference was found between the two groups in terms of the benefit subscale only ($p > .05$; Table 3).

The intragroup comparison indicated that the posttest scores in the experimental group related to the satisfaction subscale of CLES (14.0) were lower than the pretest scores (15.0; $p = .05$), whereas the difference was insignificant in the control group ($p = .775$). Although no difference between pretest and posttest scores was identified in the experimental group relating to PCSQ ($p = .368$), a difference between pretest and posttest scores was found in the control group in terms of mean PCSQ scores, with mean posttest scores higher than pretest scores ($p < .001$). PCSQ-harm subscale posttest scores in the experimental group were higher than pretest scores ($p = .006$). In the control group, PCSQ threat ($p < .001$) and harm ($p < .001$) subscale posttest scores were found to be higher than pretest scores. Although no difference was found between mean SS pretest and posttest scores in the experimental group ($p = .621$), a difference was found between the pretest and posttest scores in terms of mean SS scores, with the mean posttest scores higher in the control group than in the experimental group ($p = .012$; Table 4).

Discussion

The main goals of nursing education is to produce nurses who are able to incorporate theory into practice and think critically in the process of learning and who have gained effective problem-solving skills (Akyuz, 2011). Simulation training is one application that may help achieve these goals. In this study, it was found that posttest scores for the satisfaction subscale of CLES in the experimental group were statistically significantly lower than pretest scores ($p \leq .05$), whereas no pretest–posttest difference was identified in the control group ($p > .05$). Concurrently, the posttest scores on the satisfaction subscale of CLES in the experimental group were statistically significantly lower than the posttest

Table 3

Distribution of CLES, PCSQ, and SS Scale Pretest and Posttest Scores, by Group (N = 112)

Scale	Pretest				*p*	Posttest				*p*
	Experimental Group (*n* = 58)		Control Group (*n* = 64)			Experimental Group (*n* = 58)		Control Group (*n* = 64)		
	Median		Median			Median		Median		
CLES-satisfaction subscale	15.0		15.5		.556	14.0		15.0		**.046** [a]
PCSQ (*M* and *SD*)	26.68	10.53	27.23	10.80	.779	27.79	8.47	33.32	10.12	**.001** [b]
Threat	7.0		7.0		.656	8.0		9.5		**.019** [a]
Challenge	12.5		13.5		.522	12.5		14.5		**.048** [a]
Harm	2.0		2.0		.605	4.5		6.0		**.005** [a]
Benefit	3.0		3.0		.988	3.0		3.0		.716
SS (*M* and *SD*)	126.53	13.28	124.58	18.27	.481	127.09	14.36	128.83	17.11	.557

Note. Bold values indicate statistical significance was $p \leq .05$. CLES = Clinical Learning Environment Scale; PCSQ = Pagana Clinical Stress Questionnaire; SS = Self-Confidence Scale.
[a] Mann–Whitney *U* test. [b] Independent sample *t* test.

Table 4

Pretest and Posttest Scores of CLES, PCSQ, and SS Scales (N = 112)

Scale	Experimental Group (*n* = 58)				*p*	Control Group (*n* = 64)				*p*
	Pretest		Posttest			Pretest		Posttest		
	Median		Median			Median		Median		
CLES-satisfaction subscale	15.0		14.0		**.050** [a]	15.5		15.0		.775
PCSQ (*M* and *SD*)	26.68	10.53	27.79	8.47	.368	27.23	10.80	33.33	10.12	**< .001** [b]
Threat	7.0		8.0		.170	7.0		9.5		**< .001** [a]
Challenge	12.5		12.5		.175	13.5		14.5		.481
Harm	2.0		4.5		**.006** [a]	2.0		6.0		**< .001** [a]
Benefit	3.05	2.00	3.00	1.19	.840	3.0		3.0		.784
SS (*M* and *SD*)	126.53	13.28	127.09	14.36	.621	124.58	18.27	128.83	17.11	**.012** [b]

Note. Bold values indicate that statistical significance was $p \leq .05$. CLES = Clinical Learning Environment Scale; PCSQ = Pagana Clinical Stress Questionnaire; SS = Self-Confidence Scale.

[a] Wilcoxon signed-rank test. [b] Paired-sample *t* test.

scores in the control group ($p < .05$). Thus, the hypothesis that preclinical simulation training affects clinical satisfaction in students was confirmed. However, contrary to expectation, the simulation training was found to negatively affect clinical satisfaction. Studies with similar objectives have determined that simulation-based learning methods facilitate students' learning and increased satisfaction (Kim-Godwin et al., 2013; Luctkar-Flude et al., 2012; Tosterud et al., 2013). In Turkey, nursing is a profession performed by individuals with various levels of education (from high school diploma to PhD degree) who work in clinics at similar pay grades and positions (Korkmaz, 2011). In undergraduate and higher levels of nursing education, students are given a modern and systematic education that incorporates evidence-based practices and current research results (Küçük et al., 2017). However, the education provided at the high school level in Turkey does not provide this content. Moreover, nurses trained to follow research and current evidence are currently in the minority in the clinical field (Demir et al., 2012). On the other hand, high school graduate nurses, who are numerous in the clinical field, practice nursing in line with the skills acquired during their high school education and typically do not adequately update their knowledge/skills after graduation. Therefore, students often do not observe what they have learned in theoretical courses during their practice in the clinic (Karadağ et al., 2013). The results of this study may reflect the fact that clinical settings in Turkey fall short of "ideal" laboratory conditions. Students in Turkey may not be able to find opportunities to practice what they have learned in the classroom in clinical settings, which represents a gap in expectation. On the other hand, the experimental group gained more preclinical practice, which may have increased their expectations and led to a larger gap in expectation in their clinical practice.

Lack of experience may increase the fear and anxiety of students in clinical settings (Öner Altıok & Üstün, 2013; Rhodes & Curran, 2005). In this study, simulation training was found to reduce stress in terms of both PCSQ total score and the threat, challenge, and harm subscale scores ($p < .05$). Simulation training has not made any difference only in terms of PCSQ benefit subscale scores ($p > .05$). In another, similar study, preclinical simulation-based education was found to reduce stress and anxiety by increasing student performance and self-confidence (Khalaila, 2014; Terzioğlu et al., 2012). The lack of difference in PCSQ benefit subscale scores may be because of the fact that students feel useful in any case during clinical practice (regardless of the skill level).

The use of simulation in nursing education provides experience-based learning, increases students' self-confidence, and develops clinical decision-making skills. Simulation training helps students provide full care in a safe setting without fear of failing or misunderstanding the current condition of a patient and gain various strengths (Kuznar, 2007; Robertson et al., 2010). Other publications have reported that simulation education increases students' self-confidence and helps them feel more confident in clinical settings (Gardner & Raemer, 2008; Schoening et al., 2006; Terzioğlu et al., 2012). In this study, SS posttest scores in the control group were statistically significantly higher than pretest scores ($p < .05$). However, the pretest–posttest difference on the SS was not significant for this group ($p > .05$). This result does not support the hypothesis in this study that preclinical simulation training affects self-confidence. Although not statistically significant, the experimental group had a higher mean self-confidence score at pretest than the control group (experimental group: 126.53 ± 13.28, control group: 124.58 ± 18.27). Besides, although the experimental group maintained their self-confidence level through posttest (pretest: 126.53 ± 13.28, posttest: 127.09 ± 14.36; $p = .621$), the control group increased their mean self-confidence score between pretest and posttest (pretest: 124.58 ± 18.27, posttest: 128.83 ± 17.11; $p = .012$). Therefore, scenario-based simulation education may have an indirect effect on self-confidence in nursing students.

Limitations

In this study, the simulation practice and clinical practice periods for students were limited by the scope of the existing curriculum. Moreover, only the effects of the scenario-based simulation on satisfaction, clinical stress, and self-confidence were examined. Furthermore, the participants completed the three measures (CLES satisfaction subscale, SS, and PCSQ) on the first and last day of clinical practice only.

Conclusions

Simulation-based education programs foster positive educational environments that allow students to learn by doing and experiencing as well as provide opportunities for repetitive practice. In this study, simulation training was found to reduce the clinical satisfaction and clinical stress of the participants but not to influence self-confidence. In light of these findings, it is recommended that simulation training accompanied by scenarios (pregnancy, childbirth, gestational diabetes, sexual violence, infertility, and endometrial cancer) be utilized in OB-GYN nursing education. Moreover, clinically appropriate simulation scenarios should be diversified, clinical settings should be rearranged to promote satisfaction and allow students to practice what they learned during simulation training, and the current study should be replicated with different sample groups. In addition, in future studies on this subject, the effects of scenario-based simulation training on staff–student relationships and on the structuring of responsibilities within instructor–patient relationships (both of which are known indicators of student satisfaction) should be evaluated. Finally, applying the instruments before and after administering the theoretical course is recommended.

Acknowledgments

This work supported by Gazi University Scientific Research Projects Unit (Grant Number 47/2015-01). The authors wish to thank all of the students who participated in this study.

Author Contributions

Study conception and design: All authors
Data collection: All authors
Data analysis and interpretation: All authors
Drafting of the article: MUA, SYS, SPA

References

Akın, A. (2007). The development and psychometric characteristics of the self-confidence scale. *Bolu Abant Izzet Baysal University Journal of Faculty Education, 7*(2), 167–176. (Original work published in Turkish)

Akyuz, A. (2011). *Innovative applications in nursing skills training.* Paper presented at the Clinical and Communication Skills and Trainings Congress in Health Sciences, Ankara, Turkey.

Cronenwett, L., Sherwood, G., Barnsteiner, J., Disch, J., Johnson, J., Mitchell, P., Sullivan, D. T., & Warren, J. (2007). Quality and safety education for nurses. *Nursing Outlook, 55,* 122–131. https://doi.org/10.1016/j.outlook.2007.02.006

Demir, Y., Ak, B., Bilgin, N. Ç., Efe, H., Albayrak, E., Çelikpençe, Z., & Güneri, N. (2012). Barriers and facilitating factors to research utilization in nursing practice. *Journal of Contemporary Medicine, 2*(2), 94–101. (Original work published in Turkish)

Dunn, S. V., & Burnett, P. (1995). The development of a clinical learning environment scale. *Journal of Advanced Nursing, 22*(6), 1166–1173. https://doi.org/10.1111/j.1365-2648.1995.tb03119.x

Eyikara, E., & Baykara, Z. G. (2018). Effect of simulation on the ability of first year nursing students to learn vital signs. *Nurse Education Today, 60,* 101–106. https://doi.org/10.1016/j.nedt.2017.09.023

Gardner, R., & Raemer, D. B. (2008). Simulation in obstetrics and gynecology. *Obstetrics and Gynecology Clinics of North America, 35,* 97–127. https://doi.org/10.1016/j.ogc.2007.12.008

Germain, M., O'Leary-Kelley, C., Goyal, D., & Anand, S. (2018). Can clinical simulation increase confidence levels in performing postpartum care in a diverse group of baccalaureate nursing students? *Nursing Education Perspectives, 39*(2), 94–95. https://doi.org/10.1097/01.NEP.0000000000000233

Işık, B., & Kaya, H. (2014). The effect of simulation software on learning of psychomotor skills and anxiety level in nursing education. *Procedia-Social and Behavioral Sciences, 116,* 3864–3868. https://doi.org/10.1016/j.sbspro.2014.01.856

Jeffries, P. R., Rodgers, B., & Adamson, K. (2015). NLN Jeffries simulation theory: Brief narrative description. *Nursing Education Perspectives, 36*(5), 292–293. https://doi.org/10.5480/1536-5026-36.5.292

Karadağ, G., Kılıç, S. P., Ovayolu, N., Ovayolu, Ö., & Kayaaslan, H. (2013). Difficulties encountered by nursing students in practices and their views about nurses. *TAF Preventive Medicine Bulletin, 12*(6), 665–672. (Original work published in Turkish)

Khalaila, R. (2014). Simulation in nursing education: An evaluation of students' outcomes at their first clinical practice combined with simulations. *Nurse Education Today, 34,* 252–258. https://doi.org/10.1016/j.nedt.2013.08.015

Kim-Godwin, Y. S., Livsey, K. R., Ezzell, D., Highsmith, C., Winslow, H., & Aikman, A. N. (2013). Students like peer evaluation during home visit simulation experiences. *Clinical Simulation in Nursing, 9*(11), e535–e542. https://doi.org/10.1016/j.ecns.2012.06.002

Korkmaz, Ö. G. (2011). Professionalism and nursing in Turkey. *Journal of Hacettepe University Faculty of Nursing, 18*(2), 59–67. (Original work published in Turkish)

Küçük, E. Ö., Çakmak, S., Kapucu, S., Meltem, K. O. C., & Kahveci, R. (2017). Determination of nursing students' awareness of evidence-based nursing practice. *Journal of Hacettepe University Faculty of Nursing, 4*(2), 1–12. (Original work published in Turkish)

Kuznar, K. A. (2007). Associate degree nursing students' perceptions of learning using a high-fidelity human patient simulator. *Teaching and Learning in Nursing, 2,* 46–52.

Labrague, L. J., McEnroe-Petitte, D. M., Bowling, A. M., Nwafor, C. E., & Tsaras, K. (2019). High-fidelity simulation and nursing students' anxiety and self-confidence: A systematic review. *Nursing Forum, 54*(3), 358–368. https://doi.org/10.1111/nuf.12337

Luctkar-Flude, M., Wilson-Keates, B., & Larocque, M. (2012). Evaluating high-fidelity human simulators and standardized patients in an undergraduate nursing health assessment course. *Nurse Education Today, 32*, 448–452. https://doi.org/10.1016/j.nedt.2011.04.011

Maas, N. A., & Flood, L. S. (2011). Implementing high fidelity simulation in practical nursing. *Clinical Simulation in Nursing, 7*, 229–235. https://doi.org/10.1016/j.nedt.2010.10.028

Mete, M., Gümüş, F., Zengin, L., Erkan, M., Arda Sürücü, H., Yiğitalp, G., Evinç, E., Duman, M., & Durgun Ozan, Y. (2017). Evaluation of the effect of simulation method applied in occupational ability laboratory on the students' ability to solve problems. *Jaren, 3*(2), 92–96. https://doi.org/10.5222/jaren.2017.092. (Original work published in Turkish)

Oh, P. J., Jeon, K. D., & Koh, M. S. (2015). The effects of simulation-based learning using standardized patients in nursing students: A meta-analysis. *Nurse Education Today, 35*(5), e6–e15. https://doi.org/10.1016/j.nedt.2015.01.019

Öner Altıok, H., & Üstün, B. (2013). The stress sources of nursing students. *Educational Sciences: Theory & Practice, 13*(2), 760–766.

Pagana, K. D. (1989). Psychometric evaluation of the clinical stress questionnaire (CSQ). *The Journal of Nursing Education, 28*(4), 169–174.

Pınar, G., Abay, H., & Akalın, A. (2016). The effect of scenario-based simulation training technology on knowledge and skills of maternity nursing students in Turkey. *International Journal of Development Research, 6*(6), 8096–8101.

Pınar, G., & Doğan, N. (2013). Improving perinatal patient safety among Turkish nursing students using simulation training. *Procedia - Social and Behavioral Sciences, 83*, 88–93. https://doi.org/10.1016/j.sbspro.2013.06.017

Pınar, G., Knight, C. C., Gaioso, V. P., Watts, P. I., Dailey, K. D., Britt, S. E., Catron, K. S., & Zengul, F. D. (2015). The effects of high fidelity simulation on nursing students' perceptions and self-efficacy of obstetric skills. *International Archives of Nursing and Health Care, 1*(1), 1–7. https://doi.org/10.1016/j.sbspro.2013.06.017

Rhodes, M. L., & Curran, C. (2005). Use of the human patient simulator to teach clinical judgment skills in a baccalaureate nursing program. *Computers, Informatics, Nursing, 23*(5), 256–262.

Robertson, B., Kaplan, B., Atallah, H., Higgins, M., Lewitt, M. J., & Ander, D. S. (2010). The use of simulation and a modified TeamSTEPPS curriculum for medical and nursing student team training. *Simulation in Healthcare, 5*(6), 332–337. https://doi.org/10.1097/SIH.0b013e3181f008ad

Sarı, D. (2001). *The evaluation of clinical learning environment of the students of the school of nursing* [Unpublished master's thesis]. T. R. Ege University. (Original work published in Turkish)

Schoening, A. M., Sittner, B. J., & Todd, M. J. (2006). Simulated clinical experience: Nursing students' perceptions and the educators' role. *Nurse Educator, 31*(6), 253–258. https://doi.org/10.1097/00006223-200611000-00008

Şendir, M. (2013). Use of simulation in women's health nursing education. *Florence Nightingale Journal of Nursing, 21*(3), 205–212. (Original work published in Turkish)

Şendir, M., & Acaroğlu, R. (2008). Reliability and validity of Turkish version of clinical stress questionnaire. *Nurse Education Today, 28*(6), 737–743.

Skrable, L., & Fitzsimons, V. (2014). Simulation in associate degree nursing education: A literature review. *Teaching and Learning in Nursing, 9*, 120–125. https://doi.org/10.1016/j.teln.2014.03.001

Smith, R., Gray, J., Raymond, J., Catling-Paull, C., & Homer, C. S. (2012). Simulated learning activities: Improving midwifery students' understanding of reflective practice. *Clinical Simulation in Nursing, 8*(9), e451–e457. https://doi.org/10.1016/j.ecns.2011.04.007

Terzioğlu, F., Kapucu, S., Ozdemir, L., Boztepe, H., Duygulu, S., Tuna, A. Z., & Akdemir, N. (2012). Nursing students' opinions about simulation method. *Hacettepe University Faculty of Health Sciences Nursing Journal, 19*(1), 16–23. (Original work published in Turkish)

Terzioğlu, F., Yücel, C., Koç, G., Şimşek, Ş., Yaşar, B. N., Şahan, F. U., Akın, R., Öçal, S. E., Akdağ, C., Elçin, M., Mert, M., & Yıldırım, S. (2016). A new strategy in nursing education: From hybrid simulation to clinical practice. *Nurse Education Today, 39*, 104–108. https://doi.org/10.1016/j.nedt.2016.01.009

Tosterud, R., Hedelin, B., & Hall-Lord, M. L. (2013). Nursing students' perceptions of high- and low-fidelity simulation used as learning methods. *Nurse Education in Practice, 13*(4), 262–270. https://doi.org/10.1016/j.nepr.2013.02.002

Woda, A., Hansen, J., Paquette, M., & Topp, R. (2017). The impact of simulation sequencing on perceived clinical decision making. *Nurse Education in Practice, 26*, 33–38. https://doi.org/10.1016/j.nepr.2017.06.008

World Health Organization. (2013). *WHO nursing and midwifery progress report 2008–2012.* http://www.who.int/hrh/nursing_midwifery/NursingMidwiferyProgressReport.pdf?ua=1

Yuan, H. B., Williams, B. A., Fang, J. B., & Ye, Q. H. (2012). A systematic review of selected evidence on improving knowledge and skills through high-fidelity simulation. *Nurse Education Today, 32*(3), 294–298. https://doi.org/10.1016/j.nedt.2011.07.010

15

An Evolutionary Route for the Moral Development of Nursing Students: A Constructivist Grounded Theory

Hadi RANJBAR[1] • Soodabeh JOOLAEE[2]* • Abouali VEDADHIR[3] • Abbass ABBASSZADEH[4]
Colleen BERNSTEIN[5]

ABSTRACT

Background: Developing moral competency is a main aim of educational systems, especially in healthcare-related disciplines.

Purpose: The aim of this study was to explore the moral development process in nursing students.

Methods: This study used a constructivist grounded theory. Twenty-five semistructured, face-to-face interview with 22 participants were conducted to gather the data. The participants were nursing students and educators attending three nursing schools in Tehran.

Results: Moral development evolves within nursing students following a stepwise progression. Within each step or phase, students experience specific changes with regard to both their practical skills and their moral capabilities and competencies. Three main steps were identified: moral transition, moral reconstruction, and moral internalization. Techno-scientific competence, biomedical competence, and nursing competence are developed in each step, respectively.

Conclusions/Implications for Practice: Moral competency in nursing students develops along with their competency as nursing practitioners. To facilitate progress through each phase, it needs to be ensured that the learning experiences that students are exposed to during each consecutive year of study facilitate as much as possible the development of moral competence.

Key Words:
students, nursing, moral development, education, ethics.

Introduction

Healthcare professionals face moral issues on a daily basis. Taking moral decisions is an integral part of their practice (Tsai & Harasym, 2010). Moral decision-making requires that the decision-maker considers both the ethical standards of their profession and of the society (Bužgová & Sikorová, 2013). Nurses are one of the most influential workers within the healthcare system. However, they are increasingly faced with ever more complicated situations as a result of rapid techno-scientific developments in the field of medicine (Nunes, Rego, & Nunes, 2015). Hence, becoming a nurse entails both acquisition of knowledge and learning advanced techno-scientific skills. Furthermore, becoming a nurse necessitates the acquisition of specific and highly advanced professional and ethical values (Thompson, Melia, & Boyd, 2006).

Moral development has been defined as "the development of our understanding of the rules and principles that distinguish right from wrong" (Coghill, 2009), as well as prosocial behaviors that align with social norms and conventions as defined by social learning theories. Within this perspective, observational learning, reinforcement, and punishment shape these prosocial behaviors. Moral competence is evidenced when an individual has acquired a level of knowledge, skills, and values that enables him or her to understand fully the choices and actions within situations in which moral decision-making is required. In addition, moral competence is evident when the individual is prepared to be held personally accountable for the decisions he or she has made (Høivik, 2002).

According to Kälvemark Sporrong, Arnetz, Hansson, Westerholm, and Höglund (2007), competence is defined simply as the knowledge and skills needed to carry out a specific task. Locsin and Purnell (2009) note that, "while the clinical competence is acquiring and using scientific knowledge and skill in the application of therapeutic interventions in practice, nursing competence refers to possessing the suitable skill, knowledge, and experience necessary to provide adequate nursing care" (p. 39). Laak, Heymans, and Podol'skij (2013) defined moral competence as "the highest stage of moral reasoning an individual is capable of, i.e., it reflects what according to an individual should be done ideally" (p. 237).

[1]PhD, RN, Assistant Professor, Mental Health Research Center, Iran University of Medical Sciences, Tehran, Iran • [2]PhD, RN, Associate Professor, Center for Nursing Care Research, School of Nursing & Midwifery, Iran University of Medical Sciences, and Iranian Academy of Medical Sciences, Tehran, Iran • [3]PhD, Associate Professor, Faculty of Social Sciences, Department of Anthropology, University of Tehran, Tehran, Iran • [4]PhD, RN, Professor, School of Nursing & Midwifery, Shahid Beheshti University of Medical Sciences, Tehran, Iran • [5]PhD, Lecturer, Department of Psychology, School of Human and Community Development, University of the Witwatersrand, Johannesburg, South Africa.

Furthermore, it has been noted that moral competence is a psychological skill and the ability to think and act in a way that is not constrained by moral fixations or automatic reactions (Kälvemark Sporrong et al., 2007). This perspective of competence is regarded to be the effective evaluation of events and the successful conduct of moral action (Kruger, 2012) and is a crucial set of competencies required for all nurses (Bartlett, 2013).

The development of these competencies, knowledge, skills, and values must be completed by the time nursing students graduate for them to function with efficacy in the complex and demanding healthcare system (Skisland, Bjørnestad, & Söderhamn, 2012). Nursing training facilities play a crucial role in the instillation of these skills within nursing students (Grace, Robinson, Jurchak, Zollfrank, & Lee, 2014).

Training facilities need to structure their curriculum so that these facilities enable graduates to face the ethical issues and challenges in the professional practice that they will surely encounter on a daily basis (Monteverde, 2014).

A study on the moral development of nursing students in Finland showed that nursing education may exert a beneficial effect on moral development (Auvinen, Suominen, Leino-Kilpi, & Helkama, 2004). However, despite these efforts, research is still required to determine "how" moral skills are developed during nursing training and "how" nursing education may be designed to optimally facilitate this development. Little published research within the field of nursing addresses these issues.

Yeom, Ahn, and Kim (2017) examined the effects of nursing ethics education on the moral sensitivity and critical thinking disposition of nursing students in Korea. Their results indicate a need for ongoing efforts to develop innovative content, structure, and instructional methods for undergraduate nursing ethics educational programs. A study of the relationships between academic classes and the moral sensitivity and reasoning of students showed associated more hours of ethics content with higher principled thinking scores among senior students (Park, Kjervik, Crandell, & Oermann, 2012).

Therefore, the purpose of this study was to explore the process of moral development in Iranian nursing students using a constructivist grounded theory methodology (GTM). Exploring and understanding the process of moral development within nursing students may facilitate the establishment of guidelines that enhance this development during the process of nursing education.

Methods

This study utilized a qualitative approach with a constructivist GTM. GTM uses qualitative inquiry to inform strategies and procedures for exploring how individuals construct meaning from their experiences (Charmaz, 2014). A constructivist GTM assumes the relativism of multiple social realities, recognizing the mutual creation of knowledge by the viewer and the viewed. Furthermore, it allows for an interpretive understanding of subjects' meanings (Charmaz, 2014).

Sample Characteristics

The study was conducted at three major nursing schools in Tehran, the capital of Iran. Initial sampling criteria were as follows: being enrolled as a nursing student in a bachelor degree program and having some experience within situations that require moral decision-making. We constructed tentative ideas after the first interviews and examined these ideas using empirical inquiry. Participants were chosen by purposeful sampling for the first interviews. Thereafter, new participants were recruited using theoretical sampling to elaborate and refine the theoretical categories. The inclusion criteria for nursing students were as follows: either being a student in a bachelor degree program or having graduated from this program within 6 months; having experience in moral decision-making, especially in clinical settings; and passing mandatory nursing ethics courses during their college education. The inclusion criteria for instructors were as follows: teaching nursing courses in school and clinical settings and having ethics course teaching experience. We used the emerging codes and categories and memos to select the next group of participants after each interview. For example, when we identified a relationship, we noted the possible relationship between ethical and professional competencies and attempted to find new participants who reflected the relevant professional and clinical skills.

Data Collection

To explore the understanding and lived experience of nursing students, we asked students (potential participants) about their decision-making in situations requiring moral judgment. The first author, a nursing instructor, interviewed these students in various clinical settings. Students with sufficient relevant decision-making experience and an interest in participating were recruited. Three nursing instructors were also interviewed to intensify data richness, as they had "lived experiences" as students, nurses, and teachers. Theoretical saturation was accomplished when no new properties of the theoretical category were emerging from the data (Charmaz, 2014).

In general, the constructivist GTM suggests using diverse methods to gather sufficiently rich data. Rich data get beneath the surface of social and subjective life by revealing participants' views, feelings, schemas, intentions, and actions as well as the contexts and structures of their lives (Charmaz, 2014). We drew on the intensive interview format as one of the main methods of gathering rich data in the constructivist GTM. This type of interview is a gently guided, one-sided conversation that explores a person's substantial experience with the research topic (Charmaz, 2014). The interview guide developed within this study, in line with the constructivist GTM, consisted of three parts: initial open-ended, intermediate, and ending questions.

The initial open-ended questions asked about the understanding and lived experiences of the participants, with questions like "Have you ever experienced being in a situation in which you were unsure whether what you were doing was right or wrong?" The interviewer followed with probing, intermediate questions such as "How did you manage the situation?", "What decision did you make? Did you ever question your decision?", "What was your reason for making the decision that you made?", "What or who influenced your decision making?", and "From whom did you learn?"

The main part of the interview guide was thus probing, intermediate questions, after which the interviewee identified a situation or situations in which he or she was faced with making a moral decision in practice. Ending questions such as "Is there something else you think I should know in order to understand (what you have just described to me) better?" were used to conclude the interviews.

The questions for nursing instructors related to their experience with the ethical decision-making of their students. We focused on situations in which the instructor had helped her students with moral decision-making, especially in clinical settings. Example questions include "Have you had the experience of helping students in moral situations?" and "What was the reason(s) for your commenting on a student's decision?"

In addition, memo-writing was used as an analytical tool as well as a data collection method (Charmaz, 2014). Interview guides were revised according to memos after analyzing each interview. Finally, after revisions, 25 in-depth, semistructured, face-to-face interviews with 22 participants were conducted from September 2013 to October 2014. Each interview lasted between 25 and 60 minutes. Interviewing continued until the redundancy of data was evident and theoretical saturation was achieved.

Data Analysis

The first author transcribed the interviews only after listening to each one several times. All of the gathered data and evidence were analyzed along the lines of the constructivist GTM. Coding within the constructivist GTM entails two phases: initial coding and focused coding. Initial coding was begun after the first interview. The codes were simple and used the lower level of abstraction. Thereafter, focused coding took place in which codes were selected according to their frequency and significance. The codes that were of higher frequency and higher importance formed the focus codes. The focus codes in constructivist grounded theory are very similar to the categories that shape the analysis process. Analytical memos emerged from the focus codes.

The researchers constantly compared data with data, codes with data, codes with codes, codes with categories, and categories with each other. In this manner, the researchers more precisely identified, compared, and coded incidents of moral decision-makings among nursing students within their first and last years of nursing study.

We used our focused codes as the title of our successive memos. Memos were used to shape concepts and their properties. We tried to develop our memos theoretically throughout this study, making them progressively more analytical. Sorting memos in line with their importance in the process of theorizing was made during several research team meetings. The relationship between concepts was made clear by diagramming tools. All of these procedures were carried out to explore how and why Iranian nursing students construct meanings and actions in morally involved situations. The process of data analysis is presented in Figure 1.

Permission to carry out this study was obtained from the Tehran University of Medical Sciences Committee for Medical Research Ethics (Ref. 92/D/130/1781). The scholars who were involved in this study obtained permission from all of the participants to formally perform and audiotape the interviews. The confidentiality of information was guaranteed, as participants were informed that no one other than the researchers would have access to their interview data and that neither their names nor any personally identifying demographic information would be used in the published research findings. All of the participants gave written informed consent for their participation and for the audiotaping of their interviews.

To ensure the rigor and validity of the findings, the criteria outlined and asserted by Charmaz (2014) was followed; that is, this work was guided by the principles of credibility, originality, resonance, and usefulness. The credibility of research results was enhanced by focusing on the lived experience of nursing students with moral dilemmas. Analysis of in-depth interviews and observations allowed us to define the experiences of the participants as closely as possible. The findings were developed as an understanding of how nursing students develop their moral competencies rather than as an empirical truth. In this view, the emerged theory is substantive rather than formal. The results that are provided below offer detailed descriptions of these understandings. Furthermore, these results represent the processes that constructed these understandings. This study was used as a doctoral dissertation. The coding process was conducted under the direction of the lead researcher's supervisor and advisors. Regular meetings with the research team were conducted. The research team read all interviews and codes. They supervised the entire process of data analysis. After the coding of each interview, new codes were checked with the interviewee. The final categories and the model were also presented to three of the participants to canvass their thoughts and ideas regarding the results.

Results

Twenty-two participants were interviewed (19 students and 3 instructors of nursing). The mean ± *SD* age was 21.68 ±

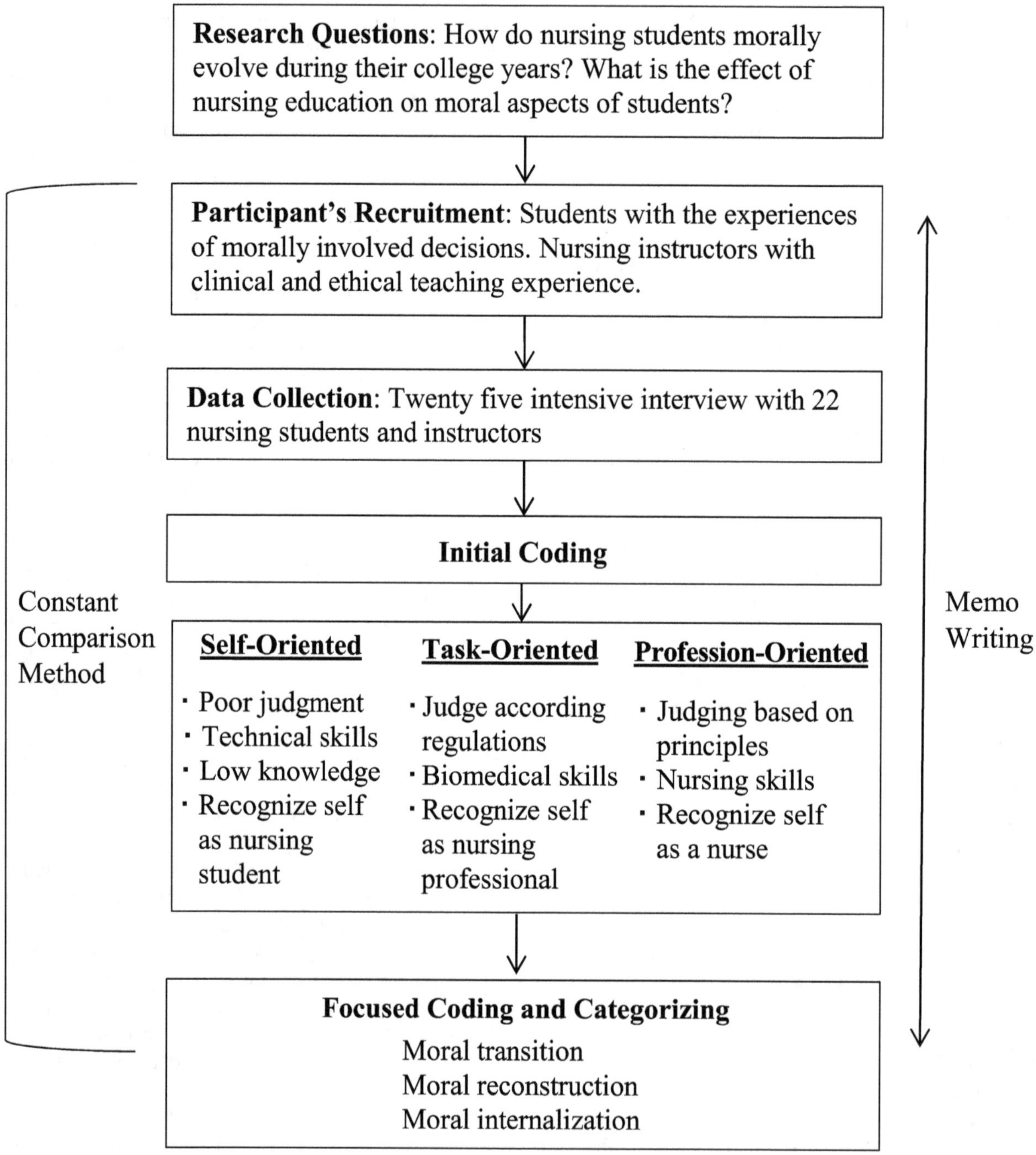

Figure 1. Analysis process for coding and category development.

3.00 years for nursing students and 43.00 ± 4.35 years for instructors. All of the nursing instructors and 8 (43%) of the nursing students were female. Participants included students in each of the four years of nursing study. All of the three instructors were fully experienced in teaching the theoretical and clinical courses of nursing across these 4 years of study. The results are presented in Figure 2 as a pyramid model.

Our initial interpretation was that the development of moral competencies of students occurred in conjunction with changes in practical capabilities. We provide a model to show the co-development of practical and moral competencies in nursing education. This model has three phases. To achieve higher levels of these competencies, the students are required to pass through the phases of development of these competencies at the lower levels. However, it is important to note that not all students will necessarily fully attain the highest, that is, the third phase of, development, as this attainment is in part a function of their inherent abilities and values. The three main phases of this evolutionary route were defined as follows: techno-scientific competence and moral transition, biomedical competence and

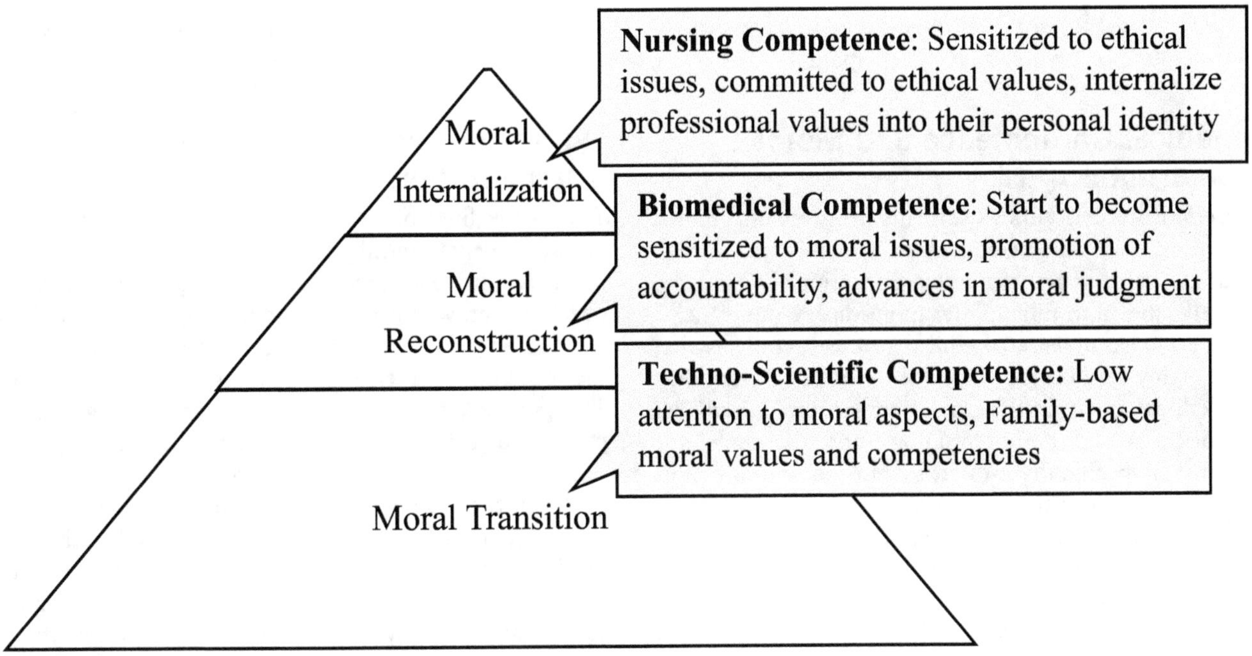

Figure 2. The pyramid of moral development.

moral reconstruction, and nursing competence and moral internalization (see Figure 2).

Techno-Scientific Competence and Moral Transition

New nursing students used their preconceived values and competencies in this phase, reflecting low sensitivity to the moral aspects of their actions. The values that the participants used were derived primarily from family and society and differed from the values and competencies that are used by nurses in the professional environment.

> *My mom told me to be smart and that if anything happens you should think of yourself, so I freaked and I did not tell my teacher about the incident.* (Participant 3)

There is evidence of two substeps within the first stage of development. The first step is gaining techno-scientific competence, and the second step is gaining awareness of ethical issues.

In the first part of this stage, this study found evidence of the growth of techno-scientific competency. As students entered into their first year and gained exposure to clinical practice, they began acquiring techno-scientific practical and technical skills. The main focus is essentially on acquiring these skills, with students holding in high regard those who evidence these skills. At this stage, students are motivated to accomplish these skills, which they see modeled by both their educators and their peers. From the student's perspective, at this stage, the highest level of attainment is to gain mastery of these skills and to be able to perform them competently and with ease. As one of the participants expressed:

> *At the time (when we first entered into clinical practice), we did not know how to do procedures. When someone could do something like IV catheterization or intubation or stitching, we were in awe of them. I think they (individuals with these skills) and our instructors were our models in the first semester…. Those who (were able teach or to quickly) learn these skills were (held in high regard).* (Participant 6)

At this early stage or step of this phase, no significant changes took place in the moral competencies of participants. Concentration focused solely on mastering procedures, with little consideration of the humanity of the subjects on which they are performing the procedures. Little attention was paid to the possible moral aspects of the decisions they were taking, and their ethical skills and competencies were not sufficiently developed. In this regard, one participant noted:

> *I paid more attention to doing the procedures correctly, I mean like giving the drugs according to the exact dosages specified. When I realized that I had made an error in administering medication, I was afraid, and, instead of reporting the error, I just wanted to pretend it did not happen and be done with the mistake I had made. I knew that if I reported the error, it would get me in trouble, so I*

> *still chose not to, not questioning the "rightness or wrongness" of my decision.* (Participant 12)

Biomedical Competence and Moral Reconstruction

This second phase occurs as students progress into higher levels within their nursing education, which is within their second and third years of nursing education. During this period, they begin to fully master biomedical competencies, and there is also a sense of ethical reconstruction as they become highly cognizant of their role as both a practitioner and an ethical agent. In this stage, they acquire knowledge about diseases and pathophysiology and the signs and symptoms of specific diseases. They also become far more knowledgeable about the drugs utilized in relation to these disease and their potential side effects.

Throughout this phase, the awareness of nursing students of discipline undergoes an extensive transition as they realize that nursing is not merely a constellation of techno-scientific procedures and that ethics within practice is of fundamental and equal importance. Eager to enhance both their biomedical knowledge and clinical skills, students aspire to be more like nurses who are so knowledgeable that they have imbued themselves with skills often ascribed only to physicians. Some nursing students expressed an even greater interest in going beyond the prescribed biomedical and ethical skills, desiring to acquire knowledge that is traditionally the preserve of physicians. In this regard, a participant noted:

> *Nursing is not simply cannulation or writing a nursing report. You should act like a physician. You should diagnose the patient problem. You should know the physical examination and drugs as well.* (Participant 7)

Thus, some of the students choose nurses who are more "like" physicians as their role model. There is also greater evidence of accountability as compared with the first stage of "Techno-scientific Competence and Moral Transition." The greater their experience and exposure to clinical knowledge, the greater the evidence of their increased accountability. A participant remembered her first experience this way:

> *I reported it quickly as I knew that the 100 IU of insulin (administered?) is much stronger than 10 IU. I called the ward several times that night. I was extremely concerned, as I knew it was my responsibility.* (Participant 14)

The participants exhibited greater sensitivity to moral issues and greater accountability for their actions in this phase. Involvement in moral decision-making improved their moral judgment abilities.

> *I think more about the consequences of my work. I think I am responsible here.* (Participant 21)

Nursing Competence and Moral Internalization

This is the final phase or step in development. Although not all students typically fully accomplish this stage, within this study, it was evident that most did attain this stage of development, whereas a few did not. For those who did not, it was apparent that they were only interested in learning the procedures prescribed within their university education. Thus, these participants were only interested in attaining the prescribed minimum with regard to their knowledge and skills. For those who did fully accomplish this stage, it was apparent that they wanted to acquire knowledge that went beyond that prescribed within their nursing education. These participants expressly indicated a desire to gain a greater and more precise understanding of nursing and its disciplinary culture and acknowledged that nursing requires that one goes above and beyond the minimum of one's prescribed duties. This subset of participants realized that nursing is more than simply the administration of medication and the application of procedures and involves striving toward the ultimate development of their identity as a professional nurse. They showed a strong commitment to internalize each and every aspect of the professional values and the ethos of nursing into their personal identity and indicated that they remained continually cognizant of their role as a nurse at all times. As one participant noted:

> *Nursing is more than medication or even curing patients. It has principles that you should always bear in mind.* (Participant 18)

Students or nurses, who have accomplished the required professional competence within this phase, are fully sensitized to ethical issues and dilemmas in the field. Their moral judgments are fully honed as a result of the knowledge that they have acquired during their university training and/or during their work experience, and there is evidence that they are committed to ethical issues and patient rights that go beyond their individual interests or organization benefits. As one participant claimed:

> *The nurses did not dress the wounds properly. Because of congestion in the wards and nursing staff shortages, they did not take vital signs correctly. I appealed to them many times and even, reported their behavior to the head nurse and the nursing office. When I saw that nothing was done, I did not want to work in this ward.* (Participant 11)

Thus, this particular individual had such a strong sense of internalized moral values that he indicated that he would rather not work in a neglectful environment.

It was also apparent that nurses or students who accomplished this phase internalized the professional values of nursing in their personal and family lives, evidenced by the way that participants extended the caring role of the nurse into their personal lives, where they cared about those around them with similar levels of concern and professionalism. One participant who was a nursing instructor made this observation:

> *Students who are interested in nursing and are successful.... If you look at their personal life, there is evidence that "the nurse" is always there. I always use my nursing skills in my daily life. Being a nurse is as intrinsic to me as being a woman. That is how important (my nursing is) to me.* (Participant 19)

Some senior nursing students know themselves as a nurse. They feel highly committed to professional values and even use professional values in their personal life. They have higher levels of moral values and competencies, which are requisites in their professional work.

> *I am a nurse now, I think it is very important to me. I use a lot of things that I learned from nursing. As a nurse, I use them in my life.* (Participant 22)

The participants gained greater ethical competence as they grew their skills as nurses. They described learning ethical codes and became skilled with new nursing experiences. As one of the participants said:

> *Each time I faced a moral decision, I thought I had more skills in ethical decision making. When I recall my first days of clinical practice, I think about my decisions, especially ethical ones. My decisions were very simple. During these years, by making decisions and by using my instructors advice, I learned to make suitable decisions.* (Participant 21)

The Role of Nursing Instructors

Nursing instructors have two evident roles in the development of nursing students. Along with their providing a role model in clinical practice, they help students make ethical decisions by providing support in the educational process. The participants expressed that their instructors taking a supportive attitude toward students positively affects and expedites the moral development of students.

> *Our instructor's attitude had a very special effect. She was very ethical herself and she stood behind me after I uncovered my drug mistake. It helped me make a new decision based on my conscience.* (Participant 15)

Discussion

This study extended the existing body of knowledge by exploring the unfolding of moral development within nursing students undergoing nursing education in Iran and by elucidating that this unfolding is intrinsically interlinked with their learning of both clinical and practical competencies. The developed model is based on an interpretation of the interactions between the research team and the participants. Findings enabled us to build a simple, applicable, and comprehensive model with three phases. In this evolutionary model, the process of moral development follows a linear progression, with students unable to attain the highest levels of development without progressing through each of the prior phases in succession.

In comparing our model with that of others in the literature, it is evident that, although attaining clinical competence was taken into consideration within several studies and within a number of models across different settings, the steps that were described in the prior models differ from those described in this study. For instance, the novice to expert model, developed by Benner, Tanner, and Chesla (2009), is one of the most prominent models of competency development in nursing. The novice to expert model uses five stages to describe and interpret skill acquisition and clinical judgment in nursing practice and education (Benner et al., 2009).

This study presents an evolutionary model that reflects our interpretation of the data. The data were derived from our interviews and interactions with participants. With this model, we explained the relationship between the development of moral competencies with the "meanings" of practical nursing, which participants derived from their experience. This attained meaning is of great importance as it does play a role in determining whether students complete their education and whether they remain in the nursing profession (Jalal, Hajibabaee, Farahaninia, Joolaee, & Hosseini, 2014). A possible relationship has also been identified between moral development and the formation of nursing students' professional identity (Ranjbar, Joolaee, Vedadhir, Abbaszadeh, & Bernstein, 2017).

From our interpretation of the data derived from first-year students, it was apparent that their development was in the earliest phase of moral transition. During this early phase, students lack sufficient knowledge about nursing. They may know of the nursing profession, but this knowledge does not result from direct experience. As Tayebi, Dehghan-Nayeri, Negarandeh, and Shahbazi (2013) observed, nursing students in Iran have poor knowledge about nursing at the commencement of their academic life. The results of other studies also show that students have limited knowledge about nursing, which is not a consequence of their academic experience (Miligi & Selim, 2014; Poreddi, Ramachandra, Konduru, & Math, 2012; Sharpless et al., 2015). Their first encounter with the nursing profession focuses on the learning of technical skills. As a result, during this phase, nursing students perceive the profession as a series of procedures.

From this perspective, the meaning of nursing for students is a set of techno-scientific skills and procedures, with a nurse being a person who is able to perform these procedures successfully. This phase is analogous to the "novice" and "advanced beginner" in Benner et al.'s model. As Benner et al. (2009) explained, novices have no experiential background to base their approach to or understanding of a clinical situation. Skills for a range of medical and nursing interventions on particular patients will be new. Clinical situations are perceived by advanced beginners as a set of tasks that must be accomplished.

Thus, although students have moral values, these values are derived from their prenursing life experiences. Similarly, the model that was developed in this study notes that moral competencies of students in the first phase are the ones that they entered with into nursing school. Personal knowledge and attributes that are derived from their family and life experiences are used in their moral decision-making. Students at this phase, which coincides with their first year of study, lack familiarity with the clinical environment and their professional role. At this time, they are under immense pressure to master techno-scientific competencies and do not as yet realize the importance of making morally appropriate and professional decisions (Sharif & Masoumi, 2005). However, as mentioned, this phase contains two steps. Thus, as nursing students master techno-scientific skills (Step 1), they gain awareness of their need to exercise the moral competencies that are aligned with their professional role (Step 2). Consequently, in this first phase, students gradually move on to realize that their moral knowledge and skills are not sufficient to solve multiple dilemmas in the nursing practice, which leads to a moral transition that leads to the second phase of moral reconstruction.

In this second phase, which coincides with students' second to third years of study, nursing students enter the world of biomedical knowledge. Here, they learn about diseases, about disease-related pathophysiology and treatments, and about drugs and their effects. The new knowledge and the broad viewpoints introduced in this phase change student attitudes toward nursing. The dominant aspect of this phase is the focus on biomedical knowledge. The students are in the competent and proficient steps of Benner et al.'s theory. As Benner et al. described, the focus is now more on clinical issues (i.e., the clinical condition and management of the patient) and less on organizing and completing tasks. Proficiency is a transition stage because, once the nurse begins to see changing relevance, a current clinical situation may be seen in terms of a past clinical situation, complete with all its sense of salience, thus enabling a higher level of skill for perception (Benner et al., 2009).

Our interpretation of data revealed that the meaning of nursing as a profession changed for the participants during their process of education. Toward the end, they paid greater attention to the scientific aspect of nursing rather than the technical aspect. They had also paid more attention to the moral aspect of their works as they gathered further knowledge about the consequences of their decisions and actions.

The third phase was moral internalization, when students or nurses develop new professional competencies. We used current professional nurses as the participants for this phase, as most students do not reach this phase. Working as a nurse is a requisite of this phase. This phase is compatible with the expert stage in Benner et al.'s model. She explained the moral competency of nurses in this phase as follows: "The moral agency of the nurse practicing at the expert level is also a strong recurring theme. Central to expert practice is a concern for revealing and responding to patients as persons; respecting their dignity; caring for them in ways that preserve their personhood; protecting them in their vulnerability; helping them feel safe in a somewhat alien environment; and comforting their family, striving to preserve the integrity of close relationships" (Benner et al., 2009).

Nursing students or nurses reach a level of competency in this phase so that they are able to apply the existing knowledge and skills to new situations. They use their moral knowledge and skills to address and manage new moral issues in the workplace. In addition, they use their competencies in their personal life. In this view, the moral skills and competencies become personal traits. This has been considered by moral experts as an important role of education (Eriksson, Helgesson, & Höglund, 2007).

There are another two notable works in the field of moral competency development among Iranian nurses. Memarian, Salsali, Vanaki, Ahmadi, and Hajizadeh (2007) and Vanaki and Memarian (2009) showed a relationship between moral and clinical competencies. Furthermore, they concluded that nurses with moral competence have greater clinical competence. In line with these studies, this study observed that clinical and moral competencies are not detached but rather developed in concert with one another. They are neither the result nor the cause of each other. Both moral and clinical skills are developed in conjunction with one another, with increasing academic knowledge exposing students to the experience of ever new and challenging moral situations.

Nursing teachers' experiences from the field and from moral education focused more on the decisions of students. They recalled how their students handle moral issues and the decisions that these students ultimately made. They also used examples of prior experiences to teach their students. Nursing students used their own experiences as well as the experiences of their peers and teachers. Moral education, as mentioned in previous studies, plays a positive role in the development of moral competence (Park et al., 2012; Yeom et al., 2017).

Conclusions

The main aim of this study was to examine the development of moral competencies during the 4-year education of nursing students. Findings indicate a co-creation and co-evolution of moral and clinical competencies within nursing students that unfold in phases over time.

Three phases were evidenced and described. It is apparent that students cannot acquire higher levels of competence without having undergone progressive levels of training and exposure earlier in their nursing education. Their level of moral competencies evolves in co-creation with academic knowledge as their exposure and theoretical knowledge advances and they are increasingly exposed to clinical practice. It is therefore important to ensure that curricula contain the appropriate content for each level to facilitate the exposure of students to practical situations that will enhance their moral competencies. The model provided in this study may be utilized by educational program developers and nursing instructors in the future to guide students through a learning experience that enables and co-develops clinical and moral competencies.

The main limitation of this study is that it focused on the nursing students of three nursing schools in Tehran, Iran. However, academic education and professional life are the most important phases in this process. We tried to explain the higher level of ethical development by interviewing nursing instructors. They had the lived experiences of being a student, nurse, and teacher. Further study is recommended to examine the transition in ethical competence from early nursing education through the commencement of professional nursing work.

The developers of educational curricula and nursing instructors may use and validate the developed model in their future works, as this study provides rich information about the various levels of ethical development. They may also design and employ appropriate content and methods in ethics education for each level. This study may further be used as a base to assess the co-development of clinical and ethical competencies.

Acknowledgments

This was a doctoral dissertation funded by Tehran University of Medical Sciences. The authors would like to acknowledge all of those who cooperated on this research project. Furthermore, the authors also thank Tehran University of Medical Sciences for their coordination and financial support.

References

Auvinen, J., Suominen, T., Leino-Kilpi, H., & Helkama, K. (2004). The development of moral judgment during nursing education in Finland. *Nurse Education Today, 24*(7), 538–546. doi:10.1016/j.nedt.2004.07.005

Bartlett, J. L. (2013). *Developing ethical competence: The perspective of nurse educators from pre-licensure baccalaureate nursing programs accredited by the Commission on Collegiate Nursing Education* (Doctoral dissertation). University of Nevada, Las Vegas, USA.

Benner, P. E., Tanner, C. A., & Chesla, C. A. (2009). *Expertise in nursing practice: Caring, clinical judgment, and ethics* (2nd ed.). New York, NY: Springer.

Bužgová, R., & Sikorová, L. (2013). Moral judgment competence of nursing students in the Czech Republic. *Nurse Education Today, 33*(10), 1201–1206. doi:10.1016/j.nedt.2012.06.016

Charmaz, K. (2014). *Constructing grounded theory* (2nd ed.). London, UK: Sage Publications.

Coghill, D. (2009). *Child and adolescent psychiatry.* Oxford, UK: Oxford University Press.

Eriksson, S., Helgesson, G., & Höglund, A. T. (2007). Being, doing, and knowing: Developing ethical competence in health care. *Journal of Academic Ethics, 5*(2), 207–216. doi:10.1007/s10805-007-9029-5

Grace, P. J., Robinson, E. M., Jurchak, M., Zollfrank, A. A., & Lee, S. M. (2014). Clinical ethics residency for nurses: An education model to decrease moral distress and strengthen nurse retention in acute care. *The Journal of Nursing Administration, 44*(12), 640–646. doi:10.1097/NNA.0000000000000141

Høivik, H. v. W. (2002). *Moral leadership in action: Building and sustaining moral competence in European organizations* (1st ed.). Cheltenham, UK: Edward Elgar.

Jalal, E. J., Hajibabaee, F., Farahaninia, M., Joolaee, S., & Hosseini, F. (2014). Relationship between job satisfaction, absence from work and turnover among nurses. *Journal of Nursing and Midwifery Sciences, 1*(1), 12–18. doi:10.18869/acadpub.jnms.1.1.12

Kälvemark Sporrong, S., Arnetz, B., Hansson, M. G., Westerholm, P., & Höglund, A. T. (2007). Developing ethical competence in health care organizations. *Nursing Ethics, 14*(6), 825–837. doi:10.1177/0969733007082142

Kruger, T. (2012). *Moral intelligence: The construct and key correlates* (Master's thesis). University of Johannesburg, Johannesburg, South Africa.

Laak, J. J. F., Heymans, P. G., & Podol'skij, A. I. (2013). *Developmental tasks: Towards a cultural analysis of human development.* Houten, The Netherlands: Springer.

Locsin, R. C., & Purnell, M. (2009). *A contemporary nursing process: The (un) bearable weight of knowing in nursing.* New York, NY: Springer.

Memarian, R., Salsali, M., Vanaki, Z., Ahmadi, F., & Hajizadeh, E. (2007). Professional ethics as an important factor in clinical competency in nursing. *Nursing Ethics, 14*(2), 203–214. doi:10.1177/0969733007073715

Miligi, E., & Selim, A. (2014). Saudi nursing students' attitudes towards the nursing profession. *European Journal of Business and Management, 6*(29), 197–208.

Monteverde, S. (2014). Undergraduate healthcare ethics education, moral resilience, and the role of ethical theories. *Nursing Ethics, 21*(4), 385–401. doi:10.1177/0969733013505308

Nunes, S., Rego, G., & Nunes, R. (2015). The impact of economic recession on health-care and the contribution by nurses to promote individuals' dignity. *Nursing Inquiry, 22*(4), 285–295. doi:10.1111/nin.12100

Park, M., Kjervik, D., Crandell, J., & Oermann, M. H. (2012). The relationship of ethics education to moral sensitivity and moral reasoning skills of nursing students. *Nursing Ethics, 19*(4), 568–580. doi:10.1177/0969733011433922

Poreddi, V., Ramachandra, Konduru, R., & Math, S. B. (2012). Assessing the attitudes and perceptions towards nursing profession among nursing students. *The Nursing Journal of India, 103*(1), 6–8.

Ranjbar, H., Joolaee, S., Vedadhir, A., Abbaszadeh, A., & Bernstein, C. (2017). Becoming a nurse as a moral journey: A constructivist grounded theory. *Nursing Ethics, 24*(5), 583–597. doi:10.1177/0969733015620940

Sharif, F., & Masoumi, S. (2005). A qualitative study of nursing student experiences of clinical practice. *BMC Nursing, 4*, 6. doi:10.1186/1472-6955-4-6

Sharpless, J., Baldwin, N., Cook, R., Kofman, A., Morley-Fletcher, A., Slotkin, R., & Wald, H. S. (2015). The becoming: Students' reflections on the process of professional identity formation in medical education. *Academic Medicine, 90*(6), 713–717. doi:10.1097/ACM.0000000000000729

Skisland, A., Bjørnestad, J. O., & Söderhamn, O. (2012). Construction and testing of the Moral Development Scale for Professionals (MDSP). *Nurse Education Today, 32*(3), 255–260. doi:10.1016/j.nedt.2011.04.002

Tayebi, Z., Dehghan-Nayeri, N., Negarandeh, R., & Shahbazi, S. (2013). Motives for entering nursing in Iran: A qualitative study. *Iranian Journal of Nursing and Midwifery Research, 18*(1), 59–64.

Thompson, L., Melia, K., & Boyd, K. (2006). *Nursing ethics* (4th ed.). Edinburg, UK: Churchill Livingstone.

Tsai, T. C., & Harasym, P. H. (2010). A medical ethical reasoning model and its contributions to medical education. *Medical Education, 44*(9), 864–873. doi:10.1111/j.1365-2923.2010.03722.x

Vanaki, Z., & Memarian, R. (2009). Professional ethics: Beyond the clinical competency. *Journal of Professional Nursing, 25*(5), 285–291. doi:10.1016/j.profnurs.2009.01.009

Yeom, H. A., Ahn, S. H., & Kim, S. J. (2017). Effects of ethics education on moral sensitivity of nursing students. *Nursing Ethics, 24*(6), 644–652. doi:10.1177/0969733015622060

16

Reliability and Validity of the Turkish Version of the Job Performance Scale Instrument

Arzu Kader Harmanci Seren[1] • Rujnan Tuna[2]* • Feride Eskin Bacaksiz[3]

ABSTRACT

Background: Objective measurement of the job performance of nursing staff using valid and reliable instruments is important in the evaluation of healthcare quality. A current, valid, and reliable instrument that specifically measures the performance of nurses is required for this purpose.

Purpose: The aim of this study was to determine the validity and reliability of the Turkish version of the Job Performance Instrument.

Methods: This study used a methodological design and a sample of 240 nurses working at different units in four hospitals in Istanbul, Turkey. A descriptive data form, the Job Performance Scale, and the Employee Performance Scale were used to collect data. Data were analyzed using IBM SPSS Statistics Version 21.0 and LISREL Version 8.51.

Results: On the basis of the data analysis, the instrument was revised. Some items were deleted, and subscales were combined.

Conclusions/Implications for Practice: The Turkish version of the Job Performance Instrument was determined to be valid and reliable to measure the performance of nurses. The instrument is suitable for evaluating current nursing roles.

Key Words:
contextual performance, job performance, nurses, reliability and validity, task performance.

Introduction

Nursing care affects the quality of healthcare that is provided to patients in the acute care setting. Technical knowledge and skills, experience, educational level, and efficiency of service provision, that is, nursing "performance," play a very important role in achieving desired healthcare outcomes (Whyte, Lugton, & Fawcett, 2000).

Healthcare services are complex and provided by a multidisciplinary team. Nurses play critical roles within a patient care team in terms of both their number and the services that they provide. Nurses spend most of their time with patients and their relatives and affect health outcomes directly through nursing care (DeLucia, Ott, & Palmieri, 2009; Larrabee et al., 2004; Pappas, 2008). To realize this positive effect and achieve expected outcomes, nurses should perform competently, and managers should evaluate their performance (Behrenbeck, Timm, Griebenow, & Demmer, 2005; Gregg, 2002).

The job performance of nurses is a multidimensional concept (Bakker, Demerouti, & Euwema, 2005; Coleman & Borman, 2000; Griffin, Neal, & Parker, 2007). In academic studies, nurse performance is usually approached as two components, namely, task performance and contextual performance (Bakker et al., 2005; Borman & Motowidlo, 1993; Coleman & Borman, 2000). Task performance includes the roles of employees within an organization in terms of their main jobs and tasks (Coleman & Borman, 2000) and activities that support the main functions of healthcare institutions (mostly hospitals) and contribute to the achievement of primary targets, with their content usually revealed through business analyses (Borman & Motowidlo, 1993). The second component, contextual performance, is stated as an employee's willingness to help colleagues, ability to achieve collaboratively, and willingness to exert extra effort to complete the work (Coleman & Borman, 2000).

Although nurse performance has a significant impact on the delivery of qualified healthcare services, only a few instruments have been developed for use in this field. The most commonly known are the "Schwirian Six-D Scale" (Schwirian, 1978) and the "Slater Nursing Competencies Rating Scale" (Wandelt & Stewart Slater, 1975). Both were developed in the 1960s and 1970s (Redfern & Norman, 1990; Wandelt & Phaneuf, 1972). These instruments have largely met the need to evaluate nurse performance for many years. However, the role of nurses within the health system today has expanded, the delivery of qualified healthcare services continues to grow in importance, and new concepts such as the satisfaction with and expectations of patients and healthy individuals regarding healthcare services have come into play. Evaluation of the performance levels of nurses who play main roles in the delivery of healthcare services is of critical importance. In light of all these developments and changes, new methods and instruments to evaluate the job performance of nurses are required (Hamilton et al., 2007; Pelletier et al., 2000). Although healthcare institutions have their own performance scales to conduct this evaluation, there is no valid and reliable performance scale for measuring the performance of nurses in Turkey.

[1]PhD, RN, Assistant Professor, Florence Nightingale Faculty of Nursing, Department of Nursing Administration, Istanbul University, Istanbul, Turkey • [2]PhD, RN, Research Assistant, Faculty of Health Sciences, Department of Nursing, Istanbul Medeniyet University, Istanbul, Turkey • [3]PhD, RN, Research Assistant, Florence Nightingale Faculty of Nursing, Department of Nursing, Administration, Istanbul University, Istanbul, Turkey.

In this study, all of the abovementioned scales that had been developed for the purpose of measuring nurses' performance were evaluated in terms of their validity and reliability. The Turkish adaptation of the scale that was developed by Greenslade and Jimmieson (2007) was preferred, as it was developed after 2000 and seemed to more effectively address the concepts currently used in the field of nursing care.

Methods

Design

A cross-sectional and methodological study design was used for the purposes of adapting the Job Performance Scale (JPS) into Turkish and evaluating its psychometric properties.

Sample

The sample consisted of 240 volunteers, all of whom were nurses working at four hospitals (a public hospital, a public university hospital, a private hospital, and a private university hospital) in Istanbul, Turkey.

Data Collection

Data were collected at the hospitals between March and June 2015. A descriptive data collection form, the JPS, and the Employee Performance Scale (EPS), which was used to show criterion validity, were used for data collection.

Descriptive data collection form

This form consists of seven questions regarding the respondent's age, gender, educational level, unit position, and tenure both in the hospital and the nursing profession.

Job Performance Scale

The original version of the JPS, developed by Greenslade and Jimmieson (2007), was based on the job performance model of Borman and Motowidlo (1993) and intended to measure the performance of nurses. Greenslade and Jimmieson aimed to develop a performance scale to be used on nurses and based it on a structure that approached the job performance concept of Borman and Motowidlo as two different domains: task performance and contextual performance. In the JPS, task performance is an aspect of performance that directly contributes to the organization's technical competence and is related to the employee's work, whereas contextual performance is examined as a performance aspect that expands the organization's social environment and impact and includes the employee's voluntary behaviors (Borman & Motowidlo, 1993). The original scale for which the authors determined the items according to focus group interviews consists of two subscales. The first of these subscales is the Task Performance Scale (TPS), and the second is the Contextual Performance Scale (CPS). The TPS consists of the four subscales of information (seven items), coordination of care (five items), social support (six items), and technical care (five items), respectively, with a total of 23 items. The Cronbach's alpha internal consistency coefficients of this scale and its subscales vary between .85 and .94. The CPS consists of the four subscales of interpersonal support (six items), job task support (six items), compliance (three items), and volunteering for additional duties (four items), respectively, with a total of 18 items. The Cronbach's alpha internal consistency coefficients of the scale and its subscales vary between .80 and .90. For this scale, which was developed as a 7-point Likert-type scale, each statement is scored between 1 and 7 points, with a higher item total mean score associated with better performance on that item (Greenslade & Jimmieson, 2007).

Employee Performance Scale

The EPS, which is widely used to assess criterion validity, was developed by Erdoğan (2011). The employee performance subscale consists of seven items, and the Cronbach's alpha for the EPS was .94 in the current study. Statements in the 5-point Likert-type scale are scored on a spectrum between "absolutely disagree" (1 point) and "absolutely agree" (5 points), with higher total mean scores for an item associated with better performance on that item.

Procedures

No universal agreement exists regarding adaptation of an instrument for use in a different cultural setting (Gjersing, Caplehorn, & Clausen, 2010). Different numbers of similar steps in terms of context have been suggested for scale adaptation studies (Borsa, Damásio, & Bandeira, 2012; Gjersing et al., 2010). This study adopted the steps that were suggested by Gjersing et al. (2010) for scale adaptation studies (Table 1).

Data Analysis

The obtained data were analyzed using IBM SPSS Statistics Version 21 (IBM Inc., Armonk, NY, USA) and LISREL Version 8.51 (Scientific Software International, Skokie, IL, USA). Descriptive statistics (number, percentage, mean, standard deviation), correlations (Pearson product–moment correlation), and psychometric tests (content validity ratio, item–total correlation, Kaiser–Meyer–Olkin [KMO] measure of adequacy and Bartlett's test of sphericity, exploratory factor analysis [EFA], and confirmatory factor analysis [CFA], internal consistency coefficient) were used for the data analysis.

Ethical Consideration

The permission of the researchers who developed the original scale was received via e-mail. Ethics committee approval

TABLE 1.
The Study Procedures According to "A Suggested Cross-Cultural Adaptations Process" by Gjersing et al. (2010)

Suggested	Performed
Adaptation process	
Investigation of conceptual and item equivalence	Literature review Discussion with experts in the field and members of target population
Original instrument translated	Two independent translators Fluent in Turkish and good understanding of English
A synthesized translated version	One academician Good command of both languages
Back-translations	Two independent translators Fluent in Turkish and good understanding of English
A synthesized back-translated version	One academician Good command of both languages
Expert committee	12 experts In the area of nursing and had experiences of instrument development and adaptation
Instrument pretested	17 voluntaries Same characteristics with target population
Revised instrument	Researchers
Investigation of operational equivalence	Discussions with experts in the field of nursing
Validation process	
Main study	240 voluntary nurses
Exploratory and confirmatory factor analysis	CFA for testing the fit of the original structure on target population Item analyses regarding the reliability of each item EFA for exploring the factor structure on target population CFA for confirming the construct validity Cronbach's alpha for testing the internal consistency Correlation analyses for criterion validity
Final instrument	

Note. CFA = confirmatory factor analysis; EFA = exploratory factor analysis.

was received with the Decision no. A.07 dated January 6, 2015, from the ethics committee of a university in Istanbul. Approvals were also received from the administrative and nursing service departments of the hospitals where the data were collected.

Results

Participants

The participants were mostly female (94.6%), held a bachelor's degree (62.1%), and worked in inpatient units (79.1%) as bedside nurses (85.4%). The ages of participants varied from 19 to 52 years (mean = 31.95 years, *SD* = 7.55 years), and their experience at the hospital and in the nursing profession ranged from 1 to 33 years (mean = 8.11 years, *SD* = 7.92 years) and 1 to 33 years (mean = 10.29 years, *SD* = 8.14 years), respectively.

Adaptation Process

Language validity was conducted for both TPS and CPS. This stage was based on the method recommended by the World Health Organization for the adaptation of instruments that were developed in a language different from the target language (World Health Organization, 2008). The original scale was translated and back-translated by four language professionals. Translated and back-translated versions of the scales were then synthesized by two academicians who had a good command of both Turkish and English. Finally, the original scale and the translated version were compared by an expert committee for content validity. The Lawshe technique was used to assess content validity (Lawshe, 1975). The prepared Turkish form was evaluated by 12 experts outside the research team who both worked in the field of nursing and had experience with scale development or adaptation studies. As opinions were received from 12 experts, as suggested by the Lawshe technique, the content validity criterion was specified as .56 (Lawshe, 1975). No items were omitted at this stage, as no statement received a value below .56.

A pilot study was conducted using a 17-person group outside the sample group in February 2015. Respondents were probed for their understanding to identify potentially confusing or misleading items. On the basis of their responses, the items were finalized by the researchers and discussed with four nurse managers in terms of performance evaluation.

Validation Process

The final version of the adapted scale was given to the main sample of 240 people.

Construct Validity

The CFA was conducted for both scales primarily to evaluate construct validity. The CFA did not confirm the factor structures of the original scales. The realization of the recommended modifications did not ensure any increase at an acceptable level in the goodness-of-fit indices; whereupon, an additional CFA that approached both scales as a single subscale was conducted as an alternative. However, the results indicated that the goodness-of-fit indices did not improve but rather fell to lower levels (Table 2).

Item Analysis

When the item–total score correlations for the total of 41 items, including 23 in the TPS and 18 in the CPS, were examined, the item–total score correlation coefficients for Item 7 in the TPS and Items 2, 8, 11, 16, and 17 in the CPS were found to be $r < .45$. For this reason, these six items were omitted.

A new EFA was then conducted that considered all of the items of both scales as a single item pool (principal component analysis/varimax rotation). At this stage, a KMO test and Bartlett's test of sphericity were performed, finding a KMO value of .89 and a sphericity test result of $\chi^2 = 7206.1$ ($df = 595$, $p < .001$). The difference between the factor load values was less than .10. Thus, as the EFA results showed that three items loaded in two or more factors simultaneously, these items were also omitted from the scale. The factor loads of the 32 items remaining in the scale varied between .50 and .84, and the scale items were distributed to six factors having eigenvalues above 1 and explaining 70.6% of the total variance. Nine items were involved in the first factor, seven items were involved in the second factor, six items were involved in the third factor, four items each were involved in the fourth and fifth factors, and two items were involved in the sixth factor (Table 3).

CFA was applied again to evaluate the fit of the newly explored structure of the scale. When modification suggestions were examined, error covariance was assigned between Items 8–9 and 22–23 in the first factor, Items 13–14 and 16–18 in the second factor, and Items 24–27 in the third factor (Figure 1). Factor loadings in the subscales were found to be ≥ .64 in the first factor, ≥ .66 in the second factor, ≥ .59 in the third factor, ≥ .56 in the fourth factor, ≥ .36 in the fifth factor, and ≥ .65 in the sixth factor (Figure 1). Goodness-of-fit indices were calculated as $\chi^2 = 1828.22$, $df = 453$, root mean square error of approximation (RMSEA) = .09, goodness-of-fit index (GFI) = .91, adjusted GFI (AGFI) = .88, and comparative fit index (CFI) = .95 (Table 2).

Internal Consistency Analysis

The Cronbach's alpha reliability coefficients of the subscales that were obtained after the factor analysis and the subscales in the analysis that were conducted to evaluate the scale's total internal consistency varied between .65 and .93. The total score for the scale was $\alpha = .95$ (Table 3).

Criterion Validity

The EPS was applied on the same group simultaneously to determine the criterion validity. After testing for linearity, Pearson correlation analysis was applied, and positive (+), moderate level ($r = .617$), and advanced level significant

TABLE 2.

Goodness of Fit Indices for the Original and Adapted Version of the Scales

Scale	Factor loadings	$\chi 2$	*df*	RMSEA	GFI	AGFI	CFI
Original Scales							
Task Performance Scale							
4-Factor	≥ .66	1993.60	226	.181	.58	.49	.71
One Factor	≥ .60	4576.75	230	.281	.38	.25	.51
Contextual Performance Scale							
4-Factor	≥ .59	1794.30	131	.230	.55	.41	.65
One Factor	≥ .53	3003.42	135	.298	.42	.26	.44
Adapted Version of the Scale							
Nurse Job Performance Scale		1828.22	453	.094	.91	.88	.95

Note. df = degrees of freedom; RMSEA = root mean square error of approximation; GFI = goodness of fit index; AGFI = adjusted goodness of fit index; CFI = comparative fit index.

TABLE 3.
Results of Reliability and Structural Analyses

Factor Number	Item	*n*	% of Explained Variance	Factor Loading	Corrected Item Total Correlations	Cronbach's Alpha
F1	8, 9, 10, 11, 12, 19, 21, 22, 23	9	38.90	.562–.844	.66–.82	.93
F2	13, 14, 15, 16, 17, 18, 20	7	11.13	.593–.840	.63–.85	.93
F3	24, 25, 26, 27, 28, 29	6	8.04	.701–.836	.63–.80	.88
F4	30, 37, 38, 41	4	4.83	.631–.805	.58–.77	.82
F5	1, 2, 4, 6	4	4.17	.593–.649	.51–.73	.79
F6	33, 35	2	3.54	.504–.610	.50–.50	.65
Total		32	70.59	.504–.844	.45–.71	.95

($p < .001$) correlations were determined between the total scores obtained from both scales.

Discussion

Adaptation Process

Language validity

The scale adaptation studies referenced in the literature recommend implementing practices to diminish the psycholinguistic differences between cultures (Şencan, 2005). For this purpose, the translations of the scale first from the original English into Turkish and then from Turkish back into English were conducted in this study in accordance with the method recommended by the World Health Organization (2008) for rendering instruments into languages other than the original language.

Content validity

In scale development and adaptation studies, content validity is used to assess whether the items of a scale include the field to be measured (Öner, 2008). The Turkish form prepared within this study was submitted for the opinion of experts. The content validity criterion was found to be .56 (Lawshe, 1975), and no items were omitted in this stage, as no statement had a criterion value below this value.

Validation Process

First stage: confirmatory factor analysis

Factor analysis is the most commonly used method of analysis to test the construct validity of a scale. Factor analysis is a concept that relates to how a scale accurately measures what (Öner, 2008). CFA was conducted in this study to test the structure of the scale.

In the CFA, the various results of the GFI determine the compatibility of the model. There are numerous goodness-of-fit indices, and there is no absolute consensus as to which ones should be reported (Şimşek, 2007). Chi-square/degree of freedom, RMSEA, AGFI, GFI, and CFI results were reported in this study as the most commonly used fit indices. According to the results of the analyses, it was determined that adaptation values did not show acceptable fit (Table 2).

Second stage: item analysis

Item analysis gives information regarding the reliability of each item in a scale. Therefore, if items in a scale are equally weighted and independent, the correlation value between each item and the total score should be high (Tavşancıl, 2014). The item–total score correlations for the items in the scale's Turkish form were evaluated as part of the item analysis that was conducted for this study. Accordingly, as the correlation values for the total of 41 items in both scales were $r < .45$, six items were omitted from the study.

Third stage: exploratory factor analysis

As the CFAs did not confirm the original structure, a new EFA was carried out that considered all items of both scales, which had been reduced to 35 items after the item analysis, as a single item pool.

The literature recommends applying a KMO test and a Bartlett's test of sphericity before performing factor analysis. In this study, the KMO coefficient was evaluated as "good," and the Bartlett's test result was determined to be significant in the advanced level (Şencan, 2005).

The literature further recommends that, if each item is listed under a factor, where it receives the highest factor load value, after the EFA; however, the items receiving high factor loads are evaluated under multiple factors; and the difference between the factor load values obtained by the same item under different factors is lower than 0.10, the item in question should be omitted (Büyüköztürk, 2011). Item 5 in the TPS and Items 9 and 13 in the CPS of the original form were omitted in this study because they received similar factor load values in two or more factors. The factor load values of the remaining 32 items of the scale varied between .50 and .84 (Table 3), and the scale items were distributed across six factors, which explained 70.6% of the total variance. The items in the "coordination

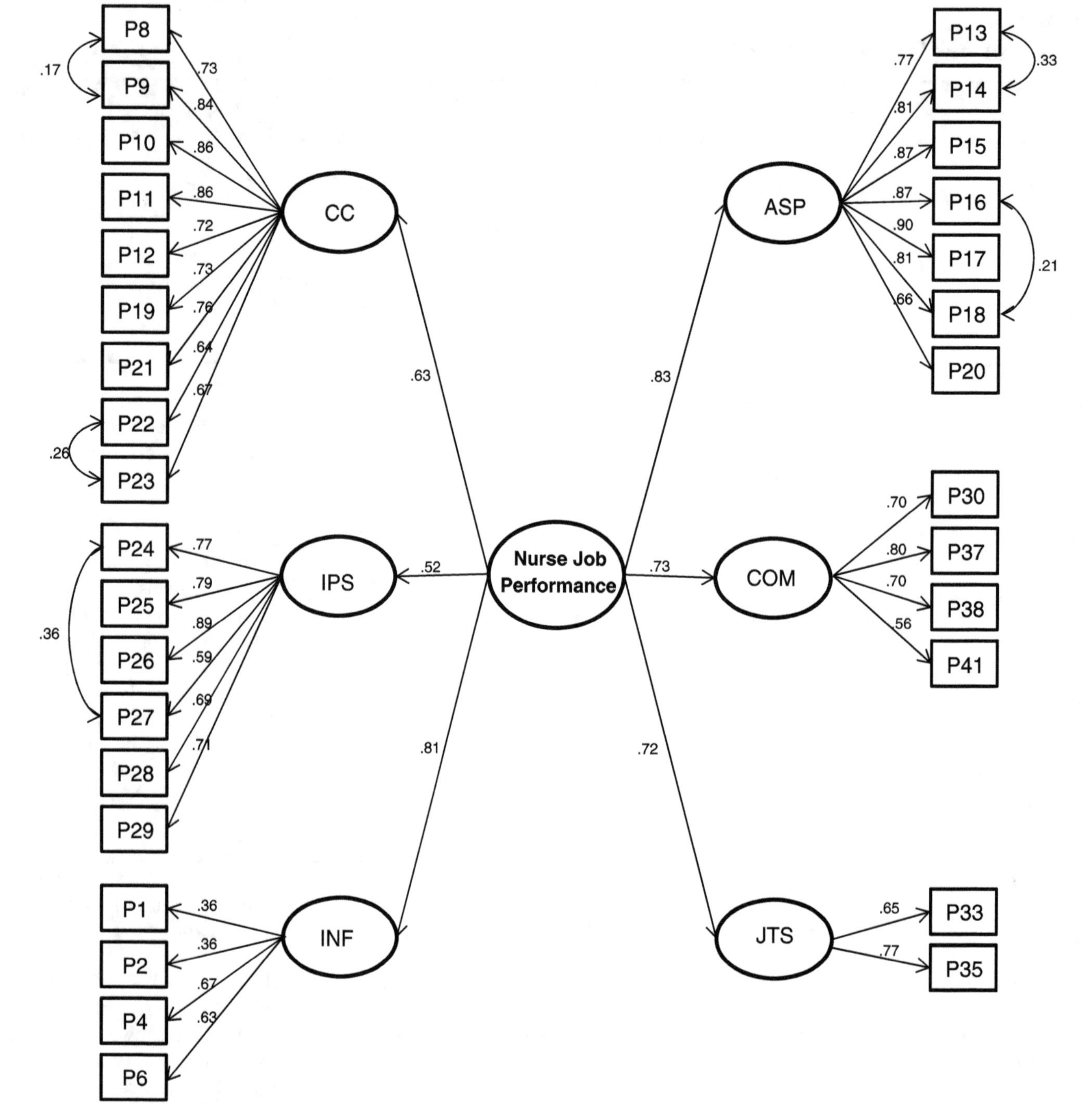

Figure 1. Confirmatory factor analysis results for the adapted version of the nurse Job Performance Scale. CC = coordination of care; ASP = assisting and supporting patients; IPS = interpersonal support; COM= compliance; INF = information; JTS = job task support.

of care" subscale in the TPS of the original scale were combined with Items 21–23 in the "technical care" subscale to create a new factor. This factor was called "coordination of care," as in the original scale, because items containing the technical aspect of care were added. All five items in the "social support" subscale of the TPS and Item 20 in the "technical care" subscale of the original scale were included in the second factor. Different from the original scale, this subscale was called "assisting and supporting patients." All items in the "interpersonal support" subscale in the CPS of the original scale were included in the third factor, and the name of the factor was kept the same. One item from the "job task support" subscale of the CPS, two items from the "compliance" subscale, and one item from the "volunteering for additional duties" subscale were included in the fourth factor to create a new factor structure. This factor was called the "compliance" subscale by considering the compliance of the items it included. Items 1, 2, 4, and 6 in the TPS of the original scale were added to the fifth factor, and the name of the subscale was kept the same as "information," as in the original scale. Items 33 and 35 in the job task support subscale in the CPS of the original scale were added to the sixth factor. The name of the subscale was kept as "job task support," as in the original scale.

It appears meaningful to emphasize the following points concerning the revised structure:

- The structure in TPS and CPS was preserved, although the items located in the subscales of both scales were moved to other subscales. For instance, the item "assisting patients with activities of daily living (e.g., showering, toileting, and feeding)" in the "technical care" subscale of the TPS in the original structure was also involved in the TPS in the Turkish version. However, the subscale in which it was involved changed and was moved to the "social support" subscale.
- Four of the five items in the subscale "technical care" of the original structure were involved in the subscale of "coordination of care," as in the Turkish version. This condition may lead us to interpret that the nurses in Turkey evaluated planning, implementation, and technical activities in the context of nursing care as a whole.
- The item "assisting patients with activities of daily living (e.g., showering, toileting and feeding)" in the "technical care" subscale of the original structure was moved to the social support subscale in the Turkish version. Despite the fact that assisting patients to carry out daily life activities is a part of nursing care, it was considered that the shifting of this item to the latter scale was justified because the meaning of "assist" in Turkish is very close to the meaning of "support."
- No change took place in the "interpersonal support" subscale that involved items pertaining to the communication and collaboration between the nurses in both the original and new structures. This may be due to the opinion that cooperation and support among nurses were realized in the Turkish sample because of their feeling of being professional colleagues.
- Three of the seven items on the "information" subscale in the original scale were omitted in the Turkish version, with four retained. The items on informing the patient and the family about discharge and out-of-hospital processes were preserved in the new version. However, it is remarkable that the items regarding care and treatment interventions administered during admission as well as the symptoms were not kept in the new version. In Turkey, physicians play the primary role in sharing information with the patients about admission procedures. Moreover, physicians tend to share information on symptoms, side effects, treatment, and care with the patients and their relatives together, rather than only with the patient (Atıcı, 2007).
- The number of items in the "compliance" subscale was three in the original scale and four in the Turkish version. Here, the item "complying with hospital rules, regulations and procedures, even when no one is watching" was omitted. In the original structure, the item "making special arrangements for a patient's family" involved in the job task support subscale of the original structure and the item "making innovative suggestions to improve the overall quality of the department" under the subscale of volunteering for additional duties were involved in the "compliance" subscale in the new version. Apparently, the matters of improving the related department and the making of special adjustments related to patient relatives by the sample in the Turkish structure were related to embracement to hospital, that is, the institution.
- In the new structure, only the items "making special arrangements for the patient" and "taking extra time to respond to a patient's needs" remained under the subscale of "job task support." The remaining three items were omitted. The item "making special arrangements for a patient's family" in the subscale of job task support and the item "making innovative suggestions to improve the overall quality of the department" in the subscale of volunteering for additional duties in the original structure were involved in the subscale of "compliance" in the new version. This result is likely associated with reasons such as intense and long working hours and the care of excessive numbers of patients by a limited number of nurses. In addition to density of the current work of nurses, these items, including extra behaviors expected to be realized, were omitted.

Fourth stage: confirmatory factor analysis

Assigning an error covariance between items in line with modification suggestions is a method that has often been applied in the literature. However, higher values for error covariance signify that a model is less confirmative, although it does not invalidate the established model's validity. What is important here is that the theoretical rationales for the assigned covariances are very explicitly ascribed (Şimşek, 2007). Five covariance assignments were conducted between the items that affected the model's structure significantly and had theoretically similar meanings in this study (Figure 1). The first two items were "explaining to nurses in the unit the nature of the patient's condition" and "reporting the critical elements of patients' situations when turning over work shift" in the subscale "coordination of care." As both items were related to patients' clinical conditions, they were perceived similarly. The second two items were "showing care and concern to families" and "listening to families' concerns" in the subscale "assisting and supporting patients." The sample evaluated these two items as being close in meaning in both English and Turkish and thus interpreted them as related to care provided by the patient's family. The third two items were "listening to patients' concerns" and "showing care and concern to patients" in the subscale "assisting and supporting patients." The concept of "concern" stood out in both items, with participants perceiving the items as having similar meanings. The fourth two items were "administering medications and treatments" and "evaluating the effectiveness of nursing care" in the subscale "coordination of care." Because nurses in Turkey do not consider the administration of medication and treatments as separate from nursing care, these two items were evaluated similarly by the sample. The last two items were "raising morale of other nurses in the unit" and "taking time to meet unit nurses' emotional needs" in the subscale "interpersonal support." These two items were related to emotional support between nurses. Therefore, the study sample perceived both items similarly.

After the corrections made during the CFA, the model showed a normal fit according to Şimşek (2007) in terms of CFI and acceptable fit in terms of χ^2/df, RMSEA, GFI, and AGFI (Table 2).

Fifth stage: internal consistency analysis

Cronbach's alpha analyses are used in scale development studies to test the internal consistency of items using Likert scales (Polit & Beck, 2012). Coefficients that score between .80 and 1.00 indicate that the related scale has a high reliability (Tavşancıl, 2014). The Cronbach's alpha reliability coefficient of the JPS in its internal consistency analysis was found to be .95 for the full scale (Table 3), showing that the scale items had a high internal consistency and internal reliability. In addition, the Cronbach's alpha reliability coefficients were highly reliable for the first four subscales and were reliable for the fifth and sixth subscales (Table 3).

Sixth stage: criterion validity

This method, which is generally used in scale development studies and is also known as equivalent form reliability, is based on examining the results, obtained by applying a scale that is developed in two forms and with equivalent qualities to the same group incessantly at the same time, or intermittently at two different times, using Pearson correlation analysis (Gözüm & Aksayan, 2002). However, as developing equivalent test forms is difficult for cases in which a scale developed for the same purposes is present, the correlation between the present scale and the newly developed scale may be examined as an alternative approach (Gözüm & Aksayan, 2002).

Akgül (2005) emphasized that an absolute linear correlation must exist between the variables to calculate the Pearson correlation coefficient, suggesting that a scatter graph should be formed to examine the presence of a linear correlation between variables. In this study, the scatter graph of the measurements that were obtained from the JPS and EPS was examined, which revealed the presence of a positive linear correlation. A correlation that was positive, strong to moderate, and statistically significant was determined between the measurements obtained from the two scales in the analysis.

Conclusions and Recommendations

The scale that was developed by Greenslade and Jimmieson (2007) following the structure of Borman and Motowidlo (1993), which approaches job performance as the two distinct domains of task performance and contextual performance, was not structurally valid in the Turkish context. The revised structure that was developed in this study, which used six subscales that related directly to performance with 32 items, was found to be a valid and reliable structure for a Turkish version of the scale.

The scope of the original English version of the scale seems to be a sufficient instrument for measuring the performance of nurses. However, the authors recommend testing scales in terms of validity and reliability before applying them in different cultures by considering that their structure is affected by intercultural differences.

Limitation

In conducting reliability analyses, a test–retest to show the scale's reliability over time was not conducted.

Acknowledgment

We would like to thank the nurses who participated in the study.

References

Akgül, A. (2005). *Statistical analysis techniques in medical researches SPSS applications* (3rd ed.). Ankara, Turkey: Emek Ofset. (Original work published in Turkish)

Atıcı, E. (2007). Factors affecting patient–physician relationship. *Uludağ Medical Journal, 33*(2), 91–96. (Original work published in Turkish)

Bakker, A. B., Demerouti, E., & Euwema, M. C. (2005). Job resources buffer the impact of job demands on burnout. *Journal of Occupational Health Psychology, 10*(2), 170–180. doi:10.1037/1076-8998.10.2.170

Behrenbeck, J. G., Timm J. A., Griebenow, L. K., & Demmer, K. A. (2005). Nursing-sensitive outcome reliability testing in a tertiary care setting. *International Journal of Nursing Terminologies and Classifications, 16*(1), 14–20. doi:10.1111/j.1744-618X.2005.00002.x

Borman, W. C., & Motowidlo, S. J. (1993). Expanding the criterion domain to include elements of contextual performance. In N. Schmitt & W. C. Borman (Eds.), *Personnel selection in organizations* (pp. 71–98). San Francisco, CA: Jossey-Bass.

Borsa, J. C., Damásio, B. F., & Bandeira, D. R. (2012). Cross-cultural adaptation and validation of psychological instruments:

Some considerations. *Paidéia, 22*(53), 423–432. doi:10.1590/S0103-863X2012000300014

Büyüköztürk, Ş. (2011). *Manual of data analysis for social sciences* (15th ed.). Ankara, Turkey: Pegem Academy. (Original work published in Turkish)

Coleman, V. I., & Borman, W. C. (2000). Investigating the underlying structure of the citizenship performance domain. *Human Resource Management Review, 10*(1), 25–44. doi: 10.1016/S1053-4822(99)00037-6

DeLucia, P. R., Ott, T. E., & Palmieri, P. A. (2009). Performance in nursing. *Reviews of Human Factors and Ergonomics, 5*(1), 1–40. doi:10.1518/155723409X448008

Erdoğan, E. (2011). *The correlation between effective leadership, organizational silence, and performance* (Unpublished master's thesis). Gebze, Turkey: Gebze Advanced Technology Institute. (Original work published in Turkish)

Gjersing, L., Caplehorn, J. R., & Clausen, T. (2010). Cross-cultural adaptation of research instruments: Language, setting, time and statistical considerations. *BMC Medical Research Methodology, 10*, 13. doi:10.1186/1471-2288-10-13

Gözüm, S., & Aksayan, S. (2002). Guideline II for intercultural scale adaptation: Psychometric features and intercultural comparison. *HEMAR-G, 4*(2), 9–20. (Original work published in Turkish)

Greenslade, J. H., & Jimmieson, N. L. (2007). Distinguishing between task and contextual performance for nurses: Development of a job performance scale. *Journal of Advanced Nursing, 58*(6), 602–611. doi:10.1111/j.1365-2648.2007.04256.x

Gregg, A. C. (2002). Performance management data systems for nursing service organizations. *Journal of Nursing Administration, 32*(2), 71–78.

Griffin, M. A., Neal, A., & Parker, S. K. (2007). A new model of work role performance: Positive behavior in uncertain and interdependent contexts. *Academy of Management Journal, 50*(2), 327–347. doi:10.5465/AMJ.2007.24634438

Hamilton, K. E., Coates, V., Kelly, B., Boore, J. R., Cundell, J. H., Gracey, J., ... Sinclair, M. (2007). Performance assessment in health care providers: A critical review of evidence and current practice. *Journal of Nursing Management, 15*(8), 773–791. doi:10.1111/j.1365-2934.2007.00780.x

Larrabee, J. H., Ostrow, C. L., Withrow, M. L., Janney, M. A., Hobbs, G. R. Jr., & Burant, C. (2004). Predictors of patient satisfaction with inpatient hospital nursing care. *Research in Nursing and Health, 27*(4), 254–268. doi:10.1002/nur.20021

Lawshe, C. H. (1975). A quantitative approach to content validity. *Personnel Psychology, 28*(4), 563–575. doi:10.1111/j.1744-6570.1975.tb01393.x

Öner, N. (2008). *Psychological tests used in Turkey: A reference guide* (2nd ed.). Istanbul, Turkey: Boğaziçi University Publishing House. (Original work published in Turkish)

Pappas, S. H. (2008). The cost of nurse-sensitive adverse events. *Journal of Nursing Administration, 38*(5), 230–236. doi:10.1097/01.NNA.0000312770.19481.ce

Pelletier, D., Duffield, C., Adams, A., Nagy, S., Crisp, J., & Mitten-Lewis, S. (2000). Australian nurse educators identify gaps in expert practice. *The Journal of Continuing Education in Nursing, 31*(5), 224–231. doi:10.3928/0022-0124-20000901-09

Polit, D. F., & Beck, C. T. (2012). *Nursing research principles and method* (6th ed.). Philadelphia, PA: Lippincott Williams & Wilkins.

Redfern, S. J., & Norman, I. J. (1990). Measuring the quality of nursing care: A consideration of different approaches. *Journal of Advanced Nursing, 15*(11), 1260–1271. doi:10.1111/j.1365-2648.1990.tb01741.x

Schwirian, P. M. (1978). Evaluating the performance of nurses: A multidimensional approach. *Nursing Research, 27*(6), 347–351.

Şencan, H. (2005). *Reliability and validity in social and behavioural measurements.* Ankara, Turkey: Seçkin. (Original work published in Turkish)

Şimşek, Ö. F. (2007). *Introduction to the structural equation modeling: Principles and LISREL applications.* Ankara, Turkey: Ekinoks. (Original work published in Turkish)

Tavşancıl, E. (2014). *Measurement of attitudes and data analysis with SPSS* (5th ed.). Ankara, Turkey: Nobel. (Original work published in Turkish)

Wandelt, M., & Phaneuf, M. (1972). Three instruments for measuring the quality of nursing care. *Hospital Topics, 50*(8), 20–29. doi:10.1080/00185868.1972.9947925

Wandelt, M. A., & Stewart Slater, D. (1975). *Slater nursing competencies rating scale.* New York, NY: Appleton- Century Croft.

Whyte, D. A., Lugton, J., & Fawcett, T. N. (2000). Fit for purpose: The relevance of masters preparation for the professional practice of nursing: A 10-year follow-up study of postgraduate nursing courses in the University of Edinburgh. *Journal of Advanced Nursing, 31*(5), 1072–1080. doi:10.1046/j.1365-2648.2000.01388.x

World Health Organization. (2008). *Process of translation and adaptation of instruments.* Retrieved from http://www.who.int/substance_abuse/research_tools/translation/en/

17

The Effects of an Educational Program on the Professional Quality of Life and Health of Nurses: A Cluster Experimental Design

Chia-Yun FU[1] • Chia-Chan KAO[2] • Ruey-Hsia WANG[3*]

ABSTRACT

Background: The complexity of the healthcare environment and intense workloads may negatively impact the health and professional quality of life (ProQOL) of nurses. Prior research has identified a significant association in nurses between ProQOL and health. Developing an intervention to improve the ProQOL and health of nurses may benefit the quality of nursing care.

Purpose: The aim of this study was to explore the effects of a compassion fatigue Resiliency, mindfulness Respiration, and Relatives and friends' support (i.e., 3Rs) educational program on ProQOL, physical health, and mental health in nurses.

Methods: A cluster experimental design was used in this study to recruit registered nurses at two regional teaching hospitals in southern Taiwan as participants. The experimental group (n = 67) attended the 4-week (2-hours-per-week) 3R educational program. The control group (n = 57) received no intervention. The outcome variables, including compassion satisfaction, burnout, secondary traumatic stress, physical health, and mental health, were measured at baseline, at the end of the intervention (immediate effect), at 4 weeks postintervention (short-term effect), and at 12 weeks postintervention (medium-term effect). The study was conducted from May 2017 to December 2017.

Results: Increases in compassion satisfaction and mental health and decreases in secondary traumatic stress were significantly greater in the experimental group than in the control group between baseline and all three posttest time points. Moreover, burnout decreased and physical health improved more significantly in the experimental group than in the control group between the baseline and end of intervention time points (p < .001).

Conclusions/Implications for Practice: The 3R educational program intervention, integrating compassion fatigue resiliency, mindfulness respiration, and support from relatives and friends, had immediate and positive effects on ProQOL as well as physical and mental health. Moreover, the intervention was shown to have short-term and medium-term positive effects on compassion satisfaction, secondary traumatic stress, and mental health. Nursing managers may apply programs that integrate compassion fatigue resiliency, mindfulness respiration, and relatives and friends' support to improve ProQOL and health in nurses.

KEY WORDS:
nurses, professional quality of life, physical health, mental health, compassion fatigue.

Introduction

The complexity of the healthcare environment and the intensity of workloads may impact negatively on the physical and mental health of nurses, causing skeletal and muscle pain, poor sleep quality, depression, and other effects (Freimann et al., 2016; Li et al., 2019; Weigl et al., 2016). Poor physical and mental health in nurses may lead to increases in sick leave requests and patient safety-related problems (Carlesi et al., 2017; Van Gerven et al., 2016). Improving the physical and mental health of nurses is a crucial issue for nursing managers. Professional quality of life (ProQOL), defined as the quality perceived by professional providers when performing work (Stamm, 2010), includes the two aspects of compassion satisfaction and compassion fatigue. Compassion satisfaction, the positive aspect of ProQOL, is the satisfaction derived from helping others (Jang et al., 2016). Compassion fatigue, the negative aspect of ProQOL, consists of burnout and secondary traumatic stress and fosters negative feelings toward clinical work and contributes to physical and mental exhaustion (Nolte et al., 2017; Ruiz-Fernández et al., 2020). Burnout is a negative emotional reaction to stressful work environments (Rayan et al., 2019), whereas secondary traumatic stress is caused by deep, vicarious traumatization associated with caring for patients (Peters, 2018). Levels of burnout and secondary traumatic stress

[1]*PhD, RN, Assistant Professor, Department of Nursing, Fooyin University, Kaohsiung, Taiwan, ROC* • [2]*PhD, RN, Associate Professor, Department of Nursing, I-Shou University, Kaohsiung, Taiwan, ROC* • [3]*PhD, RN, Professor, College of Nursing, Kaohsiung Medical University, Kaohsiung, Taiwan, ROC, and Adjunct Researcher, Department of Medical Research, Kaohsiung Medical University Hospital, Kaohsiung, Taiwan, ROC.*

have been found to be higher in nurses than other health practitioners, such as physicians, social workers, and palliative care professionals (Cavanagh et al., 2020). Intensive care unit nurses have been found to experience higher levels of burnout and secondary traumatic stress than either ward nurses (Kawar et al., 2019) or oncology nurses (Mooney et al., 2017). Higher compassion satisfaction has been significantly associated with better physical and mental health (Fu et al., 2018), whereas higher levels of burnout and secondary traumatic stress have been significantly associated with poor physical and mental health (Fu et al., 2018; Ruiz-Fernández et al., 2020). Improving ProQOL may benefit the physical and mental health of nurses.

Background

Strategies for improving ProQOL have been previously developed. Compassion fatigue resiliency refers to helping professionals enhance their resilience against compassion fatigue and, ultimately, enhance their empathy toward patients, themselves, and their peers (Figley & Figley, 2017). Gentry et al. (2002) proposed a compassion fatigue resiliency program that includes five components, as described in the following: (a) self-regulation: use muscle relaxation to activate the parasympathetic nervous system and learn to change negative perceptions into positive ones, thereby strengthening recovery ability, resiliency, and adaptability of stress; (b) intentionality: modify impulsive thinking and negative stress-related coping behaviors and cultivate the habit of thinking thoroughly before reorganizing oneself for work; (c) perceptual maturation/self-validation: change one's mood, relax when encountering stress, identify with one's own response to stressful events through self-talk, and format work-related negative feelings into normal requirements; (d) connection and support: cope with stress through interactions with an organization or support network; and (e) self-care and revitalization: balance physical and mental health by doing aerobic exercise, following appropriate dietary and sleep regimens, and strengthening professional abilities.

A compassion fatigue resiliency intervention has been shown to significantly increase compassion satisfaction, with burnout and secondary traumatic stress significantly decreased at the end of intervention (Flarity et al., 2013). Furthermore, two longer follow-up studies found significantly decreased secondary traumatic stress at 2 months (Flarity, Nash, et al., 2016) and 6 months after this intervention (Flarity et al., 2018). These findings support that compassion fatigue resiliency interventions improve compassion satisfaction, burnout, and secondary traumatic stress. Nevertheless, the effect of this compassion fatigue intervention on physical and mental health in nurses has not been investigated adequately.

"Mindfulness" refers to paying attention purposefully, being in the present moment, and nonjudgmentally unfolding experiences from moment to moment (Kabat-Zinn, 1982). Mindfulness may be achieved in a variety of scenarios, including eating meditation, breathing exercises, and meditation exercises, to activate the parasympathetic nervous system and reduce negative thinking to achieve physical and mental balance (Killingsworth & Gilbert, 2010). Mindfulness may also reduce the production of stress hormones, such as α-amylase (Duchemin et al., 2015). In addition, studies have reported significantly decreased levels of burnout and secondary traumatic stress at the conclusion of mindfulness interventions (Duarte & Pinto-Gouveia, 2016). Although meditation and breathing exercises have been shown to significantly increase levels of compassion satisfaction and significantly decrease levels of burnout and secondary traumatic stress at the conclusion of the intervention (Hevezi, 2016), the longer effects of these exercises on mindfulness have been inadequately addressed. The results of previous studies on nurses support that mindfulness training affects mental health positively but has no significant effect on physical health (Bazarko et al., 2013; Goodman & Schorling, 2012).

Social support refers to receiving emotional, intimate, material, and cognitive support from significant others (Williams et al., 2004). Social support from a supervisor has been correlated positively with compassion satisfaction and negatively with burnout and secondary traumatic stress (Hunsaker et al., 2015). Social support from relatives and friends has been found to moderate the negative effect of secondary traumatic stress on physical health (Fu et al., 2018). However, no study has examined the effect of social support on ProQOL. A social support intervention was found to significantly improve the physical health but not the mental health of nursing students at the end of the intervention (Walcott et al., 2018).

Few interventions have been developed to simultaneously improve ProQOL, physical health, and mental health in nurses. This type of intervention may require combining a variety of intervention components (Duhoux et al., 2017). Therefore, the purpose of this study was to examine the effects of an educational program that integrates compassion fatigue Resiliency, mindfulness Respiration, and Relatives and friends' support (3R) to improve ProQOL, physical health, and mental health in nurses.

Methods

Design

A cluster experimental design was adopted to prevent contamination of the sample. Two teaching hospitals in southern Taiwan were selected and respectively assigned to either the experimental group or the control group. The participants in the experimental group received a 3R educational program in the hospital. The control group did not receive any intervention. Compassion satisfaction, burnout, secondary traumatic stress, physical health, and mental health were measured at baseline and at the end of the intervention (immediate effect), at 4 weeks postintervention (short-term effect), and at 12 weeks

Figure 1

Flow of Study Recruitment, Intervention, and Measurements

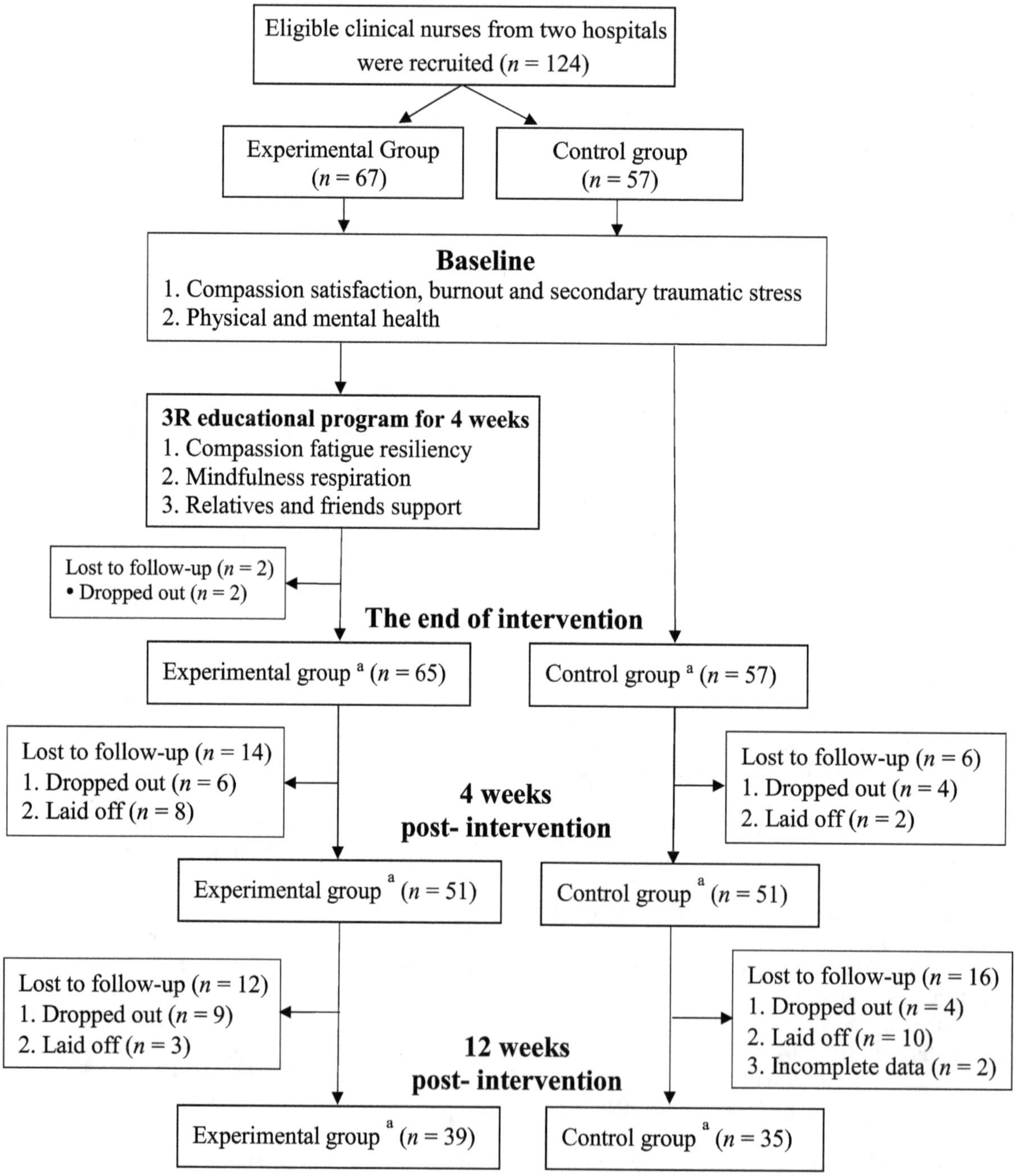

Note. [a] Outcome variables, including compassion satisfaction, burnout, secondary traumatic stress, and physical and mental health, were measured at four time points.

postintervention (medium-term effect). This study was conducted from May 2017 to December 2017.

Participants

The target population comprised clinical registered nurses. In this study, the inclusion criteria were registered nurses with at least 1 year of nursing experience. Eligible participants were recruited by the head nurses or nursing supervisors in the selected hospitals and referred to the researchers. After receiving signed consent forms from all of the participants, research assistants collected data from the two groups at baseline, at the end of the intervention, at 4 weeks postintervention, and at 12 weeks postintervention. Considering the lack of prior research on this topic, a medium effect size of 0.5 for the mean difference between the experimental and control groups was used for sample size estimation in this study (Cohen, 1988). Considering an effect size of 0.5, an alpha of .05, and a power of 0.8, 63 nurses were required for each group (Cohen, 1988). An initial group of 67 and 57 nurses were recruited for the experimental and control groups, respectively. The retention rates for the experimental group were 97.0% (n = 65) at the end of intervention, 76.1% (n = 51) at 4 weeks postintervention, and 58.2% (n = 39) at 12 weeks postintervention. The retention rates for the control group were 100% (n = 57) at the end of intervention, 89.5% (n = 51) at 4 weeks postintervention, and 61.4% (n = 35) at 12 weeks postintervention. The flow of recruitment, intervention, and measurement is shown in Figure 1.

The 3R Educational Program Intervention

The compassion fatigue resiliency (Gentry et al., 2002) and mindfulness respiration (Kabat-Zinn, 1982) components of the 3R educational program were implemented by the researcher, whereas the relatives and friends' support course component was conducted by a psychologist. The 3R educational program was implemented in once-per-week 2-hour sessions over a period of 4 weeks. The 3R educational program included several components, which are described in the following paragraphs.

Compassion fatigue resiliency

In the first week, the triggers and symptoms of compassion fatigue were introduced to the participants. Through self-evaluation, participants were taught to understand their risk levels for compassion fatigue and its adverse effects.

In the second week, self-regulation was introduced. Relaxation exercises were performed as self-regulation practice at the beginning of every class starting in the second week. Self-care and revitalization with an emphasis on better sleep and eating habits were also introduced in the second week.

In the third week, intentionality and perceptual maturation were introduced. Participants discussed the best solutions for dealing with stressful scenarios and learned to face negative situations, maintain positive mental perceptions, and avoid impulsive behaviors and reactions. Furthermore, self-validation was used to guide participants to practice talking themselves through the same stress scenario. Using self-validation, participants reflected on the appropriateness of different coping strategies. Participants were encouraged to apply appropriate strategies for managing similar, stressful situations in the future.

Mindfulness respiration

In the second week, the participants began practicing the breathing exercises associated with mindfulness respiration. In addition, the participants were encouraged to practice on their own and to record their exercise frequency and feelings in a notebook.

Relatives and friends' support

In the fourth week, the participants were encouraged to join (or organize their own) support network. The participants were asked to think about whether they had a support network and to write down the style, members, and functions of this network in their notebook.

In the first week, the participants received a pamphlet containing self-evaluation forms, information regarding compassion fatigue, and a reminder note to practice mindfulness-respiration-related breathing exercises. Beginning in the second week, participants were asked to make a weekly record in their notebook, addressing what they had learned and their reflections on how they had applied the compassion fatigue resiliency components. These records were used as subjects for discussion in each of the following weeks.

Measurements

A self-report questionnaire was used to collect the following data.

Personal characteristics

Personal characteristics data collected included age, education level, marital status, years of nursing experience, work setting, and manager (yes or no).

Physical and mental health status

The Chinese version of the SF-12v2 Physical and Mental Health Summary Scale (Ware et al., 1996) was used to assess the physical and mental health of the participants (six items each). The scale included a 3-point scale ranging from 1 (*extremely limited*) to 3 (*not limited at all*) for two items and 5-point scales ranging from 1 (*all of the time*) to 5 (*none of the time*) for eight items, 1 (*not at all*) to 5 (*extremely*) for one item, and 1 (*excellent*) to 5 (*poor*) for one item. The total scores for physical health and mental health ranged, respectively, from 6 to 26 and from 6 to 30. The original total scores for physical and mental health were standardized to create a possible score range between 1 and 100, with higher scores indicating better physical and/or mental health. In this study, the Cronbach's alpha for physical health and mental health were .62 and .63 at baseline, respectively.

Professional quality of life

The Chinese version of the ProQOL Scale Version 5 (Stamm, 2010), including compassion satisfaction, burnout, and secondary traumatic stress (10 items each), was used to measure the ProQOL of participants. Each item was rated from 1 (*never*) to 5 (*always*). The five items of the burnout subscale were reverse-scored, and the possible total score for each subscale ranged from 10 to 50, with higher scores indicating higher levels of compassion satisfaction, burnout, or secondary traumatic stress. In this study, the Cronbach's alpha values for compassion satisfaction, burnout, and secondary traumatic stress were .92, .82, and .82, respectively, at baseline.

Ethical Issues and Approval

The institutional review boards of the experimental (IRB563B) and control (20150630B) hospitals approved the protocol for this study. All of the participants were informed that their participation in this study was voluntary, that all provided information would be kept confidential, and that they could decline to participate or withdraw at any time. All of the participants signed consent forms prior to participation.

Statistical Analyses

IBM SPSS Statistics 21.0 (IBM, Inc., Armonk, NY, USA) was used to perform data analysis. Per protocol analysis was used in this study. A *t* test and a chi-square analysis were used to compare personal characteristics and outcome variables between the two groups at baseline, at the end of intervention, at 4 weeks postintervention, and at 12 weeks postintervention. Paired *t* tests were used to examine within-group differences from baseline to, respectively, the end of the intervention, 4 weeks postintervention, and 12 weeks postintervention. Generalized estimating equations were used to compare the differences in outcome variables between the experimental and control groups from baseline to the end of intervention, baseline to 4 weeks postintervention, and baseline to 12 weeks postintervention. Participants were considered to be random samples. A *p* value of less than .05 was considered statistically significant.

Results

Comparisons of Personal Characteristics and Outcome Variables Between the Experimental and Control Groups

As shown in Table 1, no significant difference in personal characteristics was indicated between the two groups. As shown in Table 2, compassion satisfaction, burnout, secondary traumatic stress, physical health, and mental health at baseline were all statistically similar between the two groups. Thus, the two groups were homogenous at baseline.

Compassion satisfaction was significantly higher in the experimental group than in the control group at the end of intervention, 4 weeks postintervention, and 12 weeks postintervention; burnout in the experimental group was significantly lower than in the control group at the end of intervention and 4 weeks postintervention; secondary traumatic stress in the experimental group was significantly

Table 1

Distributions of Personal Characteristics, With Comparisons Between Experimental and Control Groups (N = 124)

Variable	*n*	%	Experimental Group (*n* = 67)		Control Group (*n* = 57)		t/χ^2	*p*
			M	*SD*	*M*	*SD*		
Age			39.01	9.27	37.09	8.53	1.20	.23
Years of nursing experience			16.71	9.07	15.06	8.94	0.95	.34
Work setting								
Ward	52	41.9	30	44.78	22	38.60	0.66	.72
Intensive critical unit	13	10.5	6	8.96	7	12.28		
Outpatient department	59	47.6	31	46.27	28	49.12		
Education level								
Junior college	23	18.5	13	19.40	10	17.54	0.07	.79
University	101	81.5	54	80.60	47	82.46		
Manager								
Yes	6	4.8	4	5.97	2	3.51	0.41	.52
No	118	95.2	63	94.03	55	96.49		
Marital status								
Single	44	35.5	21	31.30	23	40.40	1.09	.30
Married	80	64.5	46	68.66	34	59.65		

Table 2

Intergroup Comparisons of Compassion Satisfaction, Burnout, Secondary Traumatic Stress, and Physical and Mental Health Across Different Time Points

Variable	T0		T1		T2		T3	
	M	*SD*	*M*	*SD*	*M*	*SD*	*M*	*SD*
Compassion satisfaction								
Experimental	34.85	3.79	35.23	3.65	35.18	3.18	34.62	3.30
Control	32.94	4.45	30.74	4.95	28.80	4.29	27.31	3.64
t	1.97		4.95		7.74		8.90	
p	.06		< .001		< .001		< .001	
Burnout								
Experimental	30.62	4.07	27.13	3.47	28.77	3.79	28.62	3.40
Control	31.14	3.84	30.83	3.48	30.77	3.76	30.29	3.72
t	−0.57		−4.57		−2.27		−2.01	
p	.57		< .001		.03		.05	
Secondary traumatic stress								
Experimental	29.13	3.14	27.21	3.33	27.90	3.16	27.23	3.20
Control	29.49	3.66	28.86	4.42	29.69	4.20	29.37	4.07
t	−0.45		−1.84		−2.08		−2.49	
p	.66		.07		.04		.02	
Physical health								
Experimental	63.00	8.97	68.31	8.91	59.10	8.81	56.34	8.62
Control	59.00	10.15	54.78	10.01	54.64	10.31	53.93	12.68
t	1.78		6.11		1.96		0.96	
p	.08		< .001		.05		.34	
Mental health								
Experimental	52.82	7.93	64.87	9.08	58.95	8.25	55.82	8.34
Control	54.33	7.73	54.63	8.36	55.01	5.82	54.32	7.72
t	−0.83		5.05		2.39		0.80	
p	.41		< .001		.02		.42	

Note. T0 = baseline; T1 = end of intervention; T2 = 4 weeks postintervention; T3 = 12 weeks postintervention.

lower than in the control group at 4 weeks and 12 weeks postintervention; physical health in the experimental group was significantly higher than in the control group at the end of intervention; and mental health in the experimental group was significantly higher than in the control group at the end of intervention and 4 weeks postintervention.

Difference in Outcome Variables in the Experimental and Control Groups

As shown in Table 3, although compassion satisfaction did not significantly differ from baseline to the end of intervention, baseline to 4 weeks postintervention, or baseline to 12 weeks postintervention in the experimental group, it significantly decreased over all three time periods in the control group. Burnout significantly decreased from baseline to the end of intervention, baseline to 4 weeks postintervention, and baseline to 12 weeks postintervention in the experimental group but did not change significantly over these three time periods in the control group. Secondary traumatic stress significantly decreased from baseline to the end of intervention, baseline to 4 weeks postintervention, and baseline to 12 weeks postintervention in the experimental group and significantly decreased only between baseline and the end of intervention in the control group, with the baseline to 4 weeks postintervention and baseline to 12 weeks postintervention values unchanged. Physical health significantly increased from baseline to the end of intervention and significantly decreased from baseline to 4 weeks postintervention and baseline to 12 weeks postintervention in the experimental group, whereas it significantly decreased across all three time periods in the control group. Mental health significantly increased from baseline to the end of intervention, baseline to 4 weeks postintervention, and baseline to 12 weeks postintervention in the experimental group but did not significantly change over any of the three time periods in the control group.

Differences in the Changes in Outcome Variables Between Experimental and Control Groups

Personal characteristics data were adjusted using generalized estimating equations, with results showing the increases in

Table 3

Within-Group Comparisons of Compassion Satisfaction, Burnout, Secondary Traumatic Stress, and Physical and Mental Health Across Postintervention Time Points

Variable	T1–T0		T2–T0		T3–T0	
	Pair *t*	*p*	Pair *t*	*p*	Pair *t*	*p*
Compassion satisfaction						
Experimental	1.38	.18	1.40	.17	−0.70	.49
Control	−9.23	< .001	−17.05	< .001	−14.88	< .001
Burnout						
Experimental	−9.60	< .001	−4.85	< .001	−5.31	< .001
Control	−1.11	.28	−0.97	.34	−2.13	.05
Secondary traumatic stress						
Experimental	−11.06	< .001	−3.83	< .001	−9.46	< .001
Control	−2.39	< .001	0.68	.50	−0.30	.77
Physical health						
Experimental	4.63	< .001	−2.62	.01	−4.97	< .001
Control	−5.24	< .001	−4.05	< .001	−5.68	< .001
Mental health						
Experimental	16.28	< .001	4.76	< .001	2.45	.02
Control	0.26	.80	1.02	.31	−0.10	.99

Note. T0 = baseline; T1 = end of intervention; T2 = 4 weeks postintervention; T3 = 12 weeks postintervention.

level of compassion satisfaction in the experimental group from baseline to the end of intervention, baseline to 4 weeks postintervention, and baseline to 12 weeks postintervention to be significantly greater than those in the control group over the same time periods (Table 4). The decline in burnout in the experimental group from baseline to the end of intervention was significantly greater than in the control group. Furthermore, the decline in secondary traumatic stress in the experimental group from baseline to the end of intervention, baseline to 4 weeks postintervention, and baseline to 12 weeks postintervention was significantly greater than in the control group over the same time periods.

Physical health improved significantly more in the experimental group than in the control group from baseline to the end of intervention. Also, the respective amounts of increase in mental health from baseline to the end of intervention, baseline to 4 weeks postintervention, and baseline to 12 weeks postintervention were significantly greater in the experimental group than in the control group.

Discussion

Compassion satisfaction did not differ significantly from baseline to the end of intervention in the experimental group. This finding is in line with previous studies that applied compassion fatigue resiliency (Potter, Deshields, & Rodriguez, 2013) or mindfulness (Horner et al., 2014) interventions. Moreover, compassion satisfaction in the experimental group did not significantly increase from baseline to either 4 weeks or 12 weeks postintervention. Similarly, no significant effects on compassion satisfaction were found in prior compassion fatigue resiliency intervention studies at 2 months (Horner et al., 2014), 3 months (Potter, Deshields, Berger et al., 2013), or 6 months (Flarity et al., 2018) postintervention. Nevertheless, in this study, compassion satisfaction in the control group had significantly decreased during each of the three time periods. The 3R educational program in this study, though not improving compassion satisfaction, may have prevented its decline, which is consistent with the postintervention results at 3 weeks of a previous study that applied yoga and mindfulness programs (Gregory, 2015).

The different change patterns between baseline and the three postintervention time points between the experimental and control groups contributed to increasing compassion satisfaction in the experimental group significantly more than in the control group. Compassion fatigue resiliency and mindfulness respiration are highly related to the modification of negative perceptions, which may limit the improvement effect on compassion satisfaction. Positive psychological interventions that encourage people to develop positive emotions and perceptions toward events have been shown to improve well-being in nurses (Macfarlane & Carson, 2019). Further studies may integrate positive psychology interventions into the 3R educational program and examine the effect on improving compassion satisfaction.

Burnout in the experimental group significantly decreased from baseline to the end of intervention, which was consistent with previous studies that had used compassion fatigue resiliency (Potter, Deshields, & Rodriguez, 2013) and mindfulness interventions (Duarte & Pinto-Gouveia, 2016). The 3R educational program had an immediate and positive effect on burnout. In this study, burnout in the experimental

Table 4

Changes in Compassion Satisfaction, Burnout, Secondary Traumatic Stress, Physical Health, and Mental Health Between the Experimental and Control Groups Across Postintervention Time Points

Outcome Variable	β	*SE*	*p*	QIC	QICC
Compassion satisfaction				4,062.81	4,062.68
Intercept	29.52	2.65	< .001		
Group	1.68	0.87	.05		
Time			< .001		
Group × Time			< .001		
Group × Time (T1 vs. T0)	2.59	0.36	< .001		
Group × Time (T2 vs. T0)	4.48	0.34	< .001		
Group × Time (T3 vs. T0)	5.40	0.49	< .001		
Burnout				4,061.25	4,061.23
Intercept	36.00	2.88	< .001		
Group	−0.25	0.90	.78		
Time			< .001		
Group × Time			< .001		
Group × Time (T1 vs. T0)	−2.80	0.47	< .001		
Group × Time (T2 vs. T0)	−0.82	0.53	.13		
Group × Time (T3 vs. T0)	−0.69	0.53	.20		
Secondary traumatic stress				3,826.18	3,826.90
Intercept	31.16	2.32	< .001		
Group	−0.03	0.77	.97		
Time			< .001		
Group × Time			< .001		
Group × Time (T1 vs. T0)	−1.30	0.31	< .001		
Group × Time (T2 vs. T0)	−1.43	0.43	< .001		
Group × Time (T3 vs. T0)	−1.78	0.43	< .001		
Physical health				28,057.44	28,057.26
Intercept	65.48	6.51	< .001		
Group	4.67	2.15	.07		
Time			< .001		
Group × Time			< .001		
Group × Time (T1 vs. T0)	9.52	1.38	< .001		
Group × Time (T2 vs. T0)	0.46	1.81	.80		
Group × Time (T3 vs. T0)	−1.60	1.59	.31		
Mental health				1,834.71	18,347.81
Intercept	54.33	1.29	< .001		
Group	−1.51	1.80	.40		
Time			< .001		
Group × Time			.001		
Group × Time (T1 vs. T0)	11.74	1.37	< .001		
Group × Time (T2 vs. T0)	5.45	1.43	< .001		
Group × Time (T3 vs. T0)	3.02	1.42	.03		

Note. Personal characteristics were adjusted. QIC = quasi-likelihood under independence model criterion; QICC = corrected quasi-likelihood under independence model criterion; T0 = baseline; T1 = end of intervention; T2 = 4 weeks postintervention; T3 = 12 weeks postintervention.

group significantly decreased between baseline and both 4 and 12 weeks postintervention. Previous studies that had adopted only the compassion fatigue resiliency program reported finding no significant changes in burnout at 8 weeks (Flarity, Nash, et al., 2016) or 12 weeks (Potter, Deshields, Berger et al., 2013) postintervention. Social support was found to decrease burnout (Chou et al., 2014). The 3R educational program integrating social support may help sustain the reduction effects on burnout through the 4 and 12 weeks postintervention assessments.

Burnout in the experimental group increased significantly between the end of the intervention and 4 weeks (paired $t = 3.48$, $p < .001$) and 12 weeks (paired $t = 3.68$, $p < .001$) postintervention, respectively. Thus, although burnout decreased more significantly between baseline and the end of the intervention in the experimental group than in the control group, the intergroup difference was not significant for either the baseline-to-4-weeks or the baseline-to-12-weeks postintervention period. Burnout is highly associated with external stressors, such as excessive workload (Stamm, 2010). Therefore, the lack of improvement in external stressors may lead to the lack of short-term and medium-term effects of the 3R educational program on burnout.

Secondary traumatic stress in the experimental group had decreased significantly at the end of the 3R educational program, which is consistent with previous studies that had applied compassion fatigue resiliency interventions (Potter, Deshields, & Rodriguez, 2013) and mindfulness interventions (Duarte & Pinto-Gouveia, 2016). Secondary traumatic stress in the experimental group was also significantly lower at the 4-week and 12-week postintervention time points. This finding is similar to a previous study that found significantly lower secondary traumatic stress at 2 months after the completion of a compassion fatigue resiliency program (Flarity, Rhodes, et al., 2016). By contrast, secondary traumatic stress in the control group, though significantly lower at the end of intervention, was not significantly lower at the 4-week or 12-week postintervention time points. Therefore, declines in secondary traumatic stress were significantly greater in the experimental group than in the control group at the three postintervention time points. The 3R educational program had immediate, short-term, and medium-term ameliorating effects on secondary traumatic stress.

Physical health in the experimental group had significantly increased at the end of the intervention but had significantly decreased at the 4 weeks and 12 weeks postintervention. In this study, the 3R educational program had an immediate improvement effect on physical health, which differs from previous studies, which found no positive effect of mindfulness interventions on physical health (Bazarko et al., 2013; Goodman & Schorling, 2012). The physical health of the control group in this study decreased significantly at all three postintervention time points. Physical health may worsen over time in the absence of intervention. Differences in patterns of change between the two groups resulted in the experimental group having significantly better physical health than the control group at the end of the intervention. Social support interventions have been shown to positively affect physical health (Walcott et al., 2018). Support from relatives and friends may also moderate the negative effects of secondary traumatic stress on physical health (Fu et al., 2018). 3R educational programs that incorporate support from friends and relatives may provide a stronger, immediate effect on physical health in nurses.

Mental health in the experimental group had increased significantly at the end of the intervention, which is in line with the finding of prior studies that mindfulness interventions had short-term, improvement effects on mental health (Bazarko et al., 2013; Goodman & Schorling, 2012). The mental health of the experimental group at 4 weeks and 12 weeks postintervention had significantly increased over the baseline. Nevertheless, the mental health of the experimental group at 4 weeks (pair $t = -4.33$, $p < .001$) and 12 weeks (pair $t = -6.07$, $p < .001$) after the intervention was significantly lower than immediately after the end of the intervention. The 3R educational program had the most significant impact on mental health at the end of intervention. However, this effect diminished afterward. Because mental health scores in the control group remained unchanged across all of the three postintervention time points, the experimental group had significantly better mental health scores than the control group at each time point. The 3R educational program had immediate, short-term, and medium-term effects on improving mental health. Secondary traumatic stress is known to be associated more with mental health than with physical health (Fu et al., 2018). The demonstrated ability of the 3R educational program to ameliorate secondary traumatic stress may improve the mental health of nurses over the immediate, short, and medium terms.

Limitation and Future Direction

The low retention rates in both the experimental (58.2%) and control groups (61.4%) at 12 weeks postintervention may be attributed to the time demand required to participate in the 4-week program. Developing online courses may be a feasible strategy to increase the retention rate. The results of a post hoc power analysis indicate that the intergroup powers of differences for secondary traumatic stress at the end of the intervention and for physical and mental health at 12 weeks postintervention were smaller than 0.8. The sample size in this study may have been insufficient to effectively examine the effects of the 3R educational program on secondary traumatic stress at the end of intervention and physical and mental health at 12 weeks postintervention. Furthermore, this study recruited participants from two hospitals in Taiwan only, which may have introduced a selection bias and limited the generalizability of the findings. Future studies should recruit nurses from a variety of hospitals and increase the sample size. In addition, the Cronbach's alpha of the physical and mental health scale was relatively low in this study. Further studies should use scales to measure physical and mental health that offer better internal consistency. The three components of the 3R educational program were distributed evenly over the 4 weeks of the intervention and delivered in sessions lasting only 2 hours per week. The dose and frequency of the three components may not have been sufficient to demonstrate the short-term and medium-term effects on improving burnout and physical health. Future studies may increase the doses and frequencies of each component of the 3R educational program and examine their respective effects. In addition, the long-term effects of the 3R educational program on the ProQOL, physical health, and mental health of nurses should be assessed in future studies. We were unable to exclude the possibility of a Hawthorne effect in the experimental group, which may have overestimated the actual impact of the 3R educational program. Further studies may use a placebo group to more accurately examine the effect of the program.

Conclusions

In this study, the 3R educational program was shown to provide positive effects on ProQOL, physical health, and mental health in the immediate term and to provide positive effects on compassion satisfaction, secondary traumatic stress, and mental health through the short and medium terms. The combined effects of the 3R educational program were better than the effects achieved by applying the components of 3R individually.

Relevance to Clinical Practice

Nursing managers may apply a program in workplace settings that integrates compassion fatigue resiliency, mindfulness respiration, and relatives and friends' support. The 3R educational program may be incorporated into on-the-job education programs. To overcome the challenges of shift work, this program may be distributed on compact disc or via asynchronous distance learning to achieve similar results. Finally, nursing managers should provide more resources to help clinical nurses build and sustain supportive groups of relatives and friends.

Acknowledgment

We are extremely grateful to all of the clinical nurses who participated in this study.

Author Contributions

Study conception and design: RHW, CYF
Data collection: CYF
Data analysis and interpretation: RHW, CCK
Drafting of the article: All authors
Critical revision of the article: RHW, CCK

References

Bazarko, D., Cate, R. A., Azocar, F., & Kreitzer, M. J. (2013). The impact of an innovative mindfulness-based stress reduction program on the health and well-being of nurses employed in a corporate setting. *Journal of Workplace Behavioral Health, 28*(2), 107–133. https://doi.org/10.1080/15555240.2013.779518

Carlesi, K. C., Padilha, K. G., Toffoletto, M. C., Henriquez-Roldan, C., & Juan, M. A. (2017). Patient safety incidents and nursing workload. *Revista Latino-Americana de Enfermagem, 25,* Article e2841. https://doi.org/10.1590/1518-8345.1280.2841

Cavanagh, N., Cockett, G., Heinrich, C., Doig, L., Fiest, K., Guichon, J. R., Page, S., Mitchell, I., & Doig, C. J. (2020). Compassion fatigue in healthcare providers: A systematic review and meta-analysis. *Nursing Ethics, 27*(3), 639–665. https://doi.org/10.1177/0969733019889400

Chou, L.-P., Li, C.-Y., & Hu, S. C. (2014). Job stress and burnout in hospital employees: Comparisons of different medical professions in a regional hospital in Taiwan. *BMJ Open, 4*(2), Article e004185. https://doi.org/10.1136/bmjopen-2013-004185

Cohen, J. (1988). *Statistical power analysis for the behavioral sciences.* Routledge Academic.

Duarte, J., & Pinto-Gouveia, J. (2016). Effectiveness of a mindfulness-based intervention on oncology nurses' burnout and compassion fatigue symptoms: A non-randomized study. *Internaional Journal of Nursing Studies, 64,* 98–107. https://doi.org/10.1016/j.ijnurstu.2016.10.002

Duchemin, A. M., Steinberg, B. A., Marks, D. R., Vanover, K., & Klatt, M. (2015). A small randomized pilot study of a workplace mindfulness-based intervention for surgical intensive care unit personnel: Effects on salivary alpha-amylase levels. *Journal of Occupaional and Environmenal Medicine, 57*(4), 393–399. https://doi.org/10.1097/jom.0000000000000371

Duhoux, A., Menear, M., Charron, M., Lavoie-Tremblay, M., & Alderson, M. (2017). Interventions to promote or improve the mental health of primary care nurses: A systematic review. *Journal of Nursing Management, 25*(8), 597–607. https://doi.org/10.1111/jonm.12511

Figley, C. R., & Figley, K. R. (2017). *Compassion fatigue resilience.* Oxford University Press. https://doi.org/10.1093/oxfordhb/9780190464684.013.28

Flarity, K., Gentry, J. E., & Mesnikoff, N. (2013). The effectiveness of an educational program on preventing and treating compassion fatigue in emergency nurses. *Advanced Emergency Nursing Journal, 35*(3), 247–258. https://doi.org/10.1097/TME.0b013e31829b726f

Flarity, K., Moorer, A., & Jones, W. R. (2018). Longitudinal study of a compassion fatigue resiliency intervention in nurse residents. *Journal of Nursing Education and Practice, 8*(9), 61–67. https://doi.org/10.5430/jnep.v8n9p61

Flarity, K., Nash, K., Jones, W., & Steinbruner, D. (2016). Intervening to improve compassion fatigue resiliency in forensic nurses. *Advanced Emergency Nursing Journal, 38*(2), 147–156. https://doi.org/10.1097/TME.0000000000000101

Flarity, K., Rhodes, W. J., & Reckard, P. (2016). Intervening to improve compassion fatigue resiliency in nurse residents. *Journal of Nursing Education and Practice, 6*(12), 99–104. https://doi.org/10.5430/jnep.v6n12p99

Freimann, T., Paasuke, M., & Merisalu, E. (2016). Work-related psychosocial factors and mental health problems associated with musculoskeletal pain in nurses: A cross-sectional study. *Pain Research and Management, 2016,* Article 9361016. https://doi.org/10.1155/2016/9361016

Fu, C. Y., Yang, M. S., Leung, W., Liu, Y. Y., Huang, H. W., & Wang, R. H. (2018). Associations of professional quality of life and social support with health in clinical nurses. *Journal of Nursing Management, 26*(2), 172–179. https://doi.org/10.1111/jonm.12530

Gentry, J. E., Baranowsky, A. B., & Dunning, K. (2002). The accelerated recovery program (ARP) for compassion fatigue. In C. R. Figley (Ed.), *Psychosocial stress series, no. 24. Treating compassion fatigue* (pp. 123–137). Brunner-Routledge.

Goodman, M. J., & Schorling, J. B. (2012). A mindfulness course decreases burnout and improves well-being among healthcare providers. *The Internaional Journal of Psychiatry in Medicine, 43*(2), 119–128. https://doi.org/10.2190/PM.43.2.b

Gregory, A. (2015). Yoga and mindfulness program: The effects on compassion fatigue and compassion satisfaction in social workers. *Journal of Religion & Spirituality in Social Work: Social Thought, 34*(4), 372–393. https://doi.org/10.1080/15426432.2015.1080604

Hevezi, J. A. (2016). Evaluation of a meditation intervention to reduce the effects of stressors associated with compassion fatigue among nurses. *Journal of Holist Nursing, 34*(4), 343–350. https://doi.org/10.1177/0898010115615981

Horner, J. K., Piercy, B. S., Eure, L., & Woodard, E. K. (2014). A pilot study to evaluate mindfulness as a strategy to improve inpatient nurse and patient experiences. *Applied Nursing Research, 27*(3), 198–201. https://doi.org/10.1016/j.apnr.2014.01.003

Hunsaker, S., Chen, H. C., Maughan, D., & Heaston, S. (2015). Factors that influence the development of compassion fatigue, burnout, and compassion satisfaction in emergency department nurses. *Journal of Nursing Scholarship, 47*(2), 186–194. https://doi.org/10.1111/jnu.12122

Jang, I., Kim, Y., & Kim, K. (2016). Professionalism and professional quality of life for oncology nurses. *Journal of Clinical Nursing., 25*, 2835–2845. https://doi.org/https://doi.org/10.1111/jocn.13330

Kabat-Zinn, J. (1982). An outpatient program in behavioral medicine for chronic pain patients based on the practice of mindfulness meditation: Theoretical considerations and preliminary results. *General Hospial Psychiatry, 4*(1), 33–47. https://doi.org/10.1016/0163-8343(82)90026-3

Kawar, L. N., Radovich, P., Valdez, R. M., Zuniga, S., & Rondinelli, J. (2019). Compassion fatigue and compassion satisfaction among multisite multisystem nurses. *Nursing Administration Quarterly, 43*(4), 358–369. https://doi.org/10.1097/naq.0000000000000370

Killingsworth, M. A., & Gilbert, D. T. (2010). A wandering mind is an unhappy mind. *Science, 330*(6006), 932. https://doi.org/10.1126/science.1192439

Li, Y., Fang, J., & Zhou, C. (2019). Work-related predictors of sleep quality in Chinese nurses: Testing a path analysis model. *The Journal of Nursing Research, 27*(5), Article e44. https://doi.org/10.1097/jnr.0000000000000319

Macfarlane, J., & Carson, J. (2019). Positive psychology: An overview for use in mental health nursing. *British Journal of Mental Health Nursing, 8*(1), 34–39. https://doi.org/10.12968/bjmh.2019.8.1.34

Mooney, C., Fetter, K., Gross, B. W., Rinehart, C., Lynch, C., & Rogers, F. B. (2017). A preliminary analysis of compassion satisfaction and compassion fatigue with considerations for nursing unit specialization and demographic factors. *Journal of Trauma Nursing, 24*(3), 158–163. https://doi.org/10.1097/jtn.0000000000000284

Nolte, A. G., Downing, C., Temane, A., & Hastings-Tolsma, M. (2017). Compassion fatigue in nurses: A metasynthesis. *Journal of Clinical Nursing, 26*(23–24), 4364–4378. https://doi.org/10.1111/jocn.13766

Peters, E. (2018). Compassion fatigue in nursing: A concept analysis. *Nursing Forum, 53*(4), 466–480. https://doi.org/10.1111/nuf.12274

Potter, P., Deshields, T., Berger, J. A., Clarke, M., Olsen, S., & Chen, L. (2013). Evaluation of a compassion fatigue resiliency program for oncology nurses. *Oncology Nursing Forum, 40*(2), 180–187. https://doi.org/10.1188/13.onf.180-187

Potter, P., Deshields, T., & Rodriguez, S. (2013). Developing a systemic program for compassion fatigue. *Nursing Administration Quarterly, 37*(4), 326–332. https://doi.org/10.1097/NAQ.0b013e3182a2f9dd

Rayan, A., Sisan, M., & Baker, O. (2019). Stress, workplace violence, and burnout in nurses working in king Abdullah Medical City during Al-hajj season. *The Journal of Nursing Research, 27*(3), Article e26. https://doi.org/10.1097/jnr.0000000000000291

Ruiz-Fernández, M. D., Ortíz-Amo, R., Ortega-Galán, Á., Ibáñez-Masero, O., Rodríguez-Salvador, M. M., Ramos-Pichardo, J. D., Ibáñez-Masero, O., Rodríguez-Salvador, M. D. M., & Ramos-Pichardo, J. D. (2020). Mindfulness therapies on health professionals. *International Journal of Mental Health Nursing, 29*(2), 127–140. https://doi.org/10.1111/inm.12652

Stamm, B. H. (2010). *The concise ProQOL manual* (2nd ed.). ProQOL.org

Van Gerven, E., Vander Elst, T., Vandenbroeck, S., Dierickx, S., Euwema, M., Sermeus, W., & Vanhaecht, K. (2016). Increased risk of burnout for physicians and nurses involved in a patient safety incident. *Medical Care, 54*(10), 937–943. https://doi.org/10.1097/mlr.0000000000000582

Walcott, R. L., Murcia, A. M., Berry, G. M., Juna, C. F., Roldós, M. I., & Corso, P. S. (2018). The impact of nursing students on the health-related quality of life and perceived social support of a rural population in Ecuador: Effects of a service-based learning course. *International Journal for Equity in Health, 17*(1), Article No. 16. https://doi.org/10.1186/s12939-018-0734-z

Ware, J. Jr., Kosinski, M., & Keller, S. D. (1996). A 12-item short-form health survey: Construction of scales and preliminary tests of reliability and validity. *Medical Care, 34*(3), 220–233. https://doi.org/10.1097/00005650-199603000-00003

Weigl, M., Stab, N., Herms, I., Angerer, P., Hacker, W., & Glaser, J. (2016). The associations of supervisor support and work overload with burnout and depression: A cross-sectional study in two nursing settings. *Journal of Advanced Nursing, 72*(8), 1774–1788. https://doi.org/10.1111/jan.12948

Williams, P., Barclay, L., & Schmied, V. (2004). Defining social support in context: A necessary step in improving research, intervention, and practice. *Qualitaive Health Research, 14*(7), 942–960. https://doi.org/10.1177/1049732304266997

18

How Do Hospitalized Adolescents Feel Safe?

Neda JAMALIMOGHADAM[1] • Shahrzad YEKTATALAB[2]* • Marzieh MOMENNASAB[3] • Abbas EBADI[4] • Najaf ZARE[5]

ABSTRACT

Background: The feeling of safety makes an important contribution to the sense of well-being and quality of care for hospitalized adolescents, who are at a higher risk of feeling unsafe. Feeling unsafe during hospitalization may have a negative impact on recovery. Nurses must be sensitive to the possibility that patients feel unsafe, even in the absence of obvious direct physical threat.

Purpose: This study explores the experiences of hospitalized adolescents to obtain an understanding of psychological safety.

Methods: A qualitative study using unstructured interviews was conducted to explore the sense of psychological safety of hospitalized adolescents aged 12–18 years and registered in a general medical or surgical pediatric unit. Purposive sampling was used to recruit new qualified participants until data saturation was reached (*N* = 16).

Results: Psychological safety is reflected by the four themes of receiving comprehensive support, protection of human dignity, relaxing environment, and attempts to adapt.

Conclusions: Hospitalized adolescents stated that healthcare services should provide comprehensive support in a relaxing environment that allows them to retain their human dignity and that elicits feelings of psychological safety.

Key Words:
psychological safety, adolescent, hospitalization.

Introduction

Adolescents compose a significant proportion of the population of hospitalized patients. They want control over their lives, friendships, and some level of privacy during hospitalization. However, hospitalization entails separation from family and friends, who are often important sources of support and security, requiring the adolescent to significantly change daily life and routines, live in an unfamiliar environment, and face invasive and painful medical procedures and new stressors (Moura de Moura, Costa Junior, de Amorim Silva, da Silva Reichert, & Collet, 2015). The unfamiliar hospital environment and procedures and the changes to daily routines often conflict with the developmental needs of adolescents (Hutton, 2002; Smith, 2004). Needs-based care for adolescents is important because adolescence is a time of transition from childhood to adulthood and is associated with profound biological, mental, and psychosocial changes (Smith, 2004). If security needs are not met, then higher needs cannot be fulfilled (Maslow, 1987). Psychological safety is a subjective concept that is achieved as a result of direct and indirect experiences relative to one's environment (Huisman, Morales, Van Hoof, & Kort, 2012).

Feeling safe is different from being safe (Mollon, 2014). Psychological safety and feeling safe are important to a sense of well-being and important aspects of quality of care (Aro, Pietilä, Vehviläinen-Julkunen, 2012; Hupcey, 2000; Krevers & Milberg, 2014; Lasiter, 2011). Exposure to new places such as hospitals may engender feelings of fear, insecurity, anxiety, lack of comfort, fatigue, insomnia, and depression in patients (Avdagic & Carlström, 2014). As the largest group of healthcare professionals, nurses must understand the needs of adolescents, including the need for psychological safety. Nurses should be sensitive to patient perceptions regarding level of safety (Stenhouse, 2013). However, the emphasis of previous clinical studies has largely been on the physical safety of patients, with few studies addressing the topic of emotional or psychological safety (Lasiter, 2011; Stenhouse, 2013). The significance of psychological safety in adolescents, especially in qualitative studies, is rarely mentioned. Whereas there has been little research on psychological safety in Iran, studies have been conducted in other countries such as Sweden (Avdagic & Carlström, 2014; Fagerström, Gustafson, Jakobsson, Johansson, & Vartiainen,

[1]PhD, RN, Assistant Professor, Department of Nursing, Community Based Psychiatric Care Research Center, School of Nursing and Midwifery, Shiraz University of Medical Sciences, Shiraz, Iran • [2]PhD, RN, Associate Professor, Department of Mental Health and Psychiatric Nursing, School of Nursing and Midwifery, Shiraz University of Medical Sciences, Shiraz, Iran • [3]PhD, RN, Associate Professor, Department of Nursing, School of Nursing and Midwifery, Shiraz University of Medical Sciences, Shiraz, Iran • [4]PhD, RN, Professor, Faculty of Nursing, Behavioral Sciences Research Center, Life Style Institute, Baqiyatallah University of Medical Sciences, Tehran, Iran • [5]PhD, Associate Professor, Department of Biostatistics, Shiraz School of Public Health, Shiraz University of Medical Sciences, Shiraz, Iran.

2011; Krevers & Milberg, 2014) and the United States (Hupcey, 2000; Lasiter, 2011). However, the cultural, religious, and clinical contexts of these studies differ significantly from Iran. Furthermore, most research on psychological safety has been done on patients in intensive care units (Wassenaar, Schouten, & Schoonhoven, 2014) and with chronic illness (Krevers & Milberg, 2014) older than 18 years.

As an abstract, context-dependent concept, psychological safety is not particularly amenable to quantitative research, and qualitative techniques are typically preferred. The aim of this study was to describe and explore the sense of psychological safety in adolescents using naturalistic and qualitative techniques that provide insight into subjective perceptions and provide information about the phenomenon.

Methods

Design

This exploratory descriptive study gathered naturalistic and descriptive data (Burns & Grove, 2005) and analyzed qualitative data using conventional content analysis.

Participants

A purposive sample of 16 Persian-speaking adolescents who were 12–18 years old participated in this study between March 2015 and May 2016. The participants were recruited from a hospital in Shiraz (southwestern Iran), which is one of Iran's largest healthcare centers and regularly treats clients referred from all over the country. This hospital has four medical wards and two surgical wards for children. There are no separate wards for adolescents, who are thus hospitalized with other children in rooms with two to six beds. This study recruited adolescents who had been admitted to either a medical or surgical ward in the target hospital, were physically and psychologically fit to be interviewed, and had been hospitalized for at least 2 days. Interviews were arranged by the first author, who went to the hospital on a weekly basis to interview potential participants.

Data Collection

Data were collected using face-to-face, audiotaped, unstructured interviews conducted in a quiet environment. Unstructured interviews start with a general question in the broad area of study. Except for the very beginning of the interview, no predetermined questions were used, which allowed the interview process to be flexible. Researchers followed the interests and thoughts of the participants rather than the researchers' assumptions. Subsequent questions were based on responses to earlier questions. Participants were free to answer at length, providing great depth and detail (Holloway & Wheeler, 2010; Speziale, Streubert, & Carpenter, 2011). Interviews began with the general question, "How do you feel about being in the hospital?" Examples of subsequent questions include "Since your hospitalization, please describe some situations that affected your sense of safety"; "What situations make you feel safer?"; "What situations make you feel unsafe?"; "What or who helps you to relax while in the hospital?"; and "Can you explain that/explain it/give an example?" The first interview was treated as preliminary and used to identify potential areas of interest or concern. We used maximized variation sampling because this approach searches for individuals with widely differing respective experiences and for variations in settings (Holloway & Wheeler, 2010). Participants included men and women with a broad range of ages and diagnoses to maximize variation.

Purposive sampling continued until data saturation was achieved. Interviews lasted between 25 and 65 minutes and were digitally recorded (Hyundai), converted to audio files on a portable computer, and then transcribed verbatim.

Ethical Considerations

Ethical approval for this study was granted by the ethics committee of Shiraz University of Medical Sciences (no. 94-7495). Written and oral consent was obtained from both the target hospital and participants before data collection. Interviews took place in conditions that ensured the privacy and comfort of the participants. The participants were informed that they could stop the interview or refuse to participate at any point. Data were identified by codes, and participants were identified by pseudonyms in all reports related to this study to ensure participant anonymity and confidentiality.

Data Analysis

The data were subjected to conventional content analysis using the method developed by Graneheim and Lundman (2004). Conventional content analysis was chosen because the existing theories and literature on psychological safety in hospitalized adolescents are limited, and researchers wanted to avoid preconceptions in favor of allowing the categories and names of categories to flow from the data (Elo et al., 2014; Graneheim & Lundman, 2004). The qualitative content analysis method focuses primarily on the subject and context, emphasizing the differences between and similarities within codes and categories. It also deals with both the manifest and latent contents within a text. The manifest content (i.e., what the text says) is often presented in categories, whereas themes are seen as expressions of the latent content (i.e., what the text is talking about; Graneheim & Lundman, 2004).

The interviews were read carefully several times to gain an overall picture of the material. Next, important statements were underlined to identify initial codes or units of meaning related to psychological safety. These units of meaning were organized into themes and subthemes at different levels of abstraction. Data analysis ran concurrently with data collection and continued until saturation was achieved (i.e., until more data did not reveal new information and were considered redundant). The final step in the analysis was to extract the main themes (Graneheim & Lundman, 2004). Data classification and analysis were carried out using MAXQDA10 software (VERBI Software GmbH, Berlin, Germany).

Rigor

The validity and reliability of the study were assessed using the criteria suggested by Lincoln and Guba (1985). Long-term interaction with participants (15 months) established credibility; the investment of sufficient time in collecting data is necessary for an in-depth understanding of the group or phenomenon under study as well as to test for misinformation and distortions and ensure data saturation in key categories. In planning a qualitative study, researchers must ensure that they have adequate time and resources to stay engaged in fieldwork for a sufficiently long period (Burns & Grove, 2005). In this study, researchers transcribed interviews and sorted field notes; organized, ordered, and stored the data; repeatedly listened to and read or viewed the collected materials; and coded and categorized the data. An iterative process of data analysis meant that researchers moved between data collection and data analysis over an extended period (Holloway & Wheeler, 2010).

In addition, the participants confirmed the validity of the findings, interviews were reviewed by external supervisors, and all of the interviews were audiotaped and transcribed verbatim. The reliability of the data was assessed by reviewing the material in consultation with a supervisor and associate professors as well as through data triangulation (time, space, and person triangulation). Triangulation involves the use of multiple data sources for the purpose of validating conclusions (Holloway & Wheeler, 2010). In a qualitative study, triangulation may involve an attempt to reveal the complexity of a phenomenon by using multiple means of data collection to converge on the truth (Polit & Beck, 2010). In this study, we selected different spaces (wards), different times (shifts), and different individuals (of different ages, genders, and diagnoses). Confirmability was ensured by allocating sufficient time to collect a comprehensive set of data (15 months), transcribing all interviews immediately, sampling to maximize variation (age, gender, and time), and logging all procedures to provide an audit trail. Confirmability requires an audit or decision trail that permits readers to trace the data to their sources (Holloway & Wheeler, 2010). In this study, several classes of records constituted an adequate audit trail: (a) raw data (e.g., patient quotes), (b) data reduction and analysis products (e.g., table of main themes, subthemes, and categories), (c) process notes (e.g., methodological process), (d) materials related to researchers' intentions and dispositions (e.g., method and context), and (e) data reconstruction products (e.g., results; Polit & Beck, 2010).

Transferability means that the findings in one context are transferable to similar situations or participants (Polit & Beck, 2010). In this study, to promote transferability, information such as demographics and study setting were described clearly in terms of culture and context, selection and characteristics of participants, method of data collection, and process of analysis. A thorough presentation of findings and appropriate quotations ensure transferability (Graneheim & Lundman, 2004).

Results

Sixteen adolescents (10 boys and six girls) between 12 and 18 years old and hospitalized in the general medical or surgical pediatric wards with diagnoses including irritable bowel syndrome, appendicitis, nephrotic syndrome, pyelonephritis, and pancreatitis participated in this study.

Four main themes emerged from the content analysis: (a) receiving comprehensive support, (b) protection of human dignity, (c) relaxing environment, and (d) attempts to adapt. In addition, 12 subthemes were defined. Table 1 presents the main themes, subthemes, and primary categories.

Receiving Comprehensive Support

Receiving comprehensive support was identified as a vital and multidimensional need of patients. This main theme encompasses spiritual, psychosocial, physical, and informational support provided by family, friends, staff, God, and school personnel.

Spiritual support

The participants sought support to face new environments, procedures, and people. They viewed God as a particularly good source of support. One patient stated that his family's religious practices made him feel that he was under God's protection:

> *When my mother read the Qur'an, I felt that God was helping me and that if surgery is necessary, God will take care of me.* (P3)

Presence of supporters is another primary category. The participants said that they felt safer, more relaxed, and better able to tolerate pain in the presence of family members, especially their mothers:

> *The presence of my mother gave me a certain sense of relief. When my mum was with me, I forgot about the pain.* (P9)

Having access to nurses and physicians in an emergency was important for patients:

> *If something happens, nurses and doctors come soon and treat me quickly.* (P10)

Psychosocial support

The primary categories of psychological support were emotional support from the healthcare team, family, school

TABLE 1.
Main Themes, Subthemes, and Primary Categories

Main Theme	Subtheme	Primary Category
1. Receiving comprehensive support	1.1 Spiritual support	• God's presence and support • Others' presence and support
	1.2 Psychosocial support	• Emotional support of the healthcare team • Emotional support of the family • Support by school personnel • Friend's attention • Support by relatives
	1.3 Physical support	• Existence of security services • Participation of family in physical care • Trusting care and treatment
	1.4 Informational support	• Providing information by nurses • Providing information by physicians
2. Protection of human dignity	2.1 Protection of personal privacy	• Protection of informational privacy • Protection of physical privacy
	2.2 Respect for identity	• Respect for age identity • Respect for gender identity
	2.3 Protection of autonomy	• Adjustment of restrictive laws • Providing the sense of personal control • Attention to patients and family's idea
	2.4 Intimate communication	• Kind communication • Friendly communication • Respectful communication
3. Relaxing environment	3.1 Appropriate structural factors	• Clean environment • Appropriate visual factors • Appropriate temperature • Appropriate dimensions • Closeness to the nursing station
	3.2 Adequate facility	• Quiet environment • Recreational facilities • Welfare and sanitary facilities
4. Attempts to adapt	4.1 Problem-focused coping strategies	• Communication with peer group • Acceptance of new experiences • Patient's efforts to contribute in caring
	4.2 Emotion-focused coping strategies	• Playing and entertainment • Acceptance of God's will, trust in God

personnel, friends, and relatives. One participant related a conversation with a physician:

> *My doctor emphasized my positive characteristics. For example, they told me that I was a courageous adolescent and that I could tolerate disease more than younger children, so I could cope with my disease. If I was scared from procedures such as angiography, they would help me to be calm with their hopeful speeches.* (P6)

Social relationships with school staff and friends were a source of support for adolescent patients, as one explained:

> *My teachers and friends called on me and said I shouldn't feel stressed about my lessons. They said*

that they will be there for me. They said that I should try to be healthy as soon as possible. My principal told me when I was discharged and came back to my school, she would tell my teachers to teach me and give the exams. I realized that they supported me in any situation. (P9)

Physical support

The participants emphasized the role of guardians (i.e., family, nurses, and physicians) in supporting their physical needs. According to participants, guardians help protect them and their personal belongings such as cell phones from strangers. Furthermore, family members facilitate their physical needs such as going to the toilet and walking. Nurses and physicians provide proper and professional care and treatment of patients in the hospital. The participants noted that they felt safe when physical support needs were met and when nursing care was provided appropriately and on time:

Nurses come every half an hour. They monitor my blood pressure and body temperature and give me my medications on time. I feel safe and I think I will get better. (P10)

The participants said that the guardians in the wards gave them a sense of psychological safety, which alleviated feelings of being in danger. One participant said:

I don't feel under threat. Because the guardians are here. They stop strangers from coming into the wards. I feel safe, especially when I'm sleeping. (P7)

Informational support

Participants and families appreciated having information about the illness, treatment, medication, and recovery provided by nurses and physicians. One participant said:

When doctors tell me to undergo sonography, I'm afraid. They should explain it and its reasons to me. They should answer my questions. (P15)

Protection of Human Dignity

This main theme covers protection of personal privacy, respect for identity, protection of autonomy, and intimate communication.

Protection of personal privacy

Privacy is an important aspect of human dignity. Because the participants were all Muslim, they reported that having visitors, especially of the opposite gender, was an invasion of their hijab and of their privacy:

I was upset because when I was sleeping, my roommate's visitors came into the room without my permission. I needed to put on my scarf and cover myself with blankets. My feet were blistered, but I couldn't expose them and be calm. (P4)

The participants voiced the desire to protect their privacy:

"I can tolerate the pain, but I can't tolerate that nurses or doctors want to examine me or expose my body without my permission. If this happens, I would be angry" (P10).

Respect for identity

The participants expressed the desire for hospital staff to respect their age and gender identity. Because of legal and resource limitations, in Iran, no hospital maintains a dedicated ward for adolescents, who are hospitalized in children's wards. Given sufficient space in the pediatric wards, adolescents are typically hospitalized with their peer group in one room. If sufficient space is not available, adolescents may be hospitalized with younger children in one room.

One participant said that he did not feel it was right for him to be hospitalized in the children's ward:

They shouldn't have put me in a pediatric ward. I'm 16 years old and they admitted me in a pediatric ward. I can't sleep at night at all. When I'm sleeping, I am awakened by crying children. (P1)

Protection of autonomy

Protection of autonomy is particularly important to adolescents. The participants in this study desired control over their activities and reported that some procedures disrupted their sleep and autonomy:

We can't sleep well at nights. In the morning when we fall asleep, nurses want to do procedures such as blood test for us. This means we can't control our sleep in the hospital. (P4)

Patients in Iran are not allowed to leave their wards during hospitalization without permission from the head nurse. The participants said that this restriction on movement threatened their autonomy:

If I could go out of the ward and play around, I would feel more freedom. But, the personnel don't allow me to go there. In our home, we feel more autonomy, but I feel I'm in prison in the hospital. (P10)

Intimate communication

According to the participants, intimate communication involves kind, friendly, and respectful behavior toward patients and their families by nurses, physicians, and guardians. One participant explained the need for respect:

> *If someone doesn't communicate well, we don't feel safe. But when they communicate well, we do feel safe. It's a law of physics; every action has a reaction. It means I want friendly nurses who call me by my first name and communicate respectfully with me and my family.* (P4)

Relaxing Environment

The participants explained that a silent environment with appropriate structural factors and adequate facilities gave them comfort and was a source of psychological safety.

Appropriate structural factors

The participants said that cleanliness in the ward was an important factor in psychological safety: "*The ward is a clean environment. They use disinfectants here. The cleaning crews clean the ward regularly*" (P6).

In addition, being in a quiet environment was relaxing and made the participants feel safe. One participant said:

> *Relaxation means that there isn't much noise in the ward. For example, my roommates and visitors should speak in low voices. There shouldn't be too many visitors at any one time. Also, they shouldn't make much noise when they want to move chairs in the room.* (P10)

Adequate facilities

Recreational facilities were also important to the comfort of participants. One mentioned the adverse effects of the lack of recreational facilities:

> *I feel so bad because I don't have Internet in the ward. I cannot play and use chat forums.* (P11)

The dimensions and temperature of the room were also identified as important factors. One participant said:

> *My room is too small. When I and my roommate have visitors, there isn't enough air to breathe. Also, it is so cold when the air conditioner is turned on.* (P4)

Attempts to Adapt

Adaptation was another main theme that emerged from the data. This theme reflects the perception that external and environmental factors are not sufficient to ensure the psychological safety of a patient and that the patient must also adapt and adjust to the hospital environment and to his or her disease. The participants in this study reported that psychological safety is the motivation to adapt to stressors and that they used the two approaches of problem- and emotion-focused coping.

Problem-focused coping strategies

Problem-focused coping involves accepting new experiences, trying to participate in care, and asking peers and friends for helpful experiences and coping strategies. The participants said that asking questions might be useful in reducing their fear of surgery:

> *I had many questions about surgery, so I asked my hospitalized friend, who had undergone surgery, about his experience. He told me that a nurse got him ready and asked him some questions before he was taken to the operating room. Also, I asked my questions about pain, anesthesia, period of unconsciousness, and so on. I felt that I knew about my surgery and would have a good surgery without adverse consequences.* (P9)

Emotion-focused coping strategies

In addition to problem-focused coping, the participants also used emotion-focused coping strategies. Recreational activities such as games and entertainment and trust in God helped them stay calm and cope with stress. One participant told us that he felt he would cope better if he were able to play and have fun:

> *Look, in this ward, there is no games room. My legs are in plaster, so I can't go to the opposite ward to play. If there was a games room, I could entertain myself and the time would pass faster.* (P13)

Discussion

Interviews indicated that respecting human dignity and providing comprehensive support in a relaxing environment were important to maximize psychological safety. However, patients must also be able to adapt to new circumstances.

"Receiving comprehensive support" was one of the main themes and involves ensuring that help and support are always available to patients (Bruwer, Emsley, Kidd, Lochner, & Seedat, 2008). The participants stated that receiving "physical and psychosocial support" from family, friends, teachers, and relatives; "informational support" from nurses and physicians; and "spiritual support" from God provided a sense of psychological safety. Once a patient has been admitted to a hospital, the physical presence and mental support of trusted personnel, particularly nurses, play an important role in promoting a sense of peace and psychological safety (Burström, Brännström, Boman, & Strandberg, 2012; Hupcey, 2000). This study, like other studies, found that physical protection in the form of accessible and timely nursing care was important to psychological safety (Lasiter, 2011; Mollon, 2014). Participants in this study stressed the importance of reassurance provided by the presence and supervision of guardians. This issue has received less attention in other studies. One of the most important duties of guardians is to supervise the movement of visitors and to prevent strangers from gaining access to the wards.

The subtheme "informational support" refers to giving sufficient advice and information. It is important for patients to learn about the illness, treatment, and recovery process (Mattila, Kaunonen, Aalto, Ollikainen, & Åstedt-Kurki, 2010). Participants in this study wished to be informed about their illnesses, procedures, and medications.

Spirituality is the expressed essence of human beings made visible in relationships both vertically (with a higher power) and horizontally (humans), the consequences of which are love, faith, hope, and a purpose for being. A caring presence helps patients heal, strengthens the feeling of spiritual support, and involves an interaction wherein a reciprocal experience relates to the whole person, goes beyond the technical, and attends to the complexity of a person's needs (Rankin & DeLashmutt, 2006). A caring presence has a calming effect on the patient. Adolescents desire to have family members with them when they are in the hospital (Beresford & Sloper, 2003). Family support and family participation in patient care improve mood and reduce feelings of isolation and depression (Mattila et al., 2010; Yektatalab, Sharif, Kaveh, Khoshknab, & Petramfar, 2013). Adolescents seek independence but remain physically and psychologically dependent on their family. The problems that visiting a patient in the hospital causes for the family—travel difficulties, delays, and/or expenses—may cause patients to feel guilty and blame themselves, although they need and welcome the support. Moreover, visits from friends, a source of support that has been mentioned in other studies (Mattila et al., 2010), are helpful because these allow adolescent patients to talk about their disease, everyday problems, loneliness, and entertainment. Furthermore, the need for spiritual support was mentioned by the participants. Spirituality is an inherent quality, a connective force, and a source of cohesive strength in all humans. A patient who feels under the protection of a powerful God will improve, feel safe, and be less anxious and fearful (Jaberi, Momennasab, Yektatalab, Ebadi, & Cheraghi, 2017). The importance of spiritual support in this study relates to the religious and cultural background of the participants, who were all Muslim.

Our findings indicate that respect by the staff and others for the human dignity of patients promotes psychological safety. Human dignity is at the core of human relationships and is a fundamental human right (Narayan, Hooker, Jarrett, & Bennett, 2013). Respect for human dignity of patients is more important because they are in a particularly vulnerable position. This finding is consistent with an earlier study showing that respecting patient dignity helps give them a sense of security (Borhani, Abbaszadeh, & Rabori, 2015). Autonomy is essential to the dignity of adolescents because of its central role in this developmental stage. In fact, hospitalization robs them of control over many issues, and most adolescent patients disagree with some hospital rules (Findlay et al., 2008). Previous studies show that many adolescent patients believe that their healthcare team does not involve them in decisions about their care and that any decision made without their consent is unacceptable (Barkay & Tabak, 2002). This is consistent with the results of this study. The participants in this study expressed the belief that strict rules and procedures that disrupted their sleep undermined their autonomy and dignity. It is essential to involve patients and their families in decisions about care and treatment and to make the rules governing the care of adolescent patients more flexible.

Privacy is fundamental to human dignity. Holistic care must involve respect for the privacy of patients, especially in the case of hospitalized adolescents. Adolescence is a time when individuals try to establish their identity and autonomy, and any interference with this is perceived as a threat to their dignity (Reed, Smith, Fletcher, & Bradding, 2003). The participants in this study, especially the women, felt that having people of the opposite gender come into the ward without their permission was an invasion of their privacy, especially if these intrusions involved exposing parts of their body. Unwelcome ward visits clearly increased the anxiety of the participants and undermined their sense of safety. Perceptions of human dignity are rooted in culture. As noted above, all of the participants in this study were Muslim. In Islam, there are clear boundaries for encounters with the opposite gender. Adolescents regarded themselves as adults who were bound by Islamic rules, which made gender identity a particularly important issue in this study. However, even in non-Muslim countries, there is evidence that teenagers prefer not to have individuals of the opposite gender in their room and would prefer to be in single-gender wards (Narayan et al., 2013).

The psychological safety of adolescents is undermined when arrangements for hospital care do not take age and gender identity into account. In the target hospital, adolescents were exposed to the tantrums of younger children in their rooms. Hutton concluded that adolescents want to be hospitalized in a private room (Hutton, 2002). Others have also noted that adolescents do not feel that they belong in pediatric wards (Narayan et al., 2013), and it has been recommended that, whenever possible, adolescents should be cared for in adolescent wards or otherwise placed with their age peers (Hockenberry & Wilson, 2014).

We also found that a relaxing environment contributes to psychological safety. In fact, psychological safety is a subjective feeling that originates from environmental factors. The environmental factors that were mentioned by the participants in this study as contributors to psychological safety were silence, adequate facilities, and appropriate structural factors. Several studies have revealed that light, sound, temperature, and peripheral equipment affect the psychological safety of patients (Vogus, 2016). Attempting to adapt, although a main theme in this study, has received less attention in other studies. It is inevitable that hospitalization brings stress, concerns, and fears and that patients use both problem- and emotion-focused coping strategies (Fortinash & Worret, 2011). The participants in this study said that accepting new experiences, trying to participate in care, and communicating with peers and friends helped them to adapt. They also mentioned using emotion-focused strategies such as playing, having fun, and trusting in God. Trust in God boosted their confidence and power for enduring hardships, and performing religious practices such as prayers provided psychological safety and peace (Jaberi et al., 2017; Tartaro, Luecken, & Gunn, 2005). Our results show that the psychological safety of hospitalized adolescents depends not only on external factors such as the provision of comprehensive support, protection of human dignity, and a relaxing environment but also on an internal factor—the ability to cope with a new situation.

This study was performed in one hospital. Focus groups could not be conducted because the adolescent patients were distributed among several wards. Further qualitative and quantitative research at other locations and in other cultures is necessary to explore the concept of psychological safety. Future research should include investigations into the perceptions of healthcare providers regarding the psychological safety of their patients.

Implications

Optimal patient care cannot be achieved if hospital staffs do their best to maintain the physical safety but neglect the psychological safety of their patients. Ensuring both will help minimize the length of hospital stays as well as maximize patient comfort and well-being. Adolescence is a time of transition during which adolescents experience many physical, psychological, and social changes. Not working to ensure the psychological safety of patients during hospitalization may have irreversible consequences for their future lives. Furthermore, officials and hospital staffs should provide dedicated wards for adolescents to address the concerns that this age group typically has for self-identity.

Conclusions

This study shows that a relaxing environment that offers comprehensive support and that respects dignity promotes feelings of psychological safety in adolescents. However, the ability of adolescents to adapt is also an important factor.

Having a ward dedicated to this age group is necessary to prevent violations of dignity because adolescents have needs that differ from both children and adults. In addition, Muslim adolescents, especially female adolescents, regard themselves as adults who should wear hijabs. This issue made gender identity a particularly important issue in this study. The participants expressed a preference to be placed in single-gender hospital accommodations. In this study, female adolescents, especially the older ones, were particularly anxious about their privacy in the hospital.

Acknowledgments

This article is a part of the doctoral dissertation of Neda Jamalimoghadam, which was financially supported by the Shiraz University of Medical Sciences, no. 7495-94. The authors would like to thank the participants for their close cooperation; the Shiraz University of Medical Sciences, Shiraz, Iran; the Center for Development of Clinical Research of Nemazee Hospital; and Dr. Nasrin Shokrpour for editorial assistance.

References

Aro, I., Pietilä, A. M., & Vehviläinen Julkunen, K. (2012). Needs of adult patients in intensive care units of Estonian hospitals: A questionnaire survey. *Journal of Clinical Nursing, 21*(13–14), 1847–1858. https://doi.org/10.1111/j.1365-2702.2012.04092.x

Avdagic, M., & Carlström, E. (2014). The path to patient safety in primary health care—A study of nurses' and general practitioners' perceptions in Sweden. *Journal of Nursing Education and Practice, 4*(7), 85–94. https://doi.org/10.5430/jnep.v4n7p85

Barkay, A., & Tabak, N. (2002). Elderly residents' participation and autonomy within a geriatric ward in a public institution. *International Journal of Nursing Practice, 8*(4), 198–209. https://doi.org/10.1046/j.1440-172X.2002.00363.x

Beresford, B. A., & Sloper, P. (2003). Chronically ill adolescents' experiences of communicating with doctors: A qualitative study. *Journal of Adolescent Health, 33*(3), 172–179. https://doi.org/10.1016/S1054-139X(03)00047-8

Borhani, F., Abbaszadeh, A., & Rabori, R. M. (2015). New vision for the dignity: Understanding the meaning of patient dignity in Iran. *British Journal of Medicine and Medical Research, 9*(2), Article No. 18886. https://doi.org/10.9734/BJMMR/2015/18886

Bruwer, B., Emsley, R., Kidd, M., Lochner, C., & Seedat, S. (2008). Psychometric properties of the Multidimensional Scale of Perceived Social Support in youth. *Comprehensive Psychiatry, 49*(2), 195–201. https://doi.org/10.1016/j.comppsych.2007.09.002

Burns, N., & Grove, S. K. (2005). *The practice of nursing research: Conduct, critique, & utilization* (5th ed). St. Louis, MO: Elsevier Saunders.

Burström, M., Brännström, M., Boman, K., & Strandberg, G. (2012). Life experiences of security and insecurity among women with chronic heart failure. *Journal of Advanced Nursing, 68*(4), 816–825. https://doi.org/10.1111/j.1365-2648.2011.05782.x

Elo, S., Kääriäinen, M., Kanste, O., Pölkki, T., Utriainen, K., & Kyngäs, H. (2014). Qualitative content analysis: A focus on trustworthiness. *SAGE Open, 4*(1), 1–10. https://doi.org/10.1177/2158244014522633

Fagerström, L., Gustafson, Y., Jakobsson, G., Johansson, S., & Vartiainen, P. (2011). Sense of security among people aged 65 and 75: External and inner sources of security. *Journal of Advanced Nursing, 67*(6), 1305–1316. https://doi.org/10.1111/j.1365-2648.2010.05562.x

Findlay, S. M., Pinzon, J., Goldberg, E., Frappier, J.-Y., Baltzer, F., Elliott, A., ... Deo, D. (2008). Issues of care for hospitalized youth. *Paediatrics Child Health, Canadian Peadiatric Society, 13*(1), 61–64.

Fortinash, K. M., & Worret, P. H. (2011). *Psychiatric, mental health nursing* (5th ed.). St. Louis, MO: Mosby Elsevier.

Graneheim, U. H., & Lundman, B. (2004). Qualitative content analysis in nursing research: Concepts, procedures and measures to achieve trustworthiness. *Nurse Education Today, 24*(2), 105–112. https://doi.org/10.1016/j.nedt.2003.10.001

Hockenberry, M. J., & Wilson, D. (2014). *Wong's nursing care of infants and children* (Electronic books). London, England: Elsevier Health Sciences.

Holloway, I., & Wheeler, S. (2010). *Qualitative research in nursing and healthcare* (3rd ed.). Chichester, UK: John Wiley & Sons.

Huisman, E. R. C. M., Morales, E., Van Hoof, J., & Kort, H. S. M. (2012). Healing environment: A review of the impact of physical environmental factors on users. *Building and Environment, 58*, 70–80. https://doi.org/10.1016/j.buildenv.2012.06.016

Hupcey, J. E. (2000). Feeling safe: The psychosocial needs of ICU patients. *Journal of Nursing Scholarship, 32*(4), 361–367. https://doi.org/10.1111/j.1547-5069.2000.00361.x

Hutton, A. (2002). The private adolescent: Privacy needs of adolescents in hospitals. *Journal of Pediatric Nursing, 17*(1), 67–72. https://doi.org/10.1053/jpdn.2002.16718

Jaberi, A., Momennasab, M., Yektatalab, S., Ebadi, A., & Cheraghi, M. A. (2017). Spiritual health: A concept analysis. *Journal of Religion and Health, 56*, 1–24. https://doi.org/10.1007/s10943-017-0379-z

Krevers, B., & Milberg, A. (2014). The instrument 'Sense of Security in Care–Patients' Evaluation': Its development and presentation. *Psycho-Oncology, 23*(8), 914–920. https://doi.org/10.1002/pon.3502

Lasiter, S. (2011). Older adults' perceptions of feeling safe in an intensive care unit. *Journal of Advanced Nursing, 67*(12), 2649–2657. https://doi.org/10.1111/j.1365-2648.2011.05714.x

Lincoln, Y. S., & Guba, E. G. (1985). *Naturalistic inquiry* (1st ed.). Newbury Park, CA: Sage Publications.

Maslow, A. H. (1987). *Motivation and personality* (3rd ed.). New York, NY: Harper and Row.

Mattila, E., Kaunonen, M., Aalto, P., Ollikainen, J., & Åstedt-Kurki, P. (2010). Support for hospital patients and associated factors. *Scandinavian Journal of Caring Sciences, 24*(4), 734–745. https://doi.org/10.1111/j.1471-6712.2010.00771.x

Mollon, D. (2014). Feeling safe during an inpatient hospitalization: A concept analysis. *Journal of Advanced Nursing, 70*(8), 1727–1737. https://doi.org/10.1111/jan.123480

Moura de Moura, F., Costa Junior, á. L., de Amorim Silva, M. E., da Silva Reichert, A. P., & Collet, N. (2015). Hospitalized child and teenager with chronic diseases: Feelings about death. *Investigación y Educación en Enfermería (Nursing Research and Education), 33*(3), 565–572. http://dx.doi.org/10.17533/udea.iee.v33n3a21

Narayan, K., Hooker, C., Jarrett, C., & Bennett, D. (2013). Exploring young people's dignity: A qualitative approach. *Journal of Paediatrics and Child Health, 49*(11), 891–894. https://doi.org/10.1111/jpc.12430

Polit, D. F., & Beck, C. T. (2010). *Essentials of nursing research: Appraising evidence for nursing practice* (7th ed.). Philadelphia, PA: Wolters Kluwer Health/Lippincott Williams & Wilkins.

Rankin, E. A., & DeLashmutt, M. B. (2006). Finding spirituality and nursing presence—The student's challenge. *Journal of Holistic Nursing, 24*(4), 282–288. https://doi.org/10.1177/0898010106294423

Reed, P., Smith, P., Fletcher, M., & Bradding, A. (2003). Promoting the dignity of the child in hospital. *Nursing Ethics, 10*(1), 67–76. https://doi.org/10.1191/0969733003ne540oa

Smith, S. (2004). Adolescent units—An evidence-based approach to quality nursing in adolescent care. *European Journal of Oncology Nursing, 8*(1), 20–29. https://doi.org/10.1016/S1462-3889(03)00057-7

Speziale, H. S., Streubert, H. J., & Carpenter, D. R. (2011). *Qualitative research in nursing: Advancing the humanistic imperative* (Rev. ed.). Philadelphia, PA: Lippincott Williams & Wilkins.

Stenhouse, R. C. (2013). 'Safe enough in here?': Patients' expectations and experiences of feeling safe in an acute psychiatric inpatient ward. *Journal of Clinical Nursing, 22*(21–22), 3109–3119. https://doi.org/10.1111/jocn.12111

Tartaro, J., Luecken, L. J., & Gunn, H. E. (2005). Exploring heart and soul: Effects of religiosity/spirituality and gender on blood pressure and cortisol stress responses. *Journal of Health Psychology, 10*(6), 753–766. https://doi.org/10.1177/1359105305057311

Vogus, T. J. (2016). Safety climate strength: A promising construct for safety research and practice. *BMJ Quality & Safety, 25*, 649–652. https://doi.org/10.1136/bmjqs-2015-004847

Wassenaar, A., Schouten, J., & Schoonhoven, L. (2014). Factors promoting intensive care patients' perception of feeling safe: A systematic review. *International Journal of Nursing Studies, 51*(2), 261–273. https://doi.org/10.1016/j.ijnurstu.2013.07.003

Yektatalab, S., Sharif, F., Kaveh, M. H., Khoshknab, M. F., & Petramfar, P. (2013). Living with and caring for patients with Alzheimer's disease in nursing homes. *Journal of Caring Sciences, 2*(3), 187–195. https://doi.org/10.5681/jcs.2013.023

19

Moral Distress Model Reconstructed Using Grounded Theory

Hsun-Kuei Ko[1] • Chi-Chun Chin[2] • Min-Tao Hsu[3]*

ABSTRACT

Background: The problems of nurse burnout and manpower shortage relate to moral distress. Thus, having a good understanding of moral distress is critical to developing strategies that effectively improve the clinical ethical climate and improve nursing retention in Taiwan.

Purpose: The aim of this study was to reconstruct the model of moral distress using the grounded theory.

Methods: Twenty-five staff nurses at work units who attend to the needs of adult, pediatric, acute, and critical disease or end-of-life-care patients were recruited as participants using theoretical sampling from three teaching hospitals in Taiwan. Data were collected using intensive, 2- to 3-hour interviews with each participant. Audio recordings of the interviews were made and then converted into transcripts. The data were analyzed using the grounded theory.

Results: In the clinical setting, the perspective that nurses take toward clinical moral events reflects their moral values, which trigger moral cognition, provocation, and appraisal. The moral barriers that form when moral events that occur in clinical settings contradict personal moral values may later develop into moral distress. In handling moral barriers in the clinical environment, nurses make moral judgments and determine what is morally correct. Influenced by moral efficacy, the consequence may either be a moral action or an expression of personal emotion. Wasting National Health Insurance resources and Chinese culture are key sources of moral distress for nurses in Taiwan. The role of self-confidence in promoting moral efficacy and the role of heterodox skills in promoting moral actions represent findings that are unique to this study.

Conclusions: The moral distress model was used in this study to facilitate the development of future nursing theories. On the basis of our findings, we suggested that nursing students be encouraged to use case studies to establish proper moral values, improve moral cognition and judgment capabilities, and promote moral actions to better handle the regular pressures of moral distress in future clinical or workplace settings. Moreover, a better understanding of moral distress may help retain staff nurses.

KEY WORDS:
moral distress, grounded theory, model, ethics.

Introduction

Nurses leave their positions for a variety of reasons. One of these, moral distress, is linked closely to the personal moral values and professional work ethics of individual nurses and may contribute to work pressure (Hamric, 2012). The term "moral distress" first appeared in Jameton's book *Nursing Practice: The Ethical Issues*. He pointed out that the nurse participants in his study took care of patients in accordance with their (the nurses') values and expectations and that they may feel pressure and/or anger if the care process was perceived to be unclear or inappropriate. He found an association between these pressures and ethical issues and personal, moral reflections. Jameton named this phenomenon "moral distress" (Jameton, 1984). Wikinson (1987) further added considerations of mental and emotional responses to Jameton's description of moral distress and defined moral distress as "the psychological disequilibrium and negative feeling state experienced when a person makes a moral decision but does not follow through by performing the moral behavior indicated by that decision" (p. 16). Corley, Elswick, Gorman, and Clor (2001) developed the first moral distress scale based on Jameton's description of moral distress. The 32-item moral distress scale has been used to measure the frequency and intensity of moral distress in nurses, with findings indicating a moderate to high degree of moral distress that related to negative emotional response, which could reduce the quality of patient care and job satisfaction and increase the nursing turnover rate (McCarthy & Gastmans, 2015).

Moral distress affects the job satisfaction, retention, and burnout of nurses as well as patient safety and the quality of nursing care and is thus a significant nursing issue. However, a clear theoretical framework that describes this phenomenon clearly is still lacking (Pauly, Varcoe, & Storch, 2012). In Taiwan, only one unpublished master's thesis claiming that 61.8% of intensive care unit nurses experienced moral distress (Chen, 2013), and two descriptive articles (Ko & Wang, 2011; Ko & Yang, 2009) and one case report (Fu, Tsai, & Chen, 2011) addressed the issue of moral distress in Taiwan nurses. The small number of studies underscores that the phenomenon of moral distress in nurses is neither well understood nor adequately described in Taiwan. It is necessary, therefore, not only to improve the working environment and policies but also to make efforts to understand

[1]*PhD, RN, Instructor, College of Nursing, Kaohsiung Medical University* • [2]*PhD, RN, Associate Professor, College of Nursing, Kaohsiung Medical University* • [3]*PhD, RN, Professor, College of Nursing, Kaohsiung Medical University.*

the moral values of nurses as well as the barriers that cause distress for nurses in clinical settings.

The progression of moral distress includes situation, cognition, action, and feeling (Wilkinson, 1987). The situation refers to a clinical environment with many ethical issues. Nurses, as moral agents, are able to cognize, judge, and act when they face ethical issues in clinical situations (McCarthy & Gastmans, 2015). On the basis of Jameton (1993) and Wikinson's (1987) descriptions of moral distress, nurses (as moral agents) encounter ethical problems in clinical situations, initially undergoing moral provocation and appraisal in cognition before judging the best actions that are necessary to care for the patients.

Moral distress appears because of barriers that inhibit nurses from doing the right thing or doing a task correctly. Ethical barriers include internal constraints and external constraints. The former includes self-doubt and lack of courage, and the latter includes communication difficulties with physicians, hierarchy-related issues between physicians and nurses, work overload, nursing administrators not providing adequate support, and inappropriate national and hospital policies (Hamric, 2012; Wikinson, 1987). Not managing these barriers and not performing in an ethical manner facilitate the development of negative physical and emotional reactions. The former includes decreased appetite, headache, and insomnia, and the latter includes the formation of anger and frustration, which often progresses to guilt, sadness, depression, and then powerlessness, failure to meet obligations, and burnout (Jameton, 1993; McCarthy & Gastmans, 2015; Wilkinson, 1987).

Moral distress is an umbrella concept that refers to a series of cognitive processes from the provocation and appraisal of a nurse's moral values to the subsequent moral judgments that arise when he or she encounters clinical ethical issues. What are the moral values of nurses in Taiwan? Furthermore, does culture influence moral barriers and moral actions? To address these questions, the purposes of this study were to (a) understand the moral values of nurses in Taiwan, which is critical to forming an understanding of nurses' moral distress; (b) construct a structural model of moral distress using the grounded theory research method that organizes these moral values, barriers, and actions into a clear and logically structured manner; and (c) identify the moral actions of nurses based on a literature-based understanding of the consequences of moral distress in terms of mental and physical reactions. Therefore, this study also attempts to understand whether nurses take moral actions that may turn events around for the benefit of their patients. As the rights of patients and moral nursing are increasingly stressed in the clinic, the significance of the physical and emotional pressures that are imposed by moral distress should receive greater attention from nursing professionals. The authors hope that the results of the this research contribute significantly to the development and extension of an ethical climate in healthcare settings, nursing ethics education, and nursing theory.

Methods

The abovementioned literature review supports defining moral distress as "physical and emotional responses that arise in response to moral barriers that conflict with nurse's moral values." Thus, this is the definition that was adopted in this study.

Participants

The theoretical sampling method with elasticity was used to identify and recruit the sample, with researchers analyzing new data and then updating concepts for use in subsequent sample selection work. For example, the eighth participant told the researcher a unique story on moral distress that highlighted the value that she placed on her patient care abilities in the hospice unit. Thus, self-confidence was added to the list of concepts being analyzed. The ninth and tenth participants, who also worked in hospice units, were invited to join this study to clarify the concept of moral efficacy. When the ninth participant was interviewed, she identified the nurse leader as a significant source of her moral distress. Therefore, several individuals who worked in units that were different from the ninth participant were recruited as participants to analyze and compare different sources of moral distress. The phenomenon of moral distress was clarified and saturated only after a full cycle of data collection, analysis, and comparison. Saturation was reached at the 21st participant, when no new concepts were added, although the researcher continued to interview four subsequent participants to confirm that no new concepts would emerge. Thus, 25 participants participated in this study.

Oh and Gastmans (2015) systemically reviewed 15 quantitative literatures on moral distress and reached no definite conclusion on the relationship between personal characteristics and severity of moral distress (p. 25). To make the research materials more diverse and heterogeneous, a full range of personal characteristics was represented in this study. The participants were recruited from three teaching hospitals in Taiwan. Participants had a mean age of 27 years and an average seniority of 4.48 years. Nearly 9 in 10 (88%) were women. The working units of participants included the oncology ward, pediatric cancer ward, hospice ward, intensive care unit, emergency room, and operating room, and their working titles included nurse, case manager, nurse practitioner, and hospice nurse consultant. Each participant underwent at least one 2- to 3-hour interview.

Interview Questions

Table 1 lists the interview questions that were used in this study.

Data Analysis

Strauss and Corbin's grounded theory was used to analyze the data based on open coding, axial coding, and selective coding (Strauss & Corbin, 1998/2001). At the open coding stage, the researchers tried to keep an open mind regarding the potential underlying causes of moral distress. The data were conceptualized and categorized after a close reading of the texts. For example, when the textual data showed that "*the testicles of a male patient were removed as a result of an operation with the knowledge of his wife but unbeknownst to him. This could be considered concealment of the truth. Being fully informed of one's condition is a fundamental patient right. Concealment should never be the choice, the patient always has the right to know*" (16). This segment of textual data was conceptualized as "patient's right to know." Furthermore, the relevant conceptual groups were then classified into a subcategory named "patient rights." The comparative analysis would then proceed until all of the data with relevant properties were summed up and those with different properties were selected to serve as the precursor to theorizing.

The core categories were decided at the axial coding stage, with moral distress used as the axial. Taking the above case, for example, "patient rights" is grouped into the central category of "moral values." The central categories are then subjected to a chronological comparison and summed up into a whole that highlights causal relations. On the basis of this whole, questions including "what are the potential causes of moral distress," "who is related to moral distress," "what are the relationships," "how may situations of moral distress be judged," "how should nurses respond to situations of moral distress," and "what are the results of the interactions" were answered. Moral distress was thus structured and contextualized. This complex phenomenon is thus represented as theoretical structures.

The main aim of the selective coding stage was to integrate, rectify, and refine the theory as well as to eliminate the concepts with low explanatory power. For example, after reflection by the researcher, the concept of "origins of nurses' values" that was summed up in the open coding stage was later eliminated because of its low significance to the theory of moral distress. Comparing the initially constructed moral distress model with the texts of the original interviews proved that this model could not only explain approximately the stories of research participants but also complied with the sequences of moral distress. During data analysis and theory construction, our use of both inductive and deductive methods constantly rectified and either expanded or abridged the composition of the theoretical framework. The final result was a logical, systematic, and explanatory moral distress model that corresponded to the actual conditions in Taiwan.

Trustworthiness and Reducing Bias

To increase the trustworthiness and reduce the bias, we applied the rigor of credibility, transferability, dependability, and confirmability as described by Lincoln and Guba in 1985 (as cited in Tobin & Begley, 2004).

TABLE 1.
Research Purposes and Interview Questions

Research Purpose	Interview Question
1. Reconstructing a structural model of moral distress using the grounded theory research method.	1-1 The description of the clinical moral problems and difficulties: Please tell me the recent moral events that have bothered you in the clinical practice. Please describe the details.
	1-2 Who appeared in this event? What is your relationship with him or her or them?
	1-3 What is your perspective on this moral event?
	1-4 How did the situation distress you?
	1-5 What physical or emotional consequences were caused by this moral event?
2. Understanding nurses' moral values.	2-1 Why does this moral event bother you?
	2-2 What is the moral right in the event?
	2-3 What should be done to fit moral right?
	2-4 What are the moral reasons that support your position on this issue?
3. Finding nurses' moral actions.	3-1 Have you ever tried or done anything to turn this event in the right direction?
	3-2 Why didn't you do so? What were the relevant barriers?
	3-3 Why did you do it?
	3-4 How did you do it?
	3-5 What was the outcome?
	3-6 How do you feel about this outcome?

Credibility

The researcher explained the research purpose, method, and protection of anonymity as the ethical guarantee to each participant to obtain their trust. During the interviews, the researcher put aside all personal opinions and assumptions and did not interfere with the two parties' co-investigations of moral distress so that the descriptions would fit the participants' views and that credibility would be attained.

Transferability

After the interview, the word-by-word recordings were provided to participants to examine the correctness of transcripts. Only two participants revised the texts. The actual recordings of participants' stories would be retained and referred to during the general inquiry to attain transferability.

Dependability

The rigorous and logical process of the research methods that were used during theoretical sampling, data analysis, and result descriptions was designed and explained clearly. The researcher interviewed all of the participants personally to maximize analytical consistency. Furthermore, the researcher maintained reflexivity and a self-critical dialogue in the data analysis process to raise dependability.

Confirmability

A peer check was conducted, with all of the researchers reading the texts intensively to clarify the research data and reduce researcher subjectivity. For example, a discussion that revolved around the Chinese cultural concept of "dying peacefully in bed" was later clarified and used to facilitate a revision to the categorical composition of moral distress. During the above-stated analysis process, the texts were constantly reflected on and compared, so that the consistency and coherence between similar data entries could be highlighted and various categories could be compared and contrasted to show the chronological development of the theory. These efforts help establish the trustworthiness and reduce the bias of this study.

Ethical Approving

The study protocol and consent form were approved by the institutional review board of the Kaohsiung Medical University Chung-Ho Memorial Hospital (KMUH-IRB-980529).

Results

Figure 1 shows the moral distress model that was developed on the basis of the grounded theory. The most significant causes of moral distress include the moral values of a nurse, which guide him or her toward a provocation and appraisal of moral cognition, and moral judgment, which arises later. These moral values, which are brought into a nurse's clinical work, may contradict the ethical issues that are handled in the clinical environment, hence causing moral barriers in terms of cognition. Those barriers may subsequently induce moral distress. In the face of moral barriers, the nurses may continue making moral judgments that are based on their personal moral values, with the aim of "defining the moral right." After making moral judgments, nurses may discover the possible moral actions within their abilities or may find that they lack the required courage to act, triggering emotional reactions. Whether a nurse actually takes moral actions is dependent on moral efficacy.

Two cases were extracted from the textual data to explain and describe the research findings. Case 1 was a typical case of moral distress, illustrating the process of eliciting emotional pressures from clinical events. Case 2 shows a variation of moral distress in which individual abilities were the values and the focus was placed on moral actions. The second case revealed no significant indication of emotional pressure, thus providing an illustration of the impacts that are imposed by moral efficacy as well as enriching the theoretical construct of moral distress.

> *Case 1: I work in the emergency room. Once, I was taking care of a patient who needed to have an NG tube inserted for the first time. I tried to teach the family how to feed with the tube, which triggered their bad mood: "Isn't this part of your duties? Why are you nurses so lazy as to push everything off on family members? (moral barrier)" All of these incidents contributed to my sense of helplessness (emotional reaction). This is not what I expected from my job as a nurse (in a lower voice). In my opinion, a good nurse should be able to communicate well and have discussions with patients and their families during work (moral value). I now understand that this is impossible in clinical reality due to our endless workload and limited time (moral judgment). There are physicians who handle their cases callously in the emergency room. There was once a patient who felt weak in the right extremities. My instinct told me that this might be a stroke. When I reported to the physician, the*

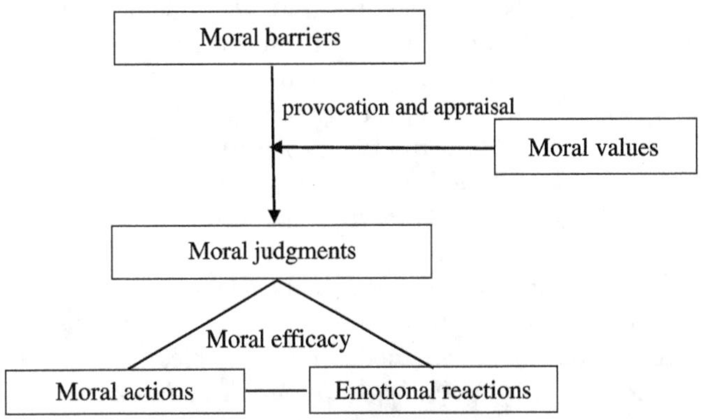

Figure 1. Moral distress model.

physician complained that I was meddling in his business (moral barrier). In cases like this when I was responsible enough to tell the physician about the patient's conditions but the physician decided not to deal with them, there was nothing further I could do (moral efficacy, self-doubt). My heart is filled with anger and frustration, I feel that the ideal of nursing is gone. I do not want to work like this anymore and have considered quitting (emotional reaction). (7)

Case 2: I have not met with too many frustrations at work, because I am aware of my abilities. I make all of my decisions from the point of view of my patients and fight for them. I care for patients on the basis of human caring (moral value). For example, there was once a terminal cancer patient who lived on a remote mountain. Since he had left home for a long time, he expressed the wish to go home for once. The team members were resistant to the idea, saying that the patient's condition was not good, and it might be dangerous for him to go home (moral barrier). I was thinking about the situation, decided to list and borrow all of the necessary things, and discussed with the physician (moral judgment). After getting the physician's approval, together with the social and volunteer workers, we sent the patient back home (moral action). I think, the biggest resistance for doing these kinds of things actually came from oneself. It depends on whether a nurse really wants to care for the patient or not. If I really want to do it, I will do it (moral efficacy / self-confidence). This job means a lot to me and I am sure that I will continue. (8)

The results of our research, which were derived using a grounded-theory-based textual analysis, are discussed below.

Category 1: Moral Values

Moral values present themselves when a nurse encounters ethical issues in the clinical environment and guide the nurse to make the "right" choices in accordance with the decision-maker's subjective appraisal. The core moral values that were highlighted in this study are patient-centered care and accountability. Patient-centered care means that attention should be paid to patient rights and that patients should always be provided with clear explanations. For example, "*The patient did not know that his testicles would be removed before the operation. I thought I should not have concealed the information from him because he had the right to know*" (16). Accountability refers to the commitment of nurses to do the right thing and to try their best to become one's own role model. For example, "*Once I cut the cuff off of a tracheal tube by accident, I admitted the mistake immediately because I believe that a nurse shouldn't shirk her responsibility*" (17) and "*While on duty, I will do all the things required of me to the best of my ability*" (14).

Category 2: Moral Barriers

If clinical moral issues that arise in the environment make nurses perceive that they cannot provide the best care based on their moral values, moral barriers appear and become sources of moral distress. Sources of moral barriers include clients, coworkers, the system, and the Chinese culture.

"Clients" refer to patients and their families. Moral barriers are easily triggered when families take a position that conflicts with a nurse's appraisal. For example, "*A family of a hospice home care patient was unwilling to change diapers regularly. This increases the area and depth of the patient's wound*" (10).

The barriers that relate to coworkers include (a) negligent coworker nurses, "*Some co-workers took their job very lightly. For example, they would turn their back when the diapers of the patients with diarrhea had to be replaced. I could not accept this*" (14); (b) trouble-avoiding nursing managers, "*When the physician came to inspect the patient, he lost his temper at seeing that the patient had not ambulated yet. The head nurse apologized to the physician immediately, called the nurses into the office and scolded her*" (12); and (c) arrogant physicians, "*Some physicians dealt with the patients' problems callously. When I gave them suggestions, they complained that I was meddling into their business*" (7).

System barriers such as nursing shortage and wastes of medical resources are related to the medical system and, although potentially dangerous for patients, lie out of the scope of nurse action. This was a source of moral distress. For example, "*The work load is great, which often delays the ending of my on-duty time. My normal off-duty time is 5:30P.M., but once I didn't get off of work until as late as 11:00P.M. Although I got home so late, I still had to get up early the next day for another day shift. It is such a vicious cycle, and may damage the patient's safety*" (21) and "*The Taiwan National Health Insurance has really spoiled patients. The registration fee for an emergency appointment for a patient with a catastrophic illness card is only 150 (NT dollars). The result is that patients make emergency appointments even when they cannot fall asleep or for a headache*" (7).

Chinese cultural barriers that were identified in this study include notorious diseases, peaceful dying on one's bed, and filial piety. Reincarnation is a prevailing concept among Chinese people. They believe that suffering in this life may be the result of evil deeds that were committed in previous lifetimes. Some diseases are thus stamped with culture stereotypes: "*AIDS is a widely discriminated-against disease in Taiwan. There was a patient diagnosed with AIDS. His mother complained in tears: 'God, what have I done wrong to put my son in this situation?'*" (19). The cultural attitudes of Chinese people mean that patients, especially the older adults, hope to spend their remaining time at home. However, this wish often cannot be met: "*A patient wished to die peacefully on his own bed (at home). Although I really wanted to fulfill his wish, there is a rule that morphine cannot be taken home. I felt bad for not being able to help him get home*" (9). Filial piety is a unique and core virtue of the Chinese culture. However, sometimes, this virtue influences the medical decisions of patients and induces moral distress in nurses: "*If there is no way to understand the patients' will, the decision must be made by his or her family members. Sometimes this is really stressful for those family members. When the choice is between DNR and CPR, and the family members decide on the former, they will be deemed as unfilial. Most family members thus tend to choose CPR even if the patient is at the terminal, end-of-life stage*" (15).

Category 3: Moral Judgments

Moral judgments are framed clearly by the question: "What should I do to determine the moral right?" The moral judgments toward clients include respect for the patients' decisions and providing necessary information: "*I once encountered a patient who would not take analgesics. I told him that terrible pain was torture. He responded that he could only feel he was still living from the pain. I therefore respected his decision*" (12). The coworker judgments included cooperative staff nurses, supportive managers, and open-minded physicians. For example, "*In terms of caring for wounds, for example, some nurses might consider this method better than the one that is preferred by others. As long as these methods are good for the patients, there should be not absolute right and wrong. The important thing is to show respect and support for each other*" (10) and "*The head nurse did interfere with our decision-making. The abilities of a nurse should be respected. It would eliminate the current hierarchy system in the hospitals*" (19).

The moral judgment coming from the system is the fair and reasonable operation of nursing manpower. In contemporary Taiwan, it has become most urgent for nurses to have sufficient manpower to uphold nursing quality: "*Work overtime and overloading are stressful. When nursing manpower faces such a shortage, nursing care quality cannot be guaranteed. Sufficient manpower is a pre-condition for good nursing quality*" (10). The Chinese cultural judgments are concerned mostly with the influence of patients' rights, including the necessity of defending these rights and respecting the medical decisions of patients. "*Although the family knew about DNR consent, they interfered with the patient's decision. I think the patient's wish should have been followed because he signed DNR consent*" (6).

Category 4: Moral Efficacy

Whether a nurse communicates adequately to solve a problem or to express the personal emotional responses after making a moral judgment is determined by moral efficacy, which includes self-doubt and self-confidence. Self-doubt indicates that a nurse is not sufficiently confident to think that she or he is capable of solving a problem and will not discuss the problem or make suggestions, even when feeling that he or she is right. "*As a new nurse, I was not confident enough to communicate with the physician. Although I thought Dopamine was better for raising the patient's blood pressure, I still recommended Epinephrine based on the physician's order. The patient's heart rate rocketed to 200 per minute. It was so scary me and I thought I was damned*" (16). Self-confidence indicates that a nurse is aware of her or his abilities and may act based on subjective moral considerations to do the right thing for a patient: "*I am actually very aggressive. I think that the biggest resistance comes from oneself. If I really want to do it, I will do it*" (8).

Category 5: Moral Actions

Moral actions such as communication and discussion are used when the nurse is aware of her or his abilities and thinks that she or he could do something that would benefit the patient. "*Because the patient spoke with a slur and felt weak in the right extremities, I suggested to the physician that the patient should be examined carefully before he was sent back home*" (7). The use of heterodox skills is one of the more interesting findings of this study: "*The visiting staff (VS) tended not to give narcotic analgesics, thus leaving the quality of life of our terminal patients' life significantly affected by pain. Under these circumstances, I used other skills, like begging the physician on duty at night to order morphine. Although it sounds strange, my intention is always to do good for the patients*" (2).

Category 6: Emotional Reactions

Emotional reactions include both explicit and nonexplicit emotions. Explicit emotions are illustrated by threats and scolding. "*The physician was unwilling to use additional analgesics. So, I told the physician that I would not administer analgesics for him in the future and informed the patient of the physician's name*" (3). Nonexplicit emotions refer to emotions that nurses keep to themselves and do not express. These emotional reactions include frustration, anger, tears, and self-blame. For example, "*In the OPD, a patient said he had no money to rent a chemotherapy pump, but the physician did not believe him. The physician insisted that the patient have a pump inserted and then told the patient to come up with his own solution. I was very angry. How could I solve the money problem?*" (11)

Discussion

Grounded theory, the research method that was applied in this study, allows the reconstruction of a logical and structure moral distress model and the comparison of this model with existing research studies to enhance general knowledge related to the theory of moral distress. Our research found results that were similar and unique to those of prior studies.

Similar Findings

Some of the research findings support the descriptions of previously published studies. The core categories such as moral values, moral barriers, moral judgments, and emotional reactions are similar to categories that were described in previous studies. Moral distress does not happen spontaneously but rather depends on the personal values and beliefs of the individual nurse (Wikinson, 1987). The moral values that nurses in Taiwan share with their counterparts in other countries include patient safety (Pauly et al., 2012) and patients' rights and accountability (Davis, Schrader, & Belcheir, 2012). This may be because of the Western-based education and training that are received by nurses in Taiwan. Moreover, this may be an underlying cause of the conflict between the moral values of nurses and Chinese culture. Only one research from Uganda, which claimed that nursing work was done in response to "the call of God" (Harrowing & Mill, 2010), differed from our finding that nurses did not perceive that religion influenced their moral values.

The moral barriers originating with clients, coworkers, and the system that were identified in this study are similar to the moral barriers that were identified in other studies. These included the family providing inappropriate patient care, the family intruding on the treatment and nursing processes (Austin, 2012; Hamric, 2012; Varcoe, Pauly, Storch, Newton, & Makaroff, 2012), differences among staff nurses in terms of nursing care philosophy (Maluwa, Andre, Ndebele, & Chilemba, 2012), nursing manager favoritism with physicians and nursing manager scolding of line nurses (Hamric, 2012), physicians' disrespect of nurse professionalism or dismissal of nurses' assessments (Varcoe et al., 2012), and staff shortages, overloading, overtime, and inappropriate work shift arrangements (Austin, 2012; Pauly et al., 2012; Varcoe et al., 2012). The results point out that nursing professionals experience a variety of moral barriers and should be respected more by clients, doctors, and coworkers.

The consequences of moral distress that are described in the literatures are described mainly as emotional reactions. The risk of emotional reactions rises significantly when a nurse doubts her or his ability to do the right thing or cannot ensure the patient's best interest (Varcoe et al., 2012). The nonexplicit emotions such as frustration, helplessness, and anger that were highlighted in this article echo the descriptions that were provided in past studies (Jameton, 1993; Maluwa et al., 2012; Varcoe et al., 2012; Wilkinson, 1987). Explicit emotions, rarely mentioned in past studies, represent an interesting finding of this study. Explicit emotions are the overt projection of negative emotions such as threats, scolds, fights, and frowns toward coworkers. Although this category of emotion may temporarily relieve personal emotional stress, it does not resolve moral distress and may undermine cooperative relationships. In addition, the participants in this study rarely mentioned physical reactions such as headaches, heart palpitations, or insomnia.

Unique Findings

Two moral barriers, namely, the National Health Insurance system and policies related to the issuance of Catastrophic Illness Cards, are worth mentioning here. The intent of the National Health Insurance in Taiwan is to provide financial support to the general public for qualified medical treatment (Bureau of National Health Insurance, 2009). The good intention of the government, however, is mistaken as a waste of national medical resources because of the abuse of this system by a small number of people. As part of this system, nurses are not able to do anything about these problems. Therefore, these problems become a source of moral distress. Another unique moral barrier is rooted in Chinese cultural mores, where the concepts of family and filial piety are central and are sometimes manifested in restrictions on patients' rights at medical facilities. The participants in this study were troubled when medical decision making was shifted from the patient to his or her family members as well as by the cultural stigmas that culture places on genetic or infectious diseases. Because it is impossible to eliminate these impacts, it is important that nurses reach a new understanding of this phenomenon. Making education-based changes from basic cognitive perspectives and accepting our own culture are critical to helping set nurses free from their moral distress on this issue.

Self-doubt is an internal constraint that has also been mentioned in past studies (Hamric, 2012; Wikinson, 1987). According to our textual analysis, self-confidence and self-doubt were incorporated under the moral efficacy category, as both factors play key roles in moral actions. Therefore, this study sets moral efficacy as a core category in the theoretical model of moral distress to reconstruct the components of the moral distress model (Figure 1). In making choices related to moral actions, nurses make an assessment of themselves (Ko & Wang, 2011). If a nurse is sure of her or his abilities (self-confidence), she or he may adopt moral actions similar to one of the participants in the study: "*I will do it as long as I really want to.*" If the nurse doubts her or his abilities (self-doubt), she or he may not have the moral courage to act, as stated by another participant: "*I am not confident enough to have discussions with the physician.*" Thus, in this study, moral efficacy plays a key role in mitigating or aggravating moral distress.

Another interesting finding is that some of the participants in this study used "heterodox skills," which have been rarely described in the literature. Heterodox skills are nonformal methods such as privately begging the doctor on duty to order some analgesics for the patient when the dosage prescribed by the chief physician is not sufficient for pain relief or privately giving advice to the patients to ensure the patients' best interests are protected. Because heterodox skills may satisfy patient needs, they are a type of moral action. Moral actions, which need moral courage to enact, do not only line up with the nurses' values of patient centrality but are also conducive to guiding patient care in the proper direction and thus is helpful in alleviating moral distress (Nickitas, 2008). Accumulating capabilities and experiences in ethical problem solving may help improve the moral efficacy of nurses, helping them to build an ethical working environment in cooperation with their colleagues (Ko & Wang, 2011).

Conclusions and Suggestions

This study attempts to reconstruct a moral distress model using the grounded theory. In the research of Lazzarin, Biondi, and Di Mauro (2012), 13.7% of the nurses make changes in their working units, 50.5% consider quitting the profession, and 15.2% have already quit because of issues of moral distress. Furthermore, Davis et al. (2012) found that 27.7% of the nurses in their study had quit because of moral distress. The effects of moral distress on burnout in nurses are significant. As may be learned from our research findings and from those of past studies, the moral distress of nurses may be attributed to multiple barriers. In clinical practice, nurses must be included in the medical decision-making process of patients so that they will understand the reasons for decisions, which would help them resolve their doubts and possibly increase their moral efficacy. It is also necessary for nurses to be respected by members of the care delivery team. The sharing of thoughts and feelings among team members would make communications as moral actions easier as well as reduce moral distress.

According to our findings, nurses make observations, appraisals, and judgments of moral issues based on their own moral values. This study confirmed that the safety and rights of patients are the core values of nursing. Respect, empathy, caring, and patient-centered care have always been the core values of nursing and implanted deeply in the hearts of nurses by education, serving as a compass for nurses in clinical practice (Davis et al., 2012; Pauly et al., 2012). In teaching nursing ethics, therefore, setting proper education goals, strategies, and content is important. On the basis of our findings, the education goals of nursing ethics include knowing one's own values, recognizing our own Chinese culture, understanding the differences in philosophy between nurses and physicians through interprofessional education, and promoting interpersonal communication skills. Teaching strategies may include small group discussions that include both nursing and medical students as well as problem-based learning, with case studies that narrate actual situations. Thus, nursing students will learn about ethical issues together with others in the healthcare team. The core values, knowledge, attitudes, and communication skills that are learned from nursing ethical education would become guides for the nurse while working, decreasing the possibility of moral distress in future clinical practice.

This was a cross-sectional study. Therefore, one limitation is that the development of nurses as professionals was not tracked. The long-term effects of moral distress, including health problems, moral outrage, burnout, and quitting the profession, could not be described in this study. Future studies on moral distress should incorporate a longitudinal perspective to contribute to a greater understanding of the long-term effects of moral distress. Our understanding of moral distress will increase significantly once more quantitative and qualitative research methods are employed in the investigation of this phenomenon, with a greater understanding offering the potential to effectively manage moral distress and to create a more positive clinical environment.

Acknowledgment

Deep appreciation is extended to the Taiwan Nurses Association for granting the research funds (TWNA1012042) necessary to complete this study.

References

Austin, W. (2012). Moral distress and the contemporary plight of health professionals. *HEC Forum, 24*(1), 27–38. doi:10.1007/s10730-012-9179-8

Bureau of National Health Insurance. (2009). *2009 introduction of national health insurance.* Taipei City, Taiwan, ROC: Author. (Original work published in Chinese)

Chen, H. C. (2013). *The associated factors of moral distress among ICU nurses* (Unpublished master's thesis). Chung Shan Medical University, Taichung City, Taiwan, ROC. (Original work published in Chinese)

Corley, M. C., Elswick, R. K., Gorman, M., & Clor, T. (2001). Development and evaluation of a moral distress scale. *Journal of Advanced Nursing, 33*(2), 250–256.

Davis, S., Schrader, V., & Belcheir, M. J. (2012). Influencers of ethical beliefs and the impact on moral distress and conscientious objection. *Nursing Ethics, 19*(6), 738–749. doi:10.1177/0969733011423409

Fu, C. Y., Tsai, M. F., & Chen, H. M. (2011). A nurse's experience caring for a patient with breast cancer who had been previously reported dead by her family. *The Journal of Nursing, 58*(3, Suppl.), 90–96. doi:10.6224/JN.58.3S.90 (Original work published in Chinese)

Hamric, A. B. (2012). Empirical research on moral distress: Issues, challenges, and opportunities. *HEC Forum, 24*(1), 39–49. doi:10.1007/s10730-012-9177-x

Harrowing, J. N., & Mill, J. (2010). Moral distress among Ugandan nurses providing HIV care: A critical ethnography. *International Journal of Nursing Studies, 47*(6), 723–731. doi:10.1016/j.ijnurstu.2009.11.010

Jameton, A. (1984). *Nursing practice: The ethical issues.* Englewood Cliffs, NJ: Prentice-Hall.

Jameton, A. (1993). Dilemmas of moral distress: Moral responsibility and nursing practice. *AWHONN's Clinical Issues in Perinatal and Women's Health Nursing, 4*(4), 542–551.

Ko, H. K., & Wang, R. H. (2011). Unity of knowing and action—Exploring moral courage in nursing practice. *The Journal of Nursing, 58*(1), 102–107. doi:10.6224/JN.58.1.102 (Original work published in Chinese)

Ko, H. K., & Yang, M. S. (2009). Moral distress and leadership in nursing. *The Journal of Nursing, 56*(3), 72–77. doi:10.6224/JN.56.3.72 (Original work published in Chinese)

Lazzarin, M., Biondi, A., & Di Mauro, S. (2012). Moral distress in nurses in oncology and haematology units. *Nursing Ethics, 19*(2), 183–195. doi:10.1177/0969733011416840

Maluwa, V. M., Andre, J., Ndebele, P., & Chilemba, E. (2012). Moral distress in nursing practice in Malawi. *Nursing Ethics, 19*(2), 196–207. doi:10.1177/0969733011414968

McCarthy, J., & Gastmans, C. (2015). Moral distress: A review of the argument-based nursing ethics literature. *Nursing Ethics, 22*(1), 131–152. doi:10.1177/0969733014557139

Nickitas, D. M. (2008). Encouragement and empowerment: Unlocking the keys to excellence. *Medsurg Nursing, 17*(6), 374, 390.

Oh, Y., & Gastmans, C. (2015). Moral distress experienced by nurses: A quantitative literature review. *Nursing Ethics, 22*(1), 15–31. doi:10.1177/0969733013502803

Pauly, B. M., Varcoe, C., & Storch, J. (2012). Framing the issues: Moral distress in health care. *HEC Forum, 24*(1), 1–11. doi:10.1007/s10730-012-9176-y

Strauss, A., & Corbin, J. (1998/2001). *Basics of qualitative research: Techniques and procedures for developing grounded theory* (C. Y. Wu & M. H. Liao, Trans.). Chiayi, Taiwan, ROC: Waterstone. (Original work published in Chinese)

Tobin, G. A., & Begley, C. M. (2004). Methodological rigour within a qualitative framework. *Journal of Advanced Nursing, 48*(4), 388–396. doi:10.1111/j.1365-2648.2004.03207.x

Varcoe, C., Pauly, B., Storch, J., Newton, L., & Makaroff, K. (2012). Nurses' perceptions of and responses to morally distressing situations. *Nursing Ethics, 19*(4), 488–500. doi:10.1177/0969733011436025

Wilkinson, J. M. (1987). Moral distress in nursing practice: Experience and effect. *Nursing Forum, 23*(1), 16–29. doi:10.1111/j.1744-6198.1987.tb00794.x

20

Person-Centered Care, Job Stress and Quality of Life Among Long-Term Care Nursing Staff

HeeKyung CHANG[1] • Chorong GIL[2] • Hyejin KIM[3] • Hanju BEA[4]*

ABSTRACT

Background: Although it has been established that person-centered care is an essential aspect in long-term care facilities, the relationship between person-centered care and job stress among nursing staff and the effect of this relationship on their quality of life are not clear.

Purpose: This study aims to investigate correlations among job stress, quality of life, and person-centered care of nurses as well as factors affecting the person-centered care abilities of nursing staff working at long-term care hospitals.

Methods: Nursing staff (N = 183) in three long-term care hospitals in South Korea completed a questionnaire on job stress, quality of life, and person-centered care. Data were analyzed using the SPSS 22.0 program for descriptive statistics, using an independent t test, a one-way analysis of variance, Pearson's correlation coefficient, and multiple stepwise regression analyses.

Results: Significant factors found to be associated with person-centered care included the quality of life ($r = .411$, $p < .001$) and job stress ($r = -.305$, $p < .001$) of the participant. The regression model with job stress and quality of life as predictor variables accounted for 29.2% of the variance in person-centered care.

Conclusions/Implications for Practice: Higher quality of life and lower job stress were found to increase the person-centered care abilities of nurses in long-term care facilities.

KEY WORDS:
job stress, long-term care facility, nurse, person-centered care, quality of life.

Introduction

South Korea is one of the world's most rapidly aging countries. In 2018, 14.3% of the population was aged 65 years or older, with this percentage expected to reach 20.8% in 2026 (Statistics Korea, 2017). This trend has led to an increased need for long-term care (LTC) settings for older adults with physical and/or mental disabilities. To deal with the higher demand for LTC services, South Korea introduced a new social insurance scheme for LTC in July 2008 (Kwon, 2009). As many families are unable to provide appropriate care for older adults affected by disabilities or frailty, the number of LTC facilities in South Korea has increased more than 7 times over a decade, from 203 in 2005 to 1,529 in 2017 (Health Insurance Review & Assessment Service, 2018).

The rapid increase in LTC facilities is causing problems such as poor management at some LTC facilities and inadequate consideration of the human rights of residents (Park & Park, 2018). Older adult residents in LTC facilities are more likely to experience declines in physical and psychosocial health than community-dwelling older adults (Lee et al., 2012). Since the 1990s, person-centered care (PCC) has been practiced widely around the world and has been set as a basic direction for LTC services in the United States and Europe (Koren, 2010). PCC, typically defined as care that is responsive to the well-being of the care recipient, includes significant social interactions; mutual choice; mutual decision making; and acceptance of the care recipient's preferences, values, and beliefs (Kogan et al., 2016). PCC is a holistic (physical–psychosocial–spiritual) approach to providing care that is respectful and individualized, allowing cooperation of care, and offering choice through a therapeutic connection where persons are empowered to be involved in health determination at whatever level is desired by the individual receiving care (Morgan & Yoder, 2012). Previous studies have reported that PCC increased well-being and reduced agitation in people with dementia after interventions based on meaningful activities and psychosocial interactions (Edvardsson et al., 2014) as well as improved bowel patterns for residents after individualized care management (Palese et al., 2010).

Job stress is defined as a harmful physical and emotional response that occurs at the workplace (Tsai et al., 2009). Nurses in LTC facilities are the primary providers of PCC, as they possess the ability to promote effective teamwork with health practitioners, foster a positive environment in the facility, and support older adults (Mueller et al., 2013). Nurses in LTC facilities face various mental and psychological problems such as emotional labor and job stress because

[1]PhD, RN, Associate Professor, College of Nursing, Gyeongsang National University, Gyeongnam, ROK • [2]MSN, RN, Researcher, Institute of Health Sciences, Gyeongsang National University, Gyeongnam, ROK • [3]MPH, RN, Assistant Professor, Department of Nursing Science, Kyungsung University, Busan, ROK • [4]PhD, RN, Assistant Professor, Department of Nursing, Keimyung College University, Daegu, ROK.

of changes in roles and workload burden (Kim & Kim, 2017; Mueller et al., 2013). In addition to the nature of the task, nurses experience secondary traumatic stress because of empathy for the pain expressed by patients in the course of their close encounters with death (Kim & Kim, 2017). Nurses at LTC facilities face specific job stressors that influence their job satisfaction and that are not experienced by acute care nurses (Stone & Harahan, 2010). In addition, with regard to the effects of outcomes of PCC on direct care staff, studies have reported that PCC led to decreased job stress and strain as well as increased personal and professional satisfaction (Jeon et al., 2012).

The World Health Organization defines quality of life as "an individual's perception of their position in life in the context of the culture and value systems in which they live, and in relation to their goals, expectations, standards, and concerns" (WHOQoL Group, 1993). For nurses, the quality of work life contributes to their turnover rate, job satisfaction, stress, organizational cohesion, organizational commitment, motivation, and quality of care (Mohamad, 2012). Different from standard medical and therapeutic nursing care, PCC is designed to improve the quality of care provided to older adults, to understand the personal characteristics of older adults, to expand the care options and autonomy of older adults, and to provide a supportive environment similar to home (Haydon et al., 2018). In addition, increased family satisfaction with LTC facilities has been associated with increased job satisfaction and lower turnover among facility employees (Brownie & Nancarrow, 2013).

Few domestic studies have evaluated the service quality (Kim & An, 2012) or examined the general stress of employees of LTC facilities (Lee & Park, 2013). Thus, little has been reported in the domestic literature on direct relationships among job stress, quality of life, and PCC in LTC settings.

The purpose of this study was to examine the job stress, quality of life, and PCC of nurses in LTC facilities in South Korea and to understand the effects of job stress and quality of life on PCC.

Methods

Design and Sample

This cross-sectional study used a descriptive correlational approach to investigate the correlations among PCC, job stress, and quality of life. One hundred eighty-nine nurses from all positions (nurse director, supervisor, and clinical nurse) working in four LTC facilities in one city in South Korea were enrolled as participants. Valid data from 183 participants were collected and used in analysis.

Measures

Job stress

The instrument used to measure the job stress of participants was a scale used in a previous study (Lee et al., 2007). A 5-point Likert-type scale was used, and four subdimensions were measured. Each subdimension used a set of items to measure job stress, including patients (four items), work (four items), interpersonal relationships (six items), and economic stress (three items). Each item was rated on a scale ranging from 1 = *not at all* to 5 = *very much*. The final score for each scale was the mean of the corresponding items, ranging from 1 to 5, with higher scores indicating higher job stress. The Cronbach's α was .82 in Lee et al. (2007) and was .90 in this study.

Quality of life

Quality of life was measured using the Korean version of the World Health Organization Quality of Life Scale abbreviated version (WHOQOL and WHOQOL-BREF; Min et al., 2000). The WHOQOL and WHOQOL-BREF both contain 26 items in the following categories: overall quality of life and health (two items), physical health (seven items), psychological (six items), social relation (three items), and environment (eight items). Each category was measured using a 5-point Likert-type scale ranging from 1 = *not at all* to 5 = *very much*. Questions 3, 4, and 26 were reversed scored. A higher total score indicates a higher quality of life. The Cronbach's α was .90 in Min et al. (2000) and was .92 in this study.

Person-centered care

The Person-centered Care Assessment Tool was developed by Edvardsson et al. (2010). It consists of three categories encompassing 13 items. The first category consists of seven items related to personalization degree, the second category consists of four items related to organization support, and the third category consists of two items related to environmental accessibility. Each item is rated using a 5-point Likert-type scale ranging from 1 = *not at all* to 5 = *very much*. Higher scores indicate higher PCC. At the time of development, Cronbach's α was .84 (Edvardsson et al., 2010) and was .78 in this study.

Personal information form

A personal information form was used in this study to gather basic demographic data on the age, gender, religion, and level of education of the participants as well as their duration working as a nurse, duration of experience in LTC facilities, and perceived health status. Perceived health status was measured by asking participants to evaluate their own health on a 4-point Likert scale ranging from 1 = *extremely good* to 4 = *extremely bad*.

Data Collection and Analysis

The study data were collected between July and August 2018 after receiving written permission from the Board of Ethics. Oral assent was sought after informing potential participants about the purpose of the study and assuring confidentiality of all of the provided data. Participants were given sufficient time (approximately 10–15 minutes) to complete the questionnaire.

One hundred eighty-nine forms were delivered to participants, and 189 forms were collected. Six of the collected forms with outliers in the sample data set were excluded from the final data analysis (Grove & Cipher, 2016). To assess the effect of excluding outliers for normal distribution and homogeneity in the characteristics of participants, we repeated all analyses after including the outliers. The exclusion of the outliers did not change the results. The final sample size (N = 183) adequacy using an F test and G*Power 3 analysis software was estimated based on an alpha level of .05, a medium effect size of 0.15, and a power of 0.90 (Faul et al., 2007). Therefore, the sample size was adequate.

The characteristics, job stress, quality of life, and PCC were analyzed using descriptive analysis. Cronbach's α reliability analyses were conducted for job stress, quality of life, and PCC among LTC nursing staff. The correlations between job stress, quality of life, and PCC were analyzed using correlation analyses and multiple stepwise regression analyses. On the basis of a general assumption used with linear regression models, a normal distribution of the residuals was assumed in this study (Kutner et al., 2005). All of the analyses were carried out using SPSS Version 23 (IBM Inc., Armonk, NY, USA), and the significance level was set to .05.

Ethical Considerations

Permission in writing was granted by the institutions where the study was conducted. In addition, ethical approval was received from the Gyeongsang National University Research Board of Ethics (Approval No. GIRB-A18-Y-0032) in South Korea. Participants were informed that all of the data would be treated as confidential and that only the researchers would have access to these data.

Results

The results of the descriptive statistics showing the differences in the mean values of PCC by participant characteristics are shown in Table 1. Nearly all (93.4%) of the participants were female. The mean age was 43.00 years (SD = 10.08), ranging from 22 to 69 years, and 30.6% were between 40 and 49 years old. Three quarters (74.9%) were married, 64.5% held a junior college degree, and 63.9% self-affiliated with a religion. The mean career duration for the participants was 11.84 (SD = 7.91) years, whereas the mean duration of LTC facility experience was 4.45 (SD = 3.52) years. Most participants (82.5%) were clinical nurses, and 56.3% self-identified as "healthy."

The descriptive statistics for job stress, quality of life, and PCC are shown in Table 2. The mean values were 2.73 (SD = 0.56) for job stress, 3.21 (SD = 0.63) for patient-related stress, 2.70 (SD = 0.67) for work-related stress, 2.48 (SD = 0.67) for interpersonal relationship stress, and 2.64 (SD = 0.77) for economic stress. The mean values were 3.48 (SD = 0.42) for quality of life, 3.44 (SD = 0.59) for overall quality of life and health, 3.52 (SD = 0.50) for the physical health category, 3.48 (SD = 0.51) for the psychological category, 3.43 (SD = 0.54) for the social relation category, and 3.48 (SD = 0.44) for the environment category. The mean values were 3.36 (SD = 0.41) for PCC, 3.26 (SD = 0.50) for extent of personalized care, 3.46 (SD = 0.67) for organizational support, and 3.50 (SD = 0.59) for environmental support.

The results for job stress, quality of life, and PCC analyzed by analysis of variance and Scheffé post hoc verification are shown in Table 3. Gender (t = −2.37, p = .019) and duration working in LTC facilities (F = 3.17, p = .026) were respectively shown to significantly impact job stress. Age

Table 1

Characteristics of Participants (N = 183)

Characteristic	*n*	%	Range
Gender			
Female	171	93.4	
Male	12	6.6	
Age (years; *M* and *SD*)	43.00	10.08	22–69
≤ 29	25	13.6	
30–39	42	23.0	
40–49	56	30.6	
≥ 50	60	32.8	
Spouse			
No	46	25.1	
Yes	137	74.9	
Education			
Junior college degree	118	64.5	
BSN	65	35.5	
Religion			
No	66	36.1	
Yes	117	63.9	
Duration working as a nurse (years; *M* and *SD*)	11.84	7.91	0.4–42.0
< 5	40	21.9	
5–9	33	18.0	
10–14	41	22.4	
15–19	37	20.2	
≥ 20	32	17.5	
Duration of experience in LTC facilities (years; *M* and *SD*)	4.45	3.52	0.3–17.0
< 2	47	25.7	
2–4	59	32.2	
5–9	52	28.4	
≥ 10	25	13.7	
Position			
Clinical nurse	151	82.5	
Manager/supervisor	32	17.5	
Perceived health status			
Bad	4	2.2	
Average	54	29.5	
Good	103	56.3	
Extremely good	22	12.0	

Note. BSN = bachelor of science in nursing; LTC = long-term care.

Table 2

Job Stress, Quality of Life, and Person-Centered Care of Participants (N = 183)

Variable	Mean	*SD*	Min	Max
Job stress	2.73	0.56	1.24	4.29
Stress related to patients	3.21	0.63	1.75	4.75
Stress related to work	2.70	0.67	1.00	4.50
Interpersonal relationship stress	2.48	0.67	1.00	4.50
Economic stress	2.64	0.77	1.00	5.00
WHOQOL-BREF	3.48	0.42	2.38	4.88
Overall quality of life and health	3.44	0.59	2.00	5.00
Physical health category	3.52	0.50	2.43	5.00
Psychological category	3.48	0.51	2.17	4.83
Social relation category	3.43	0.54	2.33	5.00
Environment category	3.48	0.44	1.75	4.88
P-CAT	3.36	0.41	2.38	4.38
Extent of personalizing care	3.26	0.50	2.00	4.71
Organizational support	3.46	0.67	1.50	5.00
Environmental support	3.50	0.59	2.00	5.00
Total score	40.33	5.07	29.00	56.00

Note. WHOQOL and WHOQOL-BREF = World Health Organization Quality of Life Scale Abbreviated Version; P-CAT = Person-centered Care Assessment Tool; Min = minimum; Max = maximum.

($F = -2.68, p = .048$), education ($F = -2.46, p = .015$), and perceived health status ($F = 17.58, p < .001$) were respectively shown to significantly impact quality of life. Age ($F = 3.19, p = .025$), spouse ($t = 2.25, p = .025$), education ($t = -2.25, p = .025$), religion ($t = -2.32, p = .022$), duration working as a nurse ($F = 3.02, p = .019$), and perceived health status ($F = 5.28, p = .006$) were respectively shown to significantly impact PCC.

The correlations among job stress, quality of life, and PCC were studied using correlation analysis, with results (Table 4) indicating PCC as positively correlated with quality of life ($r = .411, p < .001$) and negatively correlated with job stress ($r = -.305, p < .001$).

A test of the assumptions used in the regression analysis showed that all of the assumptions coincided with the required assumptions of the regression equations. First, no multicollinearity problems were identified (Durbin–Watson value = 1.947, tolerance limit = 0.91–0.97, variance inflation factor = 1.03–1.10). Second, the stepwise multiple regression analyses of quality of life and job stress were conducted using demographic variables, including duration working as a nurse, age, religion, and spouse, to identify the key factors affecting the quality of PCC provided by participants.

The analyses showed that the prediction model for PCC was significant ($F = 16.72, p < .001$). The value of the adjusted R^2 was .292, which corresponds to an explanatory power of 29.2%. The factors that were found to impact significantly on PCC included quality of life ($\beta = .33$), job stress ($\beta = -.21$), duration working as a nurse ($\beta = -.18$), age ($\beta = -.16$), religion ($\beta = .16$), and spouse ($\beta = -.15$; Table 5).

Discussion

The purpose of this study was to examine the job stress, quality of life, and PCC of nurses in LTC facilities in Korea, with results intended to provide basic data for implementing or improving PCC at LTC facilities in Korea.

In 2014, 21 older adult patients were killed in a fire accident at an LTC facility in Korea (Sagong & Lee, 2016), which brought the deteriorating quality of service at LTC facilities in the country to widespread public attention. The residential older adult care industry is facing serious difficulties in terms of maintaining and attracting a competent and stable workforce owing to the negative social image of LTCs and the unexpected shortage of personnel in this sector (Vernooij-Dasssen et al., 2009). Nurses play an important role in planning and providing patient care in LTC facilities and act as healthcare professionals who are directly involved in patient health outcomes and safety (Kang, 2015).

The results of this study show that patient-related stress was high among the participants, with a score of 3.21 for job stress. Nurses who work in LTCs require high levels of patience and attention to deal with medical disputes, poor working conditions, and low compensation and to provide safe and quality nursing care to prevent falls and safety accidents (Kim & Kim, 2016; Kim & Han, 2018). In addition, lack of regular doctor support increases the job stress of nurses because of the need to make important health and care-related decisions that affect the health and life of residents (Kennedy, 2005; Kim & Kim, 2017). Another stressor is the high number of residents with cognitive impairments who may direct physical and verbal abuse toward staff or other residents (Woodhead et al., 2016). In situations marked by the sudden deterioration of a resident's health, caregivers often direct their complaints about treatment and care to nurses. Furthermore, nurses experience considerable job stress because of the difficulties they face in building understanding and trust (Kim & Kim, 2016).

Study findings have shown that physical health has the greatest impact on the quality of life of nurses in LTC facilities. Residents in these facilities require help for incontinence and mobility-related care and for many aspects of basic care (Pekkarinen et al., 2004). A study of nurses in Mangalore, India, found that the environmental domain had the most significant impact on the quality of life (Abraham & D'silva, 2013). Nurse managers in LTC facilities should assess the principal stressors in their facilities and develop strategies to help staff effectively cope with these stressors and improve their quality of work and life.

The average score for PCC in this study of 40.33 is similar to that of a study that used the same tool to evaluate nurses in another LTC facility (Park & Park, 2018) and somewhat lower than those of studies conducted in other countries, for example, 48.8 points in Sweden (Sjögren et al., 2012) and 47 points in Spain (Martínez et al., 2016). The significant difference in PCC scores between studies done in South Korea and those done elsewhere is attributed to the early recognition of human rights issues and of the concept of PCC in many Western

Table 3

Differences in Job Stress, Quality of Life, and Person-Centered Care, by Characteristic (N = 183)

Characteristic	Job Stress					Quality of Life					Person-Centered Care				
	Mean	*SD*	*t/F*	*p*	Scheffé	Mean	*SD*	*t/F*	*p*	Scheffé	Mean	*SD*	*t/F*	*p*	Scheffé
Gender			−2.37	.019				−0.09	.927				−0.28	.779	
Female	2.76	0.54				3.48	0.43				3.36	0.41			
Male	2.37	0.68				3.47	0.32				3.33	0.40			
Age (years)			1.11	.348				2.68	.048	③ > ②			3.19	.025	① > ②
① ≤ 29	2.57	0.57				3.44	0.38				3.46	0.39			
② 30–39	2.78	0.57				3.33	0.41				3.20	0.30			
③ 40–49	2.70	0.54				3.55	0.44				3.42	0.41			
④ ≥ 50	2.80	0.55				3.53	0.41				3.38	0.46			
Spouse			−1.18	.241				−0.35	.725				2.25	.025	
No	2.65	0.55				3.46	0.34				3.48	0.38			
Yes	2.76	0.56				3.49	0.44				3.32	0.42			
Education			0.15	.879				−2.46	.015				−2.25	.025	
Vocational college	2.74	0.53				3.42	0.42				3.31	0.39			
BSN	2.72	0.61				3.58	0.39				3.45	0.44			
Religion			−0.62	.535				−0.50	.617				−2.32	.022	
No	2.69	0.64				3.46	0.40				3.27	0.37			
Yes	2.75	0.51				3.49	0.43				0	0			
Duration working as a nurse (years)			1.62	.170				0.23	.924				3.02	.019	⑤ > ④
① < 5	2.61	0.55				3.51	0.41				3.46	0.38			
② 5–9	2.80	0.53				3.43	0.37				3.32	0.34			
③ 10–14	2.86	0.56				3.49	0.49				3.32	0.46			
④ 15–19	2.77	0.51				3.46	0.40				3.21	0.41			
⑤ ≥ 20	2.60	0.62				3.49	0.41				3.50	0.41			
Duration of experience in LTC facilities (years)			3.17	.026	③ > ①			1.55	.203				2.46	.065	
① < 2	2.53	0.57				3.58	0.36				3.45	0.38			
② 2–4	2.78	0.51				3.48	0.44				3.37	0.45			
③ 5–9	2.85	0.58				3.42	0.42				3.24	0.40			
④ ≥ 10	2.73	0.51				3.42	0.46				3.42	0.36			
Position			−0.85	.395				−1.01	.313				−0.45	.651	
Clinical nurse	2.71	0.56				3.46	0.42				3.35	0.41			
Manager/supervisor	2.81	0.54				3.55	0.41				3.39	0.44			
Perceived healtd status			0.52	.595				17.58	<.001	③ > ①, ②			5.28	.006	③ >①
① Bad/average	2.79	0.55				3.30	0.36				3.22	0.36			
② Good	2.71	0.55				3.49	0.39				3.41	0.41			
③ Extremely good	2.68	0.60				3.87	0.43				3.50	0.48			

Note. BSN = bachelor of science in nursing; LTC = long-term care.

countries (Park & Park, 2018). In South Korea, the concept of PCC has not been established yet and related research has not been conducted (Sagong & Lee, 2016). Recently, PCC has become an important approach to providing care in all areas of nursing (Haydon et al., 2018). Cultural change efforts in LTC facilities have the potential to be an effective strategy for improving the quality of life of residents in institutionalized settings.

The results indicate that the female participants had a higher mean level of job stress than the male participants. LTC facilities require nursing staff to provide extensive physical care to reduce the difficulty in independent daily living caused by the development of physical disabilities and chronic diseases in old age (Kim & Kim, 2017). Moreover, cognitive impairment in patients with dementia causes violent behavior (Kim & Kim, 2016), which may also add to the job stress experienced by nursing staff and lead to higher levels of stress in female nurses than male nurses. In addition, participants who had worked in LTC facilities for less than 5–10 years reported a higher mean level of job stress than those who had

Table 4

Correlation Between Job Stress, Quality of Life, and Person-Centered Care (N = 183)

Variable	Job Stress	Quality of Life	Person-Centered Care
Job stress	1		
Quality of life	−.230, p = .005	1	
Person-centered care	−.305, p <. 001	.411, p < .001	1

worked in LTC facilities for less than 2 years. According to the National Statistical Office (Statistics Korea, 2019), the highest number of married women in their early 30s and the first birth after 2.12 years have started married. Hence, nurses with less than 5–10 years of LTC facility work experience were identified as having both high job stress and high parenting stress. In light of the above, the reason why the quality of life of 40–49 years is higher than that of 30–39 years is that the burden of raising a child is reduced.

The general characteristics of age, spouse, education, religion, duration working as a nurse, and perceived health status were all found to impact significantly on PCC. In particular, it has been shown that the relatively high-quality PCC and strong ambitions of nurses at the beginning of their professional aged-care career diminish significantly after working in this career for a long period (Zimmerman et al., 2005). In addition, a study by Kim and Kwon (2017) of 194 nurses in an LTC hospital showed a significantly higher level of geriatric nursing practice among older and married nurses. Therefore, it is possible to improve the quality of provided PCC by establishing a work environment in which married nurses may work without interruption and by providing education that improves the professionalism of old nurses with less clinical experience. In this study, perceived health status was found to relate positively with quality of life and PCC. Kim and Gu (2015), who targeted 243 nurses working in LTC hospitals, found a significantly higher level of nursing competence in nurses with good health statuses. Furthermore, in Lin et al. (2014), a moderately negative, significant correlation was found between job stress and self-perceived health status. Providing space and time for regular physical activity, hobbies, and other recreational diversions may help promote a working environment that enhances work–life balance that helps reduce physical fatigue and job stress. Reducing fatigue facilitates a better perceived health status, thereby enhancing a nurse's ability to provide PCC.

The results of the correlation analysis indicate a positive correlation between PCC and quality of life and a negative correlation between PCC and job stress. Stress management is important because it affects the quality of care and patient satisfaction provided by nurses working in LTC facilities (Aiken et al., 2002; Kim & Kim, 2016). Moreover, physical health affects quality of life, so improving the nursing work environment promotes better PCC (Park & Park, 2018).

Thus, positively influencing PCC by developing and applying a program that improves the nursing working environment is necessary. Staff in LTC settings are required to express a wide variety of emotions during their interactions with patients (Harrad & Sulla, 2018). Ciarrochi and Scott (2006) wrote that those with high levels of emotional intelligence are better able to deal with environmental demands and workplace stress.

A recent study (Chang, 2019) reported that many nursing personnel in LTC settings had experienced that PCC begins with sharing the history and personal stories of older adults. As storytelling may be applied both in older-adult care and

Table 5

Multiple Regression Analysis of Person-Centered Care With the Variables (N = 183)

Independent Variable	*B*	*SE*	β	*t*	*p*
Constant	2.77	.31		9.05	< .001
Quality of life	0.32	.06	.33	4.98	< .001
Job stress	−0.16	.05	−.21	−3.27	.002
Duration working as a nurse (< 5 years)					
15–19 years	−0.19	.07	−.18	−2.82	.004
Age (< 30 years)					
30–39 years	−0.16	.06	−.16	−2.50	.005
Religion (yes)	0.13	.05	.16	2.47	.015
Spouse (yes)	−0.14	.06	−.15	−2.33	.021

Note. Adjusted R^2 = .292, F = 16.72, p < .001.

nursing caregiver settings (Chang, 2019; Chang et al., 2018), storytelling also positively affects job stress management and the quality of relationships, which are at the core of PCC. Storytelling is cost-effective, is not dependent on being literate, and requires only the imagination and understanding of the cognitive structures in the target community (Haigh & Hardy, 2011).

On the basis of the results of stepwise multiple regression analysis, quality of life, job stress, duration working as a nurse, age, religion, and spouse together explained 29.2% of PCC. In other words, spouse, religion, age (30–39 years), and duration working as a nurse (less than 15–20 years) have affected PCC. In a study constituting 1,339 care professionals in 56 elderly nursing homes in Spain, organizational climate and employee emotional exhaustion were found to correlate positively with PCC (Martínez et al., 2016). A study conducted in South Korea yielded similar results, with PCC found to correlate positively with the nursing work environment (Park & Park, 2018). PCC not only increases the job satisfaction of employees but also enhances self-esteem and care-related satisfaction, increases professionalism, and reduces job stress (Brownie & Nancarrow, 2013). Thus, there is a need to develop organizational models based on a person-centered philosophy of care, flexible management principles, and support for nursing staff to enhance job satisfaction and employee retention. This should enable a shift of focus from the tasks and routines in LTC toward facilitating PCC at the individual, organizational, and environmental levels of care provision. Therefore, this study provides several suggestions for gerontological implementation and policymaking, especially for institutional caregiving in South Korea.

Methodological Issues and Study Limitations

There are several limitations to this study. First, in South Korea, although the necessity and importance of PCC is emphasized, the study of PCC in a domestic context remains very limited. Therefore, it is necessary to repeatedly investigate all relevant aspects of PCC. Second, job stress, quality of life, and PCC were all self-reported in this study. More-objective measurements should be employed in future studies.

Conclusions

This study examined the effects of job stress and quality of life on PCC in the context of nurses working in LTC facilities. The correlation analysis models showed that PCC decreased as stress increased and that PCC increased as quality of life increased. This finding enhances the scholarly understanding of the stressors perceived by nurses working in LTC facilities and may facilitate the development of interventions that increase quality of life and create healthier environments in LTC facilities. To improve the quality of PCC provided in LTC facilities, intervention programs should be developed to reduce job stress and improve the quality of life of nurses.

Acknowledgments

This research was supported by a National Research Foundation of Korea grant funded by the Korea government (No. 2018R1C1B6007828). We would like to thank all of the participants in this study.

Author Contributions

Study conception and design: HKC
Data collection: All authors
Data analysis and interpretation: HKC, HJB
Drafting of the article: All authors
Critical revision of the article: All authors

References

Abraham, A. K., & D'silva, F. (2013). Job satisfaction, burnout and quality of life of nurses from Mangalore. *Journal of Health Management, 15*(1), 91–97. https://doi.org/10.1177/0972063413486033

Aiken, L. H., Clarke, S. P., & Sloane, D. M. (2002). Hospital staffing, organization, and quality of care: Cross-national findings. *International Journal for Quality in Health Care, 14*(1), 5–14. https://doi.org/10.1093/intqhc/14.1.5

Brownie, S., & Nancarrow, S. (2013). Effects of person-centered care on residents and staff in aged-care facilities: A systematic review. *Clinical Interventions in Aging, 8*, 1–10. https://doi.org/10.2147/CIA.S38589

Chang, H. K. (2019). Health personnel's experience with resident-centered care in nursing homes in Korea: A qualitative study. *International Journal of Nursing Sciences, 6*(2), 176–181. https://doi.org/10.1016/j.ijnss.2019.03.012

Chang, H. K., Bea, H. J., Kim, H. J., & Gil, C. R. (2018). Storytelling interventions to realize the person-centered care for the elderly in long-term care facilities. *Korean Journal of Converging Humanities, 6*(4), 87–110. https://doi.org/10.14729/converging.k.2018.6.4.87 (Original work published in Korean)

Ciarrochi, J., & Scott, G. (2006). The link between emotional competence and well-being: A longitudinal study. *British Journal of Guidance & Counselling, 34*(2), 231–243. https://doi.org/10.1080/03069880600583287

Edvardsson, D., Fetherstonhaugh, D., Nay, R., & Gibson, S. (2010). Development and initial testing of the Person-Centered Care Assessment Tool (P-CAT). *International Psychogeriatrics, 22*(1), 101–108. https://doi.org/10.1017/S1041610209990688

Edvardsson, D., Sandman, P. O., & Borell, L. (2014). Implementing national guidelines for person-centered care of people with dementia in residential aged care: Effects on perceived person-centeredness, staff strain, and stress of conscience. *International Psychogeriatrics, 26*(7), 1171–1179. https://doi.org/10.1017/S1041610214000258

Faul, F., Erdfelder, E., Lang, A. G., & Buchner, A. (2007). G* power 3: A flexible statistical power analysis program for the social, behavioral, and biomedical sciences. *Behavior Research Methods, 39*(2), 175–191.

Grove, S. K., & Cipher, D. J. (2016). *Statistics for nursing research-e-book: A workbook for evidence-based practice* (2nd ed.). Elsevier Health Sciences.

Haigh, C., & Hardy, P. (2011). Tell me a story—A conceptual exploration of storytelling in healthcare education. *Nurse Education Today, 31*(4), 408–411. https://doi.org/10.1016/j.nedt.2010.08.001

Harrad, R., & Sulla, F. (2018). Factors associated with and impact of burnout in nursing and residential home care workers for the elderly. *Acta Bio-Medica, 89*(7, Suppl.), 60–69. https://doi.org/10.23750/abm.v89i7-S.7830

Haydon, G., Browne, G., & van der Riet, P. (2018). Narrative inquiry as a research methodology exploring person centred care in nursing. *Collegian, 25*(1), 125–129. https://doi.org/10.1016/j.colegn.2017.03.001

Health Insurance Review & Assessment Service. (2018). *2017 medical expenses statistics indicators.* http://www.hira.or.kr/bbsDummy.do?pgmid=HIRAA020045010000&brdScnBltNo=4&brdBltNo=2296&pageIndex=1#none

Jeon, Y. H., Luscombe, G., Chenoweth, L., Stein-Parbury, J., Brodaty, H., King, M., & Haas, M. (2012). Staff outcomes from the caring for aged dementia care resident study (CADRES): A cluster randomised trial. *International Journal of Nursing Studies, 49*(5), 508–518. https://doi.org/10.1016/j.ijnurstu.2011.10.020

Kang, H. (2015). Geriatric hospital nurses' perceived barriers to research utilization and empowerment. *Asian Nursing Research, 9*(1), 65—72. https://doi.org/10.1016/j.anr.2014.11.005

Kennedy, B. R. (2005). Stress and burnout of nursing staff working with geriatric clients in long-term care. *Journal of Nursing Scholarship, 37*(4), 381–382. https://doi.org/10.1111/j.1547-5069.2005.00065

Kim, E. J., & Gu, M. O. (2015). Recognition for nursing competency importance, nursing competency level, and their influencing factors of nurses in the long-term care hospitals. *Journal of the Korea Academia-Industrial Cooperation Society, 16*(3), 1989–2001. https://doi.org/10.5762/KAIS.2015.16.3.1989

Kim, H. J., & Kim, H. Y. (2016). Experience of job stress among nurses working in long-term care hospital: A phenomenological approach. *Korean Journal of Adult Nursing, 28*(5), 572–584. https://doi.org/10.7475/kjan.2016.28.5.572 (Original work published in Korean)

Kim, H. J., & Kim, H. Y. (2017). Emotional labor, job stress and professional quality of life among nurses in long-term care hospital. *Korean Journal of Adult Nursing, 29*(3), 290–301. https://doi.org/10.7475/kjan.2017.29.3.290 (Original work published in Korean)

Kim, Y., & Han, K. (2018). Longitudinal associations of nursing staff turnover with patient outcomes in long-term care hospitals in Korea. *Journal of Nursing Management, 26*(5), 518–524. https://doi.org/10.1111/jonm.12576

Kim, Y. H., & An, J. S. (2012). Stress, life satisfaction and service satisfaction of elderly and elderly family using long-term care service. *Journal of Welfare for the Aged, 57*, 161–190. https://doi.org/10.21194/kjgsw..57.201209.161

Kim, Y. K., & Kwon, S. (2017). Effects of empathy and attitude in caring for elders by nurses in geriatric nursing practice in long-term care hospitals. *Journal of Korean Gerontological Nursing, 19*(3), 203–213. https://doi.org/10.17079/jkgn.2017.19.3.203 (Original work published in Korean)

Kogan, A. C., Wilber, K., & Mosqueda, L. (2016). Person-centered care for older adults with chronic conditions and functional impairment: A systematic literature review. *Journal of the American Geriatrics Society, 64*(1), e1–e7. https://doi.org/10.1111/jgs.13873

Koren, M. J. (2010). Person-centered care for nursing home residents: The culture-change movement. *Health Affairs, 29*(2), 312–317. https://doi.org/10.1377/hlthaff.2009.0966

Kutner, M. H., Nachtsheim, C. J., Neter, J., & Li, W. (2005). *Applied linear statistical models* (5th ed.). McGraw-Hill.

Kwon, S. M. (2009). Future of long-term care financing for the elderly in Korea. *Journal of Aging & Social Policy, 20*(1), 119–136. https://doi.org/10.1300/J031v20n01_07

Lee, E. H., Chang, S. J., Kim, H. O., Roh, J., Park, E. J., & Won, J. U. (2007). Relationship between job stress and turnover of registered nurses in a university hospital. *Korean Journal of Occupational and Environmental Medicine, 19*(2), 93–104. (Original work published in Korean)

Lee, H. Y., & Park, K. S. (2013). The effect of job stress on turnover intention of the long term care workers. *Health and Social Welfare Review, 33*(2), 274–298. http://dx.doi.org/10.15709/hswr.2013.33.2.274

Lee, M., Choi, J. S., Lim, J., & Kim, Y. S. (2012). Relationship between staff-reported culture change and occupancy rate and organizational commitment among nursing homes in South Korea. *The Gerontologist, 53*(2), 235–245. https://doi.org/10.1093/geront/gns106

Lin, S. H., Liao, W. C., Chen, M. Y., & Fan, J. Y. (2014). The impact of shift work on nurses' job stress, sleep quality and self-perceived health status. *Journal of Nursing Management, 22*(5), 604–612. https://doi.org/10.1111/jonm.12020

Martínez, T., Suárez-Álvarez, J., Yanguas, J., & Muñiz, J. (2016). Spanish validation of the Person-Centered Care Assessment Tool (P-CAT). *Aging & Mental Health, 20*(5), 550–558. https://doi.org/10.1080/13607863.2015.1023768

Min, S. K., Lee, C. I., Kim, K. I., Suh, S. Y., & Kim, D. K. (2000). Development of Korean version of WHO quality of life scale abbreviated version (WHOQOL-BREF). *Journal of Korean Neuropsychiatric Association, 39*(3), 571–579.

Mohamad, M. (2012). A model of quality of work life, life satisfaction and service quality. *Asian Journal of Business Research, 2*(2), 33–46. https://doi.org/10.14707/ajbr.120009

Morgan, S., & Yoder, L. H. (2012). A concept analysis of person-centered care. *Journal of Holistic Nursing, 30*(1), 6–15. https://doi.org/10.1177/0898010111412189

Mueller, C., Burger, S., Rader, J., & Carter, D. (2013). Nurse competencies for person-directed care in nursing homes. *Geriatric Nursing, 34*(2), 101–104. https://doi.org/10.1016/j.gerinurse.2012.09.009

Palese, A., Granzotto, D., Broll, M. G., & Carlesso, N. (2010). From health organization-centred standardization work process to a personhood-centred care process in an Italian nursing home: Effectiveness on bowel elimination model. *International Journal of Older People Nursing, 5*(2), 179–187. https://doi.org/10.1111/j.1748-3743.2010.00220

Park, E. M., & Park, J. W. (2018). Influence of moral sensitivity and nursing practice environment in person-centered care in long-term care hospital nurses. *Journal of Korean Gerontological Nursing, 20*(2), 109–118. https://doi.org/10.17079/jkgn.2018.20.2.109 (Original work published in Korean)

Pekkarinen, L., Sinervo, T., Perälä, M. L., & Elovainio, M. (2004). Work stressors and the quality of life in long-term care units. *The Gerontologist, 44*(5), 633–643. https://doi.org/10.1093/geront/44.5.633

Sagong, H., & Lee, G. E. (2016). Person-centered care and nursing service quality of nurses in long-term care hospitals. *Journal of Korean Academy of Community Health Nursing, 27*(4), 309–318. https://doi.org/10.12799/jkachn.2016.27.4.309 (Original work published in Korean)

Sjögren, K., Lindkvist, M., Sandman, P. O., Zingmark, K., & Edvardsson, D. (2012). Psychometric evaluation of the Swedish version of the Person-Centered Care Assessment Tool (P-CAT). *International Psychogeriatrics, 24*(3), 406–415. https://doi.org/10.1017/S104161021100202X

Statistics Korea. (2017). *Population projections for Korea.* http://kosis.kr/statHtml/statHtml.do?orgId=101&tblId=DT_1BPA003&conn_path=I2 (Original work published in Korean)

Statistics Korea. (2019). *December 2018 population trends.* http://kostat.go.kr/portal/korea/kor_nw/1/2/1/index.board?bmode=read&aSeq=373358

Stone, R., & Harahan, M. F. (2010). Improving the long-term care workforce serving older adults. *Health Affairs, 29*(1), 109–115. https://doi.org/10.1377/hlthaff.2009.0554

Tsai, F. J., Huang, W. L., & Chan, C. C. (2009). Occupational stress and burnout of lawyers. *Journal of Occupational Health, 51*(5), 443–450. https://doi.org/10.1539/joh.L8179

Vernooij-Dasssen, M. J., Faber, M. J., Olde Rikkert, M. G., Koopmans, R. T., van Achterberg, T., Braat, D. D., & Wollersheim, H. (2009). Dementia care and labour market: The role of job satisfaction. *Aging and Mental Health, 13*(3), 383–390. https://doi.org/10.1080/13607860902861043

WHOQoL Group. (1993). Study protocol for the World Health Organization project to develop a quality of life assessment instrument (WHOQOL). *Quality of Life Research, 2*(2), 153–159. https://doi.org/10.1007/BF0043

Woodhead, E. L., Northrop, L., & Edelstein, B. (2016). Stress, social support, and burnout among long-term care nursing staff. *Journal of Applied Gerontology, 35*(1), 84–105. https://doi.org/10.1177/0733464814542465

Zimmerman, S., Williams, C. S., Reed, P. S., Boustani, M., Preisser, J. S., Heck, E., & Sloane, P. D. (2005). Attitudes, stress, and satisfaction of staff who care for residents with dementia. *The Gerontologist, 45*(1, Suppl.), 96–105. https://doi.org/10.1093/geront/45.suppl_1.96

21

Supportive Care Needs of Patients With Lung Cancer in Mainland China

Tian ZHANG[1,6] • Hongye HE[1,6] • Qunhui LIU[2] • Xiaoqing LV[3] • Yongxia SONG[4] • Jingfang HONG[5]*

ABSTRACT

Background: The diagnosis and treatment of lung cancer necessitate a variety of supportive care needs. To our knowledge, no studies have been conducted that target specifically the supportive care needs of patients with lung cancer in Mainland China. Cross-cultural studies indicate that supportive care needs vary by cultural background. Thus, it is necessary to investigate the supportive care needs of patients with lung cancer in the cultural context of China.

Purpose: This study aimed to describe the level of supportive care required by patients with lung cancer in China and to examine the relationships between supportive care needs and demographic factors and between supportive care needs and treatment variables.

Methods: A cross-sectional descriptive study design was adopted. Five hundred fifty-four patients with lung cancer were recruited using a convenience sampling method from inpatient departments in four tertiary teaching hospitals that are affiliated with a medical university in Anhui Province, China. The Nursing Professional Social Support Needs Scale and background information list were used as the data collection instruments. A Wilcoxon rank sum test and a Kruskal–Wallis rank sum test were conducted to examine the differences among the professional supportive care needs of patients of different demographic characteristics and under different treatment conditions.

Results: Participants self-reported the highest scores in the domain of informational needs (M = 3.67, interquartile range = 1.25). The most common supportive care need was "to be cared for by nurses with skilled venipuncture techniques." There were significant differences in needs across different genders, age groups, educational levels, and income levels ($p < .05$). Patients with metastasis and other illnesses had greater supportive care needs in terms of total and subscale scores in Stages III and IV ($p < .05$).

Conclusions: Patients with serious diseases and heavy socioeconomic burdens have greater supportive care needs. Therefore, healthcare providers should improve their awareness and expertise to identify the needs of their patients and to provide supportive care to patients with lung cancer. In addition, patients with high supportive care needs should be identified.

KEY WORDS:
lung cancer, need, supportive care needs.

Introduction

Lung cancer is the most prevalent form of cancer and the leading cause of cancer death both in China and around the world. About 18.1 million new cases and 9.6 million deaths were reported worldwide in 2018 (Bray et al., 2018). In China in 2015, the estimated incidence and mortality rate for lung cancer were 733.3 and 610.2 per 100,000 population, respectively (Chen et al., 2016). Lung cancer in China is typically diagnosed at a more advanced stage than most other cancers (Shao et al., 2015), and patients are frequently infected with metastatic disease at the time of diagnosis because of nonspecific symptoms and nonappropriate early screening methods (Wang et al., 2015). In addition, lung cancer progresses relatively rapidly, and the prognosis is worse than most other cancers (Shao et al., 2017), with an overall 5-year survival rate of only 18% (Siegel, Miller, & Jemal, 2015). The quality of life of patients with advanced lung cancer is poor (Dai, Yang, Chen, & Tang, 2016), as they generally experience more psychosocial and physical hardships related to their diagnosis and aggressive treatment than patients who are diagnosed with other major cancers (Iyer, Taylor-Stokes, & Roughley, 2013; Liao et al., 2011).

Reflecting the need to face these psychosocial and physical difficulties, prior research findings indicate that patients with lung cancer experience a high level of supportive care needs. Sanders, Bantum, Owen, Thornton, and Stanton (2010) used the Supportive Care Needs Survey Short Form 31 to investigate the supportive care needs of 109 patients with lung cancer, finding the greatest needs in the physical and daily living domains followed by the psychological needs, health system and informational needs, and patient care needs domains

[1]MSN, RN, School of Nursing, Anhui Medical University, Hefei, China • [2]BSN, RN, School of Nursing, Anhui Medical University, Hefei, China • [3]MSN, RN, The First Affiliated Hospital of Anhui Medical University, Hefei, China • [4]MSN, RN, Teaching Assistant, School of Nursing, Anhui Medical University, Hefei, China • [5]PhD, RN, Professor, School of Nursing, Anhui Medical University, Hefei, China • [6]contributed equally as first author.

(Sanders et al., 2010). A cross-sectional study of 152 patients with lung cancer at a medical center in Taiwan that used the Chinese version of the Cancer Needs Questionnaire found high levels of self-reported supportive care needs, with the highest needs in the three domains of health system and information, psychological, and patient care and support (Liao et al., 2011). Another study that used the Supportive Care Needs Survey Short Form 34 to investigate the supportive care needs of 89 patients with lung cancer identified health system and information, psychological, and physical as the top 3 need domains (Giuliani et al., 2016). These and other studies support the importance of providing humanistic supportive care to patients with lung cancer (Borimnejad, Mardani-Hamooleh, Seyedfatemi, & Tahmasebi, 2017).

Although previous studies indicate that demographic and disease factors influence the supportive care needs of patients, their findings are not consistent. Sanders et al. found no correlation between patient age, gender, marital status, or total score and supportive care needs (Sanders et al., 2010). In a cross-sectional survey of 830 patients with lung cancer, a logistic regression revealed several significant predictors of supportive care needs, including being female, being employed, having fewer family members, having a long period since initial cancer diagnosis, and not receiving chemotherapy (Yun et al., 2013). Liao et al. (2011) found age and educational level to relate significantly to the supportive care needs of a patient, with younger patients having relatively higher psychological needs and patients with higher levels of education having relatively higher physical and daily activities need scores (Liao et al., 2011). Jacobs-Lawson, Schumacher, Hughes, and Arnold (2009) investigated the relationship between educational level and information needs among 100 patients with lung cancer and found that patients with a lower educational level had significantly higher information needs. Li et al. (2017) studied 888 patients with lung, breast, prostate, intestinal, or skin cancer, finding that the advanced-stage patients had relatively higher supportive care needs. Furthermore, Sanson-Fisher et al. (2015) found being informed of the worse disease prognosis to be a predictor of patient psychological needs. Meanwhile, the treatment methods that patients received during the immediately preceding month were found to predict supportive care needs. Compared with patients receiving comprehensive treatment, patients receiving immunotherapy were found to have more health information needs, patients receiving chemotherapy or immunotherapy only were found to have greater sexual needs, and patients receiving surgery or radiotherapy were found to have similar sexual needs (Li & Girgis, 2006).

Supportive care needs are defined as the treatment during an illness that is necessary to manage illness-related symptoms and side effects, to enable adaptation and coping, to optimize understanding and informed decision making, and to minimize decrements in functioning (Richardson, 2003). Understanding the types and the correlation associated with supportive care needs in people diagnosed with lung cancer is an essential step toward providing effective supportive care. Despite clear evidence of the all-around supportive care needs experienced by patients with lung cancer, this population remains a neglected group because of the difficulties faced in recruiting patients and the high attrition rates (Schofield et al., 2008). With regard to China, no research has been published yet that specifically addresses the supportive care needs of patients with lung cancer. Cross-cultural studies indicate that supportive care needs vary with cultural background. Thus, it is necessary to investigate the supportive care needs of patients with lung cancer in China's cultural context. To identify the supportive care needs of patients, the accuracy of assessment is critical (Richardson, Medina, Brown, & Sitzia, 2007). At present, universal appraisal tools are often used to conduct needs assessments for patients with lung cancer. Patients with different types of cancer have needs in common as well as have needs that are disease specific. However, no instrument is currently available for measuring the specific supportive care needs of patients with lung cancer. Therefore, this study designed the Nursing Professional Social Support Needs Scale (NPSSNS), which includes general and lung-cancer-specific modules (Song, 2015), to assess the supportive care needs of patients with lung cancer.

To address the limitations in the existing research in China, this study aimed to (a) assess supportive care need levels using a questionnaire that has been qualified to assess the needs of patients with lung cancer in the cultural context of China and (b) examine the relationships between supportive care needs and, respectively, demographic factors and treatment variables. On the basis of previous research, it was hypothesized that demographic and disease factors influence patient needs for supportive care. It is hoped that the findings of this study provide a foundation to further explore the supportive care needs of patients with lung cancer and for the clinical selection of nursing interventions in China.

Methods

Design

A cross-sectional descriptive study design was adopted to assess the level of supportive care needs of patients with lung cancer and to examine the relationships between supportive care needs and demographic factors and treatment variables, respectively.

Participants and Procedure

Ethical approval was granted by the Ethical Research Committee, Anhui Medical University (Approval Number 20150328) and the directors of the participating hospitals. The inclusion criteria included (a) a histological diagnosis of lung cancer, including both non-small-cell and small cell lung cancers; (b) currently undergoing treatment; and (c) over 18 years old. To fulfill the aim of this study, patients with mental disorders, cognitive impairments, or other serious, life-threatening diseases were excluded. From June to December 2016, the research group identified and enrolled eligible patients from five inpatient departments in four tertiary teaching hospitals affiliated with a medical university in Anhui Province, China. After verbal and written information relevant to the research was presented, interested patients submitted their written consent to participate in the study. The questionnaires were reported anonymously and were collected on the spot after checking.

Data Collection

Nursing professional social support needs scale

The NPSSNS, a scale developed previously by the authors, was used to assess supportive care needs. This scale includes a general module and lung-cancer-specific modules (Song, 2015). The general module is a 49-item questionnaire in four domains, including informational needs (e.g., "tell me about my diagnosis," "tell me if my illness is hereditary"), technical needs (e.g., "to be cared for by nurses with skilled venipuncture techniques," "being able to help cope with the side effects of different treatments"), psychological needs (e.g., "support in understanding 'why me?'," "taking measures to relieve stressful situations"), care coordination and communication needs (e.g., "helping get support from family and friends," "having the security of knowing a hospital bed is available if needed [acutely]"). The lung-cancer-specific modules cover 10 items (e.g., "teaching me the methods for respiratory function training"). The NPSSNS is scored using a 5-point Likert scale, with 1 = *no need* and 5 = *always need*. The final score for each domain is derived from the average score of all of the items in that domain, and the total score for the scale is derived from the average score of all of the scale items. The psychometric properties of NPSSNS were validated previously (Song, 2015). In this study, Cronbach's alpha values were between .82 and .94 for the four domains of the general module and .86 for the lung-cancer-specific modules.

Background information list

This list included demographic characteristics (gender, age, marital status, education, occupation, income, religious belief, and the means of payment of medical expenses) and disease- and treatment-related factors (cancer metastasis, cancer stage, treatment status, and the presence of other illnesses).

Data Analysis

The data were analyzed using IBM SPSS Statistics 24.0 for Windows (IBM, Armonk, NY, USA). Demographic data and NPSSNS items were analyzed descriptively, and the median, interquartile range (IQR), and percentage were reported respectively after checking the normality of the data. Because the data were nonnormally distributed, a Wilcoxon rank sum test and a Kruskal–Wallis rank sum test were conducted to examine the differences in supportive care needs among patients with different demographic characteristics and treatment variables.

Results

Sample Characteristics

Of 585 eligible patients, 575 agreed to participate in this study and 554 completed the questionnaires (effective response rate: 96.35%). The primary reasons for not completing the questionnaires were being physically unwell and the requirement to undergo a physical examination. The age of the participants ranged from 28 to 88 years, with a median age of 62 (IQR = 14) years. Nearly three quarters of participants (n = 407, 73.47%) were men, 535 (96.57%) were married, most (73.82%) were educated to the junior high school level or less, and 341 (61.55%) were employed. Only 47 (8.48%) participants held religious beliefs.

Nearly two thirds of the participants (60.83%) had metastasis, most (45.85%) were in Stage IV, and 460 (83.03%) were receiving chemotherapy. The demographic information and disease-related characteristics are presented in Table 1.

Supportive Care Needs

The overall score for supportive care needs was 3.19 (IQR = 1.10), the score for the lung-cancer-specific modules was 2.80 (IQR = 1.53), and the scores in the four subdomains ranged from 2.77 (IQR = 1.78) to 3.67 (SD = 0.76). The greatest need was identified in the "informational needs" domain (M = 3.67, IQR = 1.25), followed by the "technical needs" domain (M = 3.55, IQR = 1.00). The distribution of supportive care needs is presented in Table 2.

In the "informational needs" domain, the greatest need was "being informed whether my treatment was effective," with only 31 (5.60%) participants reporting "no need" for this item. In addition, participants reported a high level of need for "letting me know the signs of recurrence," with 455 participants (82.13%) reporting "sometimes need" or greater. In the "technical needs" domain, the greatest need was "to be cared for by nurses with skilled venipuncture techniques," with nearly all (93.50%) reporting "sometimes need" or greater, and the second highest need was "telling me the methods to protect my veins," with half (50.50%) reporting "always need." In the lung-cancer-specific modules, the greatest self-reported need was "teaching me the methods for respiratory function training." The psychological needs domain earned the lowest score (M = 2.77, IQR = 1.78), with "being treated like a human instead of just another case" as the highest scored item in this domain. In the care coordination and communication needs domain, 493 participants (88.99%) responded with "sometimes need" or greater for the item "being allowed to have family or friends with me in hospital." The ranking of the Top 10 supportive care needs for the participants is presented in Table 3.

TABLE 1.
Participant Characteristics (N = 554)

Variable	*n*	%
Age (years)		
Median and P_{25}, P_{75}	62	54, 68
Range	28–88	
Gender		
Male	407	73.47
Female	147	26.53
Marital status		
Unmarried	2	0.36
Married	535	96.57
Widowed or divorced	17	3.07
Level of education		
Elementary school or below	225	40.61
Junior high school	184	33.21
Senior high school	80	14.44
College or above	65	11.74
Mode of paying medical expenses		
Self-payment	20	3.61
Free medical care	10	1.81
Medicare	209	37.73
New rural cooperative medical system	315	56.85
Residence		
Urban	137	24.73
County	55	9.93
Towns	81	14.62
Countryside	281	50.72
Occupation		
Employed	341	61.55
Unemployed	71	12.82
Retired	142	25.63
Income (RMB)		
≥ 5,000	35	6.31
3,000–4,999	124	22.38
1,000–2,999	249	44.96
500–999	63	11.37
≤ 499	83	14.98
Religious beliefs		
Yes	47	8.48
No	507	91.52
Cancer metastasis		
Yes	337	60.83
No	217	39.17
Combined with other illnesses		
Yes	327	50.03
No	227	49.97
Cancer stage		
I	52	9.39
II	57	10.29
III	140	25.27
IV	254	45.85
Unclear	51	9.20
Treated with chemotherapy		
Yes	460	83.03
No	94	16.97

TABLE 2.
Distribution of Supportive Care Needs (N = 554)

Variable	Range	*M*	IQR
Total score	1.41–5	3.19	1.10
Informational needs	1–5	3.67	1.25
Technical needs	1.36–5	3.55	1.00
Psychological needs	1–5	2.77	1.78
Care coordination and communication needs	1–5	3.00	1.16
Lung-cancer-specific modules	1–5	2.80	1.53

Note. IQR = interquartile range.

Relationship Between Supportive Care Needs and Demographic Factors

The female participants had more needs than their male peers ($Z = -2.590$, $p < .05$) in the domains of technical needs ($Z = -2.489$, $p < .05$), psychological needs ($Z = -4.097$, $p < .01$), and care coordination and communication needs ($Z = -2.052$, $p < .05$). In terms of age, participants who were < 40 years old earned relatively higher scores in the lung-cancer-specific modules ($\chi^2 = 8.594$, $p < .05$), whereas those 41–65 years old reported higher levels of informational needs ($\chi^2 = 8.459$, $p < .05$). Participants with a college degree or higher reported higher levels of psychological needs ($\chi^2 = 10.122$, $p < .05$). In terms of monthly income, the 249 participants (44.96%) reporting earning 1,000–2,999 RMB/month reported a higher overall level of supportive care needs ($\chi^2 = 12.243$, $p < .05$), especially in the domains of psychological needs ($\chi^2 = 10.738$, $p < .05$) and care coordination and communication needs ($\chi^2 = 13.160$, $p < .05$). However, participants who reported earning 500–999 RMB/month reported a higher level of needs in the lung-cancer-specific modules ($\chi^2 = 13.918$, $p < .01$). The relationships between supportive care needs and demographic factors are presented in Table 4.

Relationship Between Supportive Care Needs and Treatment Variables

Participants who had metastasis had more needs in total ($Z = -2.424$, $p < .05$), more informational needs ($Z = -2.087$, $p < .05$), more technical needs ($Z = -2.584$, $p < .05$), more psychological needs ($Z = -2.019$, $p < .05$), and more care coordination and communication needs ($Z = -2.000$, $p < .05$) than their nonmetastasis peers. Furthermore, half (50.03%) of the participants who experienced concomitant diseases had more needs in total ($Z = -2.060$, $p < .05$), especially in the care coordination and communication needs domain ($Z = -2.340$, $p < .05$). Participants in Stage III had higher levels of informational needs ($\chi^2 = 19.545$, $p < .01$) and care coordination and communication needs ($\chi^2 = 11.874$, $p < .05$).

TABLE 3.
Rank of Top 10 Supportive Care Needs Among Participants (N = 554)

Rank	Supportive Care Need	"Sometimes Need" or Higher		Domain
		n	%	
1	To be cared for by nurses with skilled venipuncture techniques	518	93.50	Technical needs
2	Telling me the methods to protect my veins	501	90.43	Technical needs
3	Maintain a comfortable environment and tidy beds in the ward	497	89.71	Technical needs
4	Receiving prompt nursing care	493	88.99	Technical needs
4	Being allowed to have family or friends with me in hospital	493	88.99	Care coordination and communication needs
6	Being informed whether my treatment was effective	467	84.30	Informational needs
7	Having the security of knowing a hospital bed is available if needed (acutely)	463	83.57	Care coordination and communication needs
7	Help patient make the next doctor appointment or test	463	83.57	Care coordination and communication needs
9	Teaching me the methods for respiratory function training	461	83.22	Lung-cancer-specific modules
10	Letting me know the signs of recurrence	455	82.13	Informational needs

Meanwhile, participants in Stage IV had more needs in total ($\chi^2 = 14.128$, $p < .01$), in the lung-cancer-specific modules ($\chi^2 = 12.957$, $p < .05$), and in the technical needs domain ($\chi^2 = 10.901$, $p < .05$). The relationships between supportive care needs and treatment variables are presented in Table 5.

Discussion

Supportive Care Needs

Consistent with prior research (Liao et al., 2011; Sanders et al., 2010; Yun et al., 2013), the participants in this study reported high levels of informational needs. The strongest informational need identified in this study was "being informed whether my treatment was working." In terms of age group, the middle-aged group reported the highest level of informational needs. This may be explained by the greater family responsibilities and expectations that are shouldered by middle-aged people in China, which makes them relatively more interested in being informed about the effectiveness of treatments. Moreover, having a high reported need for "letting me know the signs of recurrence" and fear of cancer recurrence have been associated with unmet supportive care needs (Sarkar et al., 2015). Therefore, clinical workers should provide information on disease progression and the effect of treatment to reduce the unmet supportive care needs of patients with lung cancer.

The second most frequently reported needs among patients were in the technical needs domain, where the Top 2 technical needs were "to be cared for by nurses with skilled venipuncture techniques" and "telling me the methods to protect my veins." This may reflect the fact that all of the participants were receiving treatment at tertiary teaching hospitals, which, in China, have many student nurses who are more likely to perform venipunctures improperly (Huang, Wu, Huang, Lu, & Wu, 2017) as well as the fact that over 80% of the participants had received chemotherapy, which is known to cause poor vascular conditions. Therefore, measures should be taken to improve the rate of venipuncture success to relieve patient pain.

The finding that the psychological needs domain earned the lowest score of all of the domains was an unexpected deviation from prior studies (Giuliani et al., 2016; Liao et al., 2011). Unwillingness to address psychological needs may reflect prevailing cultural norms (Lam, Fabrizio, Ho, Chan, & Fielding, 2009). Moreover, the findings of prior studies indicate that the prevalence of supportive care needs differs across cultures (Lam et al., 2011). A systematic review of the supportive care needs of patients with breast cancer showed that Chinese women reported more informational needs and fewer psychological needs than Western women (Fiszer, Dolbeault, Sultan, & Brédart A, 2014). This phenomenon may be because Chinese patients are more willing to share their concerns with family members. We found that most participants (88.99%) reported "sometimes need" or greater for the item "being allowed to have family or friends with me in hospital." The average nurse–bed ratio is 0.63:1 in Chinese tertiary hospitals (Xu, Wu, Zhang, Ma, & Li, 2016). Thus, most patients likely believe that nurses are very busy, with little time to address patient psychological needs, making these patients unwilling to report their psychological needs to nurses. Moreover, some nurses have reported that lack of sufficient time and the task-oriented nature of their nursing work prevent their providing psychosocial care (Chen et al., 2017). In addition, prior studies indicate that most doctors do not deem psychosocial care as their responsibility (Lam et al., 2009).

TABLE 4.

Relationship Between Supportive Care Needs and Demographic Factors (N = 554, Mean Rank)

Variable	IN	TN	PN	CCACN	LCSM	Total
Gender						
Female	278.44	305.64	323.85	300.71	293.47	306.81
Male	277.16	267.34	260.76	269.12	271.73	266.91
Z	−0.083	−2.489*	−4.097**	−2.052*	−1.412	−2.590*
Age (years)						
≤ 40	202.82	321.41	334.27	292.41	294.23	281.86
41–65	291.17	280.44	283.56	283.56	291.58	287.96
≥ 66	255.69	269.27	264.98	264.98	249.48	257.16
χ^2	8.459*	1.442	3.762	1.747	8.594*	4.538
Marital status						
Unmarried	496.00	424.50	235.75	154.75	409.25	350.00
Married	276.86	278.28	277.46	278.90	277.72	277.93
Widowed or divorced	27.88	247.91	283.62	247.91	254.94	255.32
χ^2	3.760	2.859	0.161	1.799	1.696	0.741
Education						
Elementary school	255.95	274.18	263.99	264.04	270.64	264.01
Junior high school	283.21	268.14	268.12	273.46	286.44	274.88
Senior high school	307.14	290.34	294.44	306.63	285.73	300.60
College or above	299.42	299.69	329.98	299.69	265.82	303.18
χ^2	0.823*	2.493	10.122*	5.613	1.548	4.987
Religious beliefs						
No	276.03	275.81	274.58	278.23	277.76	276.05
Yes	293.35	295.69	308.99	269.61	274.67	293.15
Z	−0.710	−0.815	−1.410	−0.354	−0.127	−0.701
Mode of paying medical expenses						
Self-payment	295.00	291.42	290.25	306.02	316.48	306.08
Free medical care	222.45	340.05	298.15	281.15	248.25	281.30
Medicare	280.32	289.89	297.89	283.52	272.94	286.27
New rural cooperative medical system	276.27	266.41	262.51	271.58	278.98	269.75
χ^2	1.507	4.449	6.452	1.369	1.718	2.009
Residence						
Urban	279.43	267.88	292.87	276.43	257.91	275.29
County	308.43	314.93	315.40	324.55	302.70	318.50
Town	274.47	293.51	265.23	271.10	296.29	280.19
Countryside	271.35	270.26	266.03	270.64	276.77	269.76
χ^2	2.519	4.895	6.273	5.408	4.557	4.313
Occupation						
Employed	287.06	287.09	284.48	288.05	292.74	292.74
Unemployed	247.34	254.96	246.93	255.01	255.01	259.44
Retired	269.61	265.74	276.04	263.41	263.41	249.94
χ^2	4.087	3.403	3.251	3.985	8.215*	4.891
Income (RMB)						
≥ 5,000	222.03	286.14	238.41	211.34	211.79	217.96
3,000–4,999	265.35	267.72	245.54	253.55	249.03	249.94
1,000–2,999	286.09	291.72	295.19	298.13	293.52	295.81
500–999	295.99	281.03	273.87	286.16	302.65	291.22
≤ 499	279.25	243.13	291.42	272.71	280.60	278.45
χ^2	6.491	6.396	10.738*	13.160*	13.918**	12.243*

Note. IN = informational needs; TN = technical needs; PN = psychological needs; CCACN = care coordination and communication needs; LCSM = lung-cancer-specific modules.
*$p < .05$. **$p < .01$.

TABLE 5.
Relationship Between Supportive Care Needs and Treatment Variables (N = 554, Mean Rank)

Variable	IN	TN	PN	CCACN	LCSM	Total
Cancer metastasis						
Yes	288.89	291.59	289.01	288.41	285.86	290.73
No	259.82	255.62	259.63	260.56	264.51	256.95
Z	−2.087*	−2.584*	−2.109*	−2.000*	−1.533	−2.424*
With other illnesses						
Yes	285.39	286.36	284.46	290.76	289.16	289.17
No	266.14	264.73	267.48	258.41	260.70	260.68
Z	−1.392	−1.566	−1.228	−2.340*	−2.060	−2.060*
Cancer stage						
I	207.99	251.65	237.44	234.48	239.18	224.81
II	289.44	279.69	266.22	278.29	288.73	279.50
III	295.21	262.85	284.60	294.86	287.78	288.19
IV	290.36	299.07	286.07	287.15	289.61	292.59
Unclear	222.37	234.19	268.78	224.84	215.50	224.46
χ^2	19.545**	10.901*	4.697	11.874*	12.957*	14.128**
Treated with chemotherapy						
Yes	280.73	276.06	279.18	278.85	272.37	278.24
No	261.70	284.53	269.28	270.90	302.61	273.24
Z	−1.051	−0.467	−0.547	−0.439	−1.670	−0.242

Note. IN = informational needs; TN = technical needs; PN = psychological needs; CCACN = care coordination and communication needs; LCSM = lung-cancer-specific modules.
**p* < .05. ***p* < .01.

Relationship Between Supportive Care Needs and Demographic Factors

This study found a significant difference in supportive care needs across genders, age groups, educational levels, and income levels. Consistent with previous research (Fitch & Steele, 2010), the female participants in this study reported having more needs than their male peers in terms of both total needs and the several NPSSNS subscales. Across the disease trajectory of lung cancer, female patients typically have more worries and face a higher incidence of psychological problems (Hill, Amir, Muers, Connolly, & Round, 2003; Sarna et al., 2006), especially in the realm of handling family tasks and self-care. This may relate to the role that women play in the home. However, Sanders et al. (2010) and Liao et al. (2011) found no significant difference in supportive care needs across genders. The different instruments used in these studies and the heterogeneity of samples may explain the differences in their findings. Sanders et al. indicated that age may not be a predictor of the supportive care needs of patients with lung cancer (Sanders et al., 2010). However, consistent with previous studies (Graves et al., 2007; Li & Girgis, 2006), this study found that participants below 40 years old had higher supportive care needs in certain dimensions. This may result from younger patients being more comfortable in expressing their needs (Sanson-Fisher et al., 2015). Therefore, clinical staff should meet the supportive care needs of their younger patients with lung cancer in a timely manner and should encourage older patients to express their needs (Liao et al., 2011). In this study, the participants holding a college degree or higher reported having higher psychological needs. This finding echoes the finding of prior studies that higher levels of education correlate with higher supportive care needs (Engelman et al., 2005; Squiers, Finney Rutten, Treiman, Bright, & Hesse, 2005; Wong et al., 2000). Receiving a diagnosis of lung cancer saddles some patients with a huge, new financial burden (Li et al., 2017). Yun et al. (2013) found that patients with lung cancer earning a monthly income of less than $2,000 faced significantly higher financial burdens. Similarly, this study found that participants with lower monthly incomes had higher supportive care needs in terms of both NPSSNS total and subscale scores. However, no significant difference in supportive care needs was found across marital statuses, which differed from previous research (Yun et al., 2013). The main reason for this inconsistency may be the very high percentage (96.57%) of participants in this study who were married.

Relationship Between Supportive Care Needs and Treatment Variables

In this study, the participants with metastasis and other illnesses reported higher total and subscale needs in Stages III and IV. This finding is similar to previous studies, which found that patients with advanced lung cancer had more supportive care needs (Li & Girgis, 2006; Sanders et al.,

2010; Sarkar et al., 2015). Nonetheless, there was no significant difference in supportive care needs between the chemotherapy and nonchemotherapy groups. This may be because of the fact that most (83.03%) participants in this study were receiving chemotherapy.

Limitations

Although results from this study provide important information for the supportive care needs of patients with lung cancer, several limitations should be taken into consideration when interpreting the data. First, this was a cross-sectional study that was not able to detect changes in supportive care needs over time. Second, the participants in this study were all being cared for in tertiary teaching hospitals. The fees and technologies applied in these hospitals may differ from hospitals of other levels, which may affect the supportive care needs of patients. Finally, to alleviate the burden of completing the questionnaires, this study only discussed the relationships between supportive care needs and demographic factors and treatment variables, respectively. However, psychosocial factors may also affect the supportive care needs of patients with lung cancer, which is an issue that should be explored in future studies.

Conclusions

Patients with lung cancer have many supportive care needs, with these needs particularly acute in the domains of informational needs and technical needs. Patients with other concurrent and serious diseases (e.g., other illnesses, metastasis) and those with high socioeconomic burdens (e.g., female, lower income levels) experience higher levels of supportive care needs. The results of this study support the hypothesis that demographic and disease-related factors influence the need for supportive care in patients with lung cancer. However, this study found that marital status, religious beliefs, and mode of medical expense payment do not significantly influence the need for supportive care.

Relevance to Clinical Practice

The results provide a basis for understanding the supportive care needs of patients with lung cancer in China. First, nurses should strengthen their awareness and expertise to effectively identify the needs of patients and provide supportive care to patients with lung cancer. Second, patients in categories that are known to have supportive care needs should be identified. Finally, culturally tailored interventions should be developed to target the supportive care needs of patients with lung cancer in China.

Acknowledgments

This study was supported by the National Natural Science Foundation of China (81573017) and the Natural Science Foundation of Anhui Provincial Universities' Key Project (KJ2015A083). We gratefully acknowledge all of the study participants.

References

Borimnejad, L., Mardani-Hamooleh, M., Seyedfatemi, N., & Tahmasebi, M. (2017). Palliative nursing for cancer patients as an abstract concept: A hermeneutic study. *The Journal of Nursing Research, 26*(4), 260–265. https://doi.org/10.1097/jnr.0000000000000232

Bray, F., Ferlay, J., Soerjomataram, I., Siegel, R. L., Torre, L. A., & Jemal, A. (2018). Global Cancer Statistics 2018: GLOBOCAN estimates of incidence and mortality worldwide for 36 cancers in 185 countries. *CA: A Cancer Journal for Clinicians, 68*(6), 394–464. https://doi.org/10.3322/caac.21492

Chen, C. S., Chan, S. W., Chan, M. F., Yap, S. F., Wang, W., & Kowitlawakul, Y. (2017). Nurses' perceptions of psychosocial care and barriers to its provision: A qualitative study. *The Journal of Nursing Research, 25*(6), 411–418. https://doi.org/10.1097/jnr.0000000000000185

Chen, W., Zheng, R., Baade, P. D., Zhang, S., Zeng, H., Bray, F., ... He, J. (2016). Cancer statistics in China, 2015. *CA: A Cancer Journal for Clinicians, 66*(2), 115–132. https://doi.org/10.3322/caac.21338

Dai, Y. L., Yang, C. T., Chen, K. H., & Tang, S. T. (2016). Changes in and determinants of quality of life in patients with advanced non-small-cell lung cancer undergoing initial chemotherapy. *The Journal of Nursing Research, 25*(3), 203–215. https://doi.org/10.1097/jnr.0000000000000148

Engelman, K. K., Perpich, D. L., Peterson, S. L., Hall, M. A., Ellerbeck, E. F., & Stanton, A. L. (2005). Cancer information needs in rural areas. *Journal of Health Communication, 10*(3), 199–208. https://doi.org/10.1080/10810730590934217

Fiszer, C., Dolbeault, S., Sultan, S., & Brédart, A. (2014). Prevalence, intensity, and predictors of the supportive care needs of women diagnosed with breast cancer: A systematic review. *Psycho-Oncology, 23*(4), 361–374. https://doi.org/10.1002/pon.3432

Fitch, M. I., & Steele, R. (2010). Supportive care needs of individuals with lung cancer. *Canadian Oncology Nursing Journal, 20*(1), 15–22. https://doi.org/10.5737/1181912x2011522

Giuliani, M. E., Milne, R. A., Puts, M., Sampson, L. R., Kwan, J. Y., Le, L. W., ... Jones, J. (2016). The prevalence and nature of supportive care needs in lung cancer patients. *Current Oncology, 23*(4), 258–265. https://doi.org/10.3747/co.23.3012

Graves, K. D., Arnold, S. M., Love, C. L., Kirsh, K. L., Moore, P. G., & Passik, S. D. (2007). Distress screening in a multidisciplinary lung cancer clinic: Prevalence and predictors of clinically significant distress. *Lung Cancer, 55*(2), 215. https://doi.org/10.1016/j.lungcan.2006.10.001

Hill, K. M., Amir, Z., Muers, M. F., Connolly, C. K., & Round, C. E. (2003). Do newly diagnosed lung cancer patients feel their concerns are being met? *European Journal of Cancer Care, 12*(1), 35–45. https://doi.org/10.1046/j.1365-2354.2003.00324.x

Huang, J. Y., Wu, X. H., Huang, C. Y., Lu, F. Y., & Wu, B. Y. (2017). Bedside observation analysis on procedure standardization of intravenous infusion among practicing nursing students. *Journal of Nursing Science, 32*(8), 81–83. https://doi.org/10.3870/j.issn.1001-4152 (Original work published in Chinese)

Iyer, S., Taylor-Stokes, G., & Roughley, A. (2013). Symptom burden and quality of life in advanced non-small cell lung cancer patients in France and Germany. *Lung Cancer, 81*(2), 288–293. https://doi.org/10.1016/j.lungcan.2013.03.008

Jacobs-Lawson, J. M., Schumacher, M. M., Hughes, T., & Arnold, S. (2009). The relationship between lung cancer patients' educational level and evaluation of their treatment information needs. *Journal of Cancer Education, 24*(4), 346–350. https://doi.org/10.1080/08858190902876601

Lam, W. W., Au, A. H., Wong, J. H., Lehmann, C., Koch, U., Fielding, R., & Mehnert, A. (2011). Unmet supportive care needs: A cross-cultural comparison between Hong Kong Chinese and German Caucasian women with breast cancer. *Breast Cancer Research and Treatment, 130*(2), 531–541. https://doi.org/10.1007/s10549-011-1592-1

Lam, W. W., Fabrizio, C., Ho, E., Chan, L., & Fielding, R. (2009). Perceived importance of evidence-based psychosocial clinical guidelines for Hong Kong Chinese women with breast cancer: Opinions of patients and health care providers. *Supportive Care in Cancer, 17*(3), 219–229. https://doi.org/10.1007/s00520-008-0500-7

Li, J., & Girgis, A. (2006). Supportive care needs: Are patients with lung cancer a neglected population? *Psycho-Oncology, 15*(6), 509–516. https://doi.org/10.1002/pon.983

Li, Y., Shi, J., Yu, S., Wang, L., Liu, J., Ren, J., ... Yao, H. (2017). Effect of socioeconomic status on stage at diagnosis of lung cancer in a hospital-based multicenter retrospective clinical epidemiological study in China, 2005–2014. *Cancer Medicine, 6*(10), 2440–2452. https://doi.org/10.1002/cam4.1170

Liao, Y. C., Liao, W. Y., Shun, S. C., Yu, C. J., Yang, P. C., & Lai, Y. H. (2011). Symptoms, psychological distress, and supportive care needs in lung cancer patients. *Supportive Care in Cancer: Official Journal of the Multinational Association of Supportive Care in Cancer, 19*(11), 1743. https://doi.org/10.1007/s00520-010-1014-7

Richardson, A. (2003). Improving supportive and palliative care for adults with cancer. *Nursing Times, 99*(39), 49.

Richardson, A., Medina, J., Brown, V., & Sitzia, J. (2007). Patients' needs assessment in cancer care: A review of assessment tools. *Supportive Care in Cancer, 15*(10), 1125–1144. https://doi.org/10.1007/s00520-006-0205-8

Sanders, S. L., Bantum, E. O., Owen, J. E., Thornton, A. A., & Stanton, A. L. (2010). Supportive care needs in patients with lung cancer. *Psycho-Oncology, 19*(5), 480–489. https://doi.org/10.1002/pon.1577

Sanson-Fisher, R., Girgis, A., Boyes, A., Bonevski, B., Burton, L., & Cook, P. (2015). The unmet supportive care needs of patients with cancer. *Cancer, 88*(1), 226–237. https://doi.org/10.1002/(SICI)1097-0142(20000101)88

Sarkar, S., Sautier, L., Schilling, G., Bokemeyer, C., Koch, U., & Mehnert, A. (2015). Anxiety and fear of cancer recurrence and its association with supportive care needs and health-care service utilization in cancer patients. *Journal of Cancer Survivorship, 9*(4), 567–575. https://doi.org/10.1007/s11764-015-0434-2

Sarna, L., Cooley, M. E., Brown, J. K., Williams, R. D., Chernecky, C., Padilla, G., & Danao, L. L. (2006). Quality of life and health status of dyads of women with lung cancer and family members. *Oncology Nursing Forum, 33*(6), 1109–1116. https://doi.org/10.1188/06.ONF.1109-1116

Schofield, P., Ugalde, A., Carey, M., Mileshkin, L., Duffy, M., Ball, D., & Aranda, S. (2008). Lung cancer: Challenges and solutions for supportive care intervention research. *Palliative & Supportive Care, 6*(3), 281–287. https://doi.org/10.1017/S1478951508000424

Shao, Q., Li, J. B., Li, F. X., Wang, S. Z., Wang, W., Liu, S. S., & Zhang, Y. J. (2015). Clinical investigation into the initial diagnosis and treatment of 1,168 lung cancer patients. *Oncology Letters, 9*(2), 563–568. https://doi.org/10.3892/ol.2014.2777

Shao, Q., Liu, S., Wang, W., Zhang, Y., Li, F., & Li, J. (2017). Clinical investigation into the initial diagnosis and treatment of 539 patients with stage IV lung cancer. *Chinese Journal of Radiological Health, 10*, 535–541. https://doi.org/10.2147/OTT.S125108

Siegel, R. L., Miller, K. D., & Jemal, A. (2015). Cancer statistics, 2015. *CA: A Cancer Journal for Clinicians, 65*(1), 11–30. https://doi.org/10.3322/caac.21254

Song, Y. X. (2015). *Development of cancer patients' Nursing Professional Social Support Needs Scale and its application* (Unpublished master's thesis). Retrieved from http://www.cnki.net/ (Original work published in Chinese)

Squiers, L., Finney Rutten, L. J., Treiman, K., Bright, M. A., & Hesse, B. (2005). Cancer patients' information needs across the cancer care continuum: Evidence from the cancer information service. *Journal of Health Communication, 10*(1, Suppl.), 15–34. https://doi.org/10.1080/10810730500263620

Wang, Y., Xu, Z., Mao, J. H., Hung, M. S., Hsieh, D., Au, A., ... You, L. (2015). Analysis of lung tumor initiation and progression in transgenic mice for Cre-inducible overexpression of Cul4a gene. *Thoracic Cancer, 6*(4), 480. https://doi.org/10.1111/1759-7714.12257

Wong, F., Stewart, D. E., Dancey, J., Meana, M., McAndrews, M. P., Bunston, T., & Cheung, A. M. (2000). Men with prostate cancer: Influence of psychological factors on informational needs and decision making. *Journal of Psychosomatic Research, 49*(1), 13–19. https://doi.org/10.1016/S0022-3999(99)00109-9

Xu, Y. M., Wu, Y., Zhang, Y., Ma, R. Y., & Li, X. H. (2016). Investigation of nursing human resources in Chinese hospitals. *Chinese Journal of Nursing, 51*(7), 819–822. (Original work published in Chinese)

Yun, Y. H., Shon, E. J., Yang, A. J., Kim, S. H., Kim, Y. A., Chang, Y. J., ... Shim, Y. M. (2013). Needs regarding care and factors associated with unmet needs in disease-free survivors of surgically treated lung cancer. *Annals of Oncology, 24*(10), 1552–1559. https://doi.org/10.1093/annonc/mdt032

Effects of Predischarge Patient Education Combined with Postdischarge Follow-Ups on Self-Care, Readmission, Sleep and Depression in Patients With Heart Failure

Hsing-Mei CHEN[1] • Shan-Tair WANG[2] • Shyh-Jong WU[3] • Chee-Siong LEE[4] • Susan J. FETZER[5] • Liang-Miin TSAI[6*]

ABSTRACT

Background: Patients with heart failure rarely engage in adequate self-care. Greater emphasis on self-care discharge readiness is needed.

Purpose: This study examined the effects of a predischarge educational program combined with 1 year of postdischarge follow-up on self-care behaviors, readmission, sleep quality, and depression in patients with heart failure.

Methods: A longitudinal, nonequivalent two-group pretest–posttest design was used. The intervention group received tailored education and follow-ups, whereas the control group received routine predischarge heart-failure education from direct care nurses only. Measurements included the self-care maintenance and self-care management subscales of the Self-Care of Heart Failure Index, Pittsburg Sleep Quality Index, Patient Health Questionnaire-9, and readmission rate. Data obtained at baseline and at 1, 3, 6, and 12 months postdischarge were analyzed using linear mixed models with both intention-to-treat and per-protocol approaches. The propensity score was used to adjust for the confounding effects of the New York Heart Association functional class and left ventricular ejection fraction.

Results: Of the 62 patients with heart failure (28 in the intervention group and 34 in the control group) who were sampled at baseline, 47 (n = 25 vs. n = 22) provided data over the entire course of this 1-year study (76% retention rate). The per-protocol analysis did not find significant differences for any variables. However, the intention-to-treat analysis showed that the intervention group significantly improved in self-care maintenance at 6 months and self-care management at 12 months after hospital discharge, with fewer, albeit not significantly fewer, first and subsequent hospital readmissions than the control group.

Conclusions/Implications for Practice: The effect of this intervention was not found to be substantial, indicating a need to design more efficacious and powerful interventions. Hospitalized patients must receive patient education before discharge to foster their self-care knowledge and skills regarding self-care at home. Strategies are needed to help nurses provide patient education in a time-efficient manner.

KEY WORDS:
heart failure, predischarge patient education, postdischarge follow-up, self-care, readmission.

Introduction

Although advanced treatments have increased the rate of survival among patients with heart failure (HF; Benjamin et al., 2017), early postdischarge readmissions are common, with 31.9% and 38.5% of patients readmitted within 6 months and 1 year of discharge, respectively (Chang et al., 2017). Many patients experience unresolved symptoms after discharge (Teo et al., 2016), including shortness of breath, difficulty in walking or climbing stairs, fatigue, edema, trouble sleeping, and depression (Huang et al., 2018). Several risk factors for HF readmission have been recognized and categorized into three factor categories, including patient factors (e.g., heart function, comorbidities, advanced age), psychosocial factors (e.g., depression, sleep quality, quality of life), and system-based factors (e.g., hospital size, limited cardiac services, low-income or minority populations; Carlson et al., 2019; Ryan et al., 2019). Active engagement in self-care facilitates symptom management and reoccurrence, which

[1]PhD, RN, Associate Professor, Department of Nursing, College of Medicine, National Cheng Kung University, Taiwan, ROC • [2]PhD, Deputy Superintendent, Ditmanson Medical Foundation Chiayi Christian Hospital, Chiayi City, Taiwan; Affiliate Professor, Institute of Gerontology, College of Medicine, National Cheng Kung University, Taiwan, ROC • [3]PhD, Associate Professor, Department of Medical Laboratory Science and Biotechnology, Kaohsiung Medical University, Taiwan, ROC • [4]MD, Lecturer, Division of Cardiology, Kaohsiung Medical University Hospital, Kaohsiung Medical University, Taiwan, ROC • [5]PhD, RN, CNL, CCRN, Professor, Department of Nursing, University of New Hampshire, USA • [6]MD, Superintendent, Department of Internal Medicine, Tainan Municipal Hospital (Managed by Show Chwan Medical Care Corporation), Taiwan, ROC.

prevents or slows deterioration, improves functional capacity, improves quality of life, and minimizes the impact of patient factors associated with readmission (Riegel et al., 2016; Ryan et al., 2019).

However, patients with HF engage only rarely in adequate self-care (Köberich et al., 2015; Tsai et al., 2015). Thus, greater emphasis on self-care readiness at discharge is needed. HF self-care includes behaviors related to medication administration, dietary choices, fluid control, exercise, symptom monitoring and management, and behaviors requiring lifestyle changes (Riegel et al., 2011). Patients must be empowered to implement self-care behaviors and be supported to integrate self-care recommendations into daily routines. For patients with HF, the challenges and obstacles begin after hospital admission and continue after their return to community and home settings (Nadrian et al., 2018; Ponikowski et al., 2016).

A well-organized predischarge educational program is important for hospitals that have limited numbers of professionals available for home-based intervention programs. Because HF is characterized by unexpected exacerbations, postdischarge telephone follow-up may contribute to the success of related predischarge educational programs (Liou et al., 2015). Domingues et al. (2011) found that hospital-based educational nursing interventions for patients with HF followed by telephone monitoring after discharge improved HF awareness and self-care knowledge scores but did not significantly reduce rates of emergency room visits, rehospitalizations, or deaths. Köberich et al. (2015) found that a single educational session coupled with consecutive telephone follow-ups improved overall self-care behaviors but had no impact on quality of life. Liou et al. (2015) found that inpatient education, using a videotape or a teaching booklet combined with telephone follow-ups, effectively promoted self-care in patients with HF but did not affect hospital readmission or the mortality rate at 3 months. Although prior studies have measured the short-term impact of educational interventions on patients with HF, a longer period of observation is necessary to advance scholarly understanding of the effects of these interventions on the self-care behaviors of patients with HF.

Therefore, the purpose of this study was to examine the effects of a predischarge educational program combined with 1 year of postdischarge follow-up on self-care behaviors, sleep quality, depression, and readmission in patients with HF. The primary outcomes were self-care maintenance, self-care management, and readmissions. The secondary outcomes were sleep quality and depression.

The readmission rate for patients with HF is higher in Taiwan than in many other countries (Chang et al., 2017). Nearly 10% (9.7%) of Taiwanese patients with HF are readmitted more than once within 1 year of discharge. This high rate of readmission suggests inadequate discharge preparations and a need to begin the predischarge planning process earlier after admission (Ryan et al., 2019). Nurses play an important role in providing predischarge education aimed at modifying self-care behaviors after discharge (Albert et al., 2015). However, many clinical practice nurses carry heavy workloads already and may lack time to provide additional patient education. Moreover, many nurses lack the confidence and teaching materials necessary to convey relevant self-care knowledge and skills (Che et al., 2016). In response to this problem, a patient-focused self-care pamphlet was developed as part of a predischarge HF educational program (Ponikowski et al., 2016). The hypothesis was that improving the quality and timing of teaching materials and conducting postdischarge nursing follow-ups would improve clinical outcomes.

Methods

Study Design

A longitudinal, nonequivalent, two-group, pretest–posttest design was used, and data were collected from November 2012 to February 2015.

Setting and Samples

Patients who were diagnosed with HF before admission to one of two medical centers in southern Taiwan were invited to participate. Adult patients 20 years or older were included if they were classified as II or higher on the New York Heart Association (NYHA) functional classification based on the *International Classification of Diseases, Ninth Revision* (Code 428) and were able to communicate in either Mandarin Chinese or Taiwanese without shortness of breath. Patients with a diagnosis of dementia, psychological impairment, or musculoskeletal limitations such as hemiplegia as noted in the medical record were excluded. Subjects were assigned to either the control group or the intervention group using computer-generated random numbers. Post hoc power analysis was calculated using Power Analysis and Sample Size 2008 software (NCSS, Kaysville, UT, USA). At a significance level of .05, with sample sizes of 22 completers in the control group and 25 completers in the intervention group, 5 points of means and standard deviations, and repeated-measures analysis of variance, the effect sizes estimated were 2.04 for self-care maintenance, 1.15 for self-care management, 0.94 for sleep quality, and 0.89 for depression. The post hoc power was calculated based on the Greenhouse–Geisser corrected *F* test (Mueller et al., 1992), and the preceding parameters were 100% for all variables except for readmission. The power for readmission achieved only 35% based on the Cox regression analysis with the log odds ratio, a standard deviation of 0.50, an anticipated event rate of 0.50, and a significance level of .05 to detect a regression coefficient equal to 1.00 (Hsieh & Lavori, 2000).

Intervention

The control group received routine, predischarge HF education from direct care nurses and were provided a one-page discharge information sheet that emphasized self-care behaviors, including medication adherence, low-salt dietary restrictions, fluid restrictions, and engaging in physical activity. The intervention group received tailored education and follow-up by either the principal investigator or a trained advanced care cardiac nurse that began on the day immediately after admission. The educators reviewed the information included in the study pamphlet, which was printed in full-color, pictorial format and a large font size for ease of reading. A previous review by two cardiologists and three advanced care cardiac nurses earned the pamphlet a content validity index of 1.0. The intervention group received five postdischarge follow-ups, which consisted of one-on-one, self-care consultations (Figure 1).

Measurements

In addition to demographic data, information related to heart status, including ejection fraction and comorbidities, was obtained from patient medical records. Dates and frequencies of readmission were simultaneously collected from the patients and their medical records at each data collection point. Three instruments were used to measure the clinical outcomes of self-care ability, sleep quality, and depression.

Self-Care

Self-care included maintenance and management and was measured using the respective subscales of the Self-Care of Heart Failure Index (Riegel et al., 2009). The 10-item self-care maintenance subscale was designed to determine the frequency of engagement in self-care behaviors that promote health maintenance such as medication adherence, body weight and edema monitoring, water and sodium intake restrictions, and regular exercise. The five-item self-care management subscale was designed to describe the participants' actions in response to HF symptoms that worsened or reoccurred during the past month. Each item on these subscales is scored from 1 to 4 (1 = *never or rarely*, 4 = *always or daily*), and subscale total scores are converted to standardized scores ranging from 0 to 100, with higher scores indicating better self-care; scores above 70 represent adequate self-care (Riegel et al., 2009). The 15 items have been translated and used in Taiwan (Tsai et al., 2015). The Cronbach's alphas for these subscales were .80 for maintenance and .68 for management in this study.

Sleep Quality

The Chinese version of the 19-item Pittsburg Sleep Quality Index (PSQI; Buysse et al., 1989) was used in this study to measure sleep quality. The PSQI consists of a patient report of sleep, including duration, latency, efficiency, and disturbances; use of medications; daytime dysfunction; and subjective sleep quality. Each component is scored on a scale ranging from 0 to 3, and the seven component scores of 18 items are summed to produce a global score ranging from 0 to 21. Higher scores indicate worse sleep quality, and a score higher than 5 indicates poor sleep quality. The Chinese version of the PSQI was translated and validated by Tsai et al. (2005), with a Cronbach's alpha of .72 for 51 primary insomniacs. The Cronbach's alpha for this measure was .79 in this study.

Depression

The Chinese version of the nine-item Patient Health Questionnaire (PHQ-9) developed by Kroenke et al. (2001) was used in this study to measure depression. The nine symptoms include little interest or pleasure in doing things; feeling down, depressed, or hopeless; feeling tired or having little energy; and having a poor appetite or overeating. These factors are ranked from 0 (*not at all*) to 3 (*nearly every day*), for a possible total score ranging from 0 to 27. A higher score indicates a greater tendency toward depression, and a score ≥ 10 is indicative of clinical depression. In a previous study on 76 cardiac surgery patients, the Chinese version of the PHQ-9 earned a Cronbach's alpha of .78 (Liao et al., 2018). In this study, the Cronbach's alpha for this measure was .84.

Procedure

After obtaining approval to conduct the study from the participating hospitals (KMUH-IRB-20120209 and A-ER-102-176), hospitalized patients with HF were referred to the study by cardiologists and nurse practitioners, and their informed consent was obtained. To minimize both expectation and answer bias, questionnaire collection and patient education were performed by different personnel. Research assistants, trained by the principal investigator to ensure the integrity of the research, recruited participants, obtained informed consent, and collected the data. Patients who agreed to participate then completed the pretest questionnaires. Participants in the intervention group were contacted by one of the cardiac educators, and a mutually agreeable time was set for the educational program. After the one-on-one education, the HF booklet was left with the participant. Five telephone follow-ups were completed by the cardiac educators. Data collection interviews were completed at 1, 3, 6, and 12 months after discharge during participant visits to the outpatient department or during home visits. If the participants were readmitted and agreed to continue, data collection continued. All of the participants were compensated the equivalent of 6 USD during each visit.

Data Analysis

The demographic characteristics of patients with HF in each group were summarized and compared using Chi-square and Mann-Whitney *U* tests. Self-care maintenance and management as well as the PHQ-9 and PSQI scores at baseline and at 1, 3, 6, and 12 months postdischarge were analyzed using linear mixed models with two factors (intervention method and time) and their interactions, whereas propensity scores were estimated using logistic regression analysis adjusted for NYHA functional classification and left ventricular ejection fraction. All of the enrolled participants were examined for the outcome variables using intention-to-treat (ITT) analysis. Participants who did not provide data at each of the four follow-ups were excluded from the per-protocol (PP) analysis. Model-building strategies followed the steps suggested by Amorim and Cai (2015). Multiple imputation methods (the Markov chain Monte Carlo method and regression) were applied to address the missing data. The final data set was based on 100 imputations. When interactions were significant, post hoc comparisons of change over time compared with the baseline were performed. Characteristics of the first three readmissions for HF were evaluated using the Cox proportional hazards model; the Anderson and Gill (AG) model; the Prentice, Williams, and Peterson total time model; and the Prentice, Williams, and Peterson gap time (PWP GT) model (Sun & Cotton, 2010). Kaplan–Meier survival curves were plotted to

Figure 1
Study Flow Chart

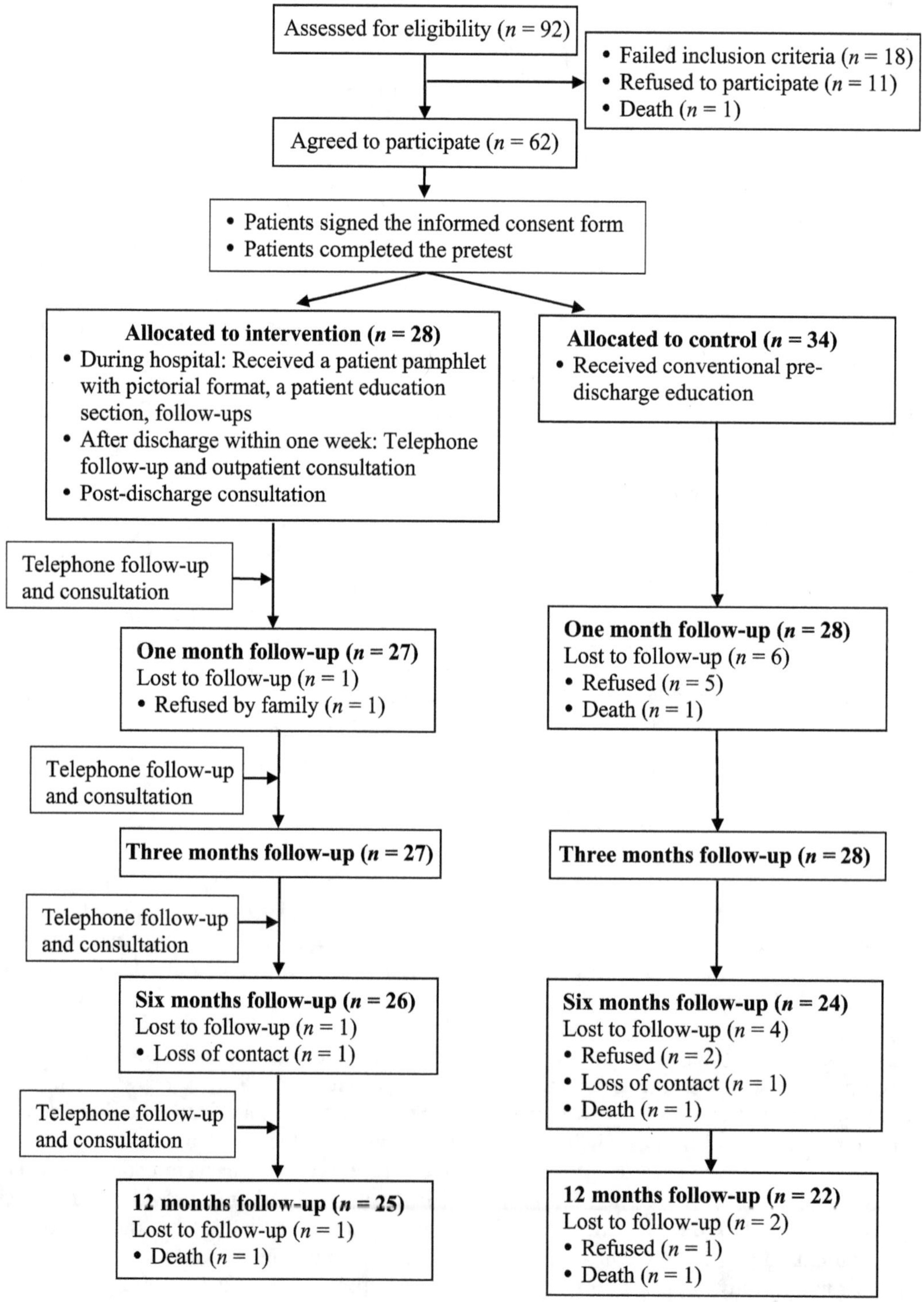

compare the times of first readmission between the two groups. SAS 9.4 (SAS Institute Inc., Cary, NC, USA) was utilized for data analysis, with the significance value set at < .05.

Results

Ninety-two patients were referred by cardiologists and nurse practitioners and screened for eligibility, with 73 patients meeting the inclusion criteria. Eleven patients declined to participate, leaving 62 eligible participants. However, after assignment and informed consent, three participants assigned to the intervention group asked to be part of the control group. At baseline data collection, the control group (n = 34) and intervention group (n = 28) were not equivalent. There was no difference between the groups in terms of mean age, gender, living arrangements, financial status, or education (Table 1). However, the control group included an insignificantly higher number of participants classified as NYHA Class IV and an insignificantly higher mean ejection fraction score than the intervention group. There was no difference between groups at baseline in terms of self-care maintenance or management, sleep quality, or depression (Table 2). Fifteen participants withdrew over the course of the study (76% retention rate). Baseline data between the withdrawn group and the completed group were compared. The results showed only gender to be significantly different between the two groups (χ^2 = 7.47, p < .01), with women (n = 10) withdrawing at a higher rate than men.

Self-Care Maintenance

After discharge, the intervention group reached a cutoff score of 70 for each time point. The ITT and PP analyses provided different results for the linear mixed model analysis of self-care maintenance. Whereas the PP approach did not find a significant interaction effect (F = 2.35, p = .057) after adjusting for the propensity score, ITT revealed that the changes over time from the baseline to 12 months differed between the intervention group and the control group (F = 4.22, p = .003). Post hoc comparisons showed that group differences over time were significant at 1, 3, and 6 months, indicating that the intervention affected the self-care maintenance of participants. However, the effect did not persist after 6 months posttest (Table 3).

Of the 10 self-care maintenance behaviors, four (monitoring weight daily, avoiding illness, eating a low-sodium diet, and asking for low-sodium food when eating out) exhibited significant intervention–time interactions (p < .05) in the linear mixed model analyses, showing the improvement in the intervention group in these four self-care maintenance behaviors.

Table 1

Demographic Characteristics and Disease Variables of Participants, by Group (N = 62)

Characteristic	Intervention Group (n = 28)		Control Group (n = 34)		χ^2 or Z	p
	n	%	n	%		
Age (years; *M* and *SD*)	56.4	13.6	58.2	13.1	−0.59	.552
Range	35.1–80.4		28.4–79.7			
Male	21	75.0	18	52.9	1.71	.220
Married	15	53.6	21	61.8	0.42	.608
Living with family	23	82.1	32	94.1	2.20	.228
Employed	18	64.3	22	64.7	0.001	1.000
Adequate financial status	21	75.0	19	55.9	2.45	.182
Education					2.21	.191
Elementary	8	28.6	16	47.1		
High school or above	20	71.4	18	52.9		
NYHA class					3.13	.209
II	14	50.0	15	44.1		
III	12	42.9	11	32.3		
IV	2	7.1	8	23.5		
Left ventricular ejection fraction (%; *M* and *SD*)	39.9	13.3	47.5	18.4	−1.52	.128
Range	19.6–70.8		13.0–76.8			
Interquartile range	31.0–45.7		31.5–62.9			
Charlson Comorbidity Index	2.8	2.4	3.5	2.5	−1.18	.239

Note. Chi-square test was used for categorical variables; Mann–Whitney *U* test was used for continuous variables. NYHA = New York Heart Association.

Table 2

Self-Care, Sleep Quality, and Depression in Participants, by Group and Time

Variable/Group	Baseline		Follow-Up							
			1 Month		3 Months		6 Months		12 Months	
	M	*SD*	*M*	*SD*	*M*	*SD*	*M*	*SD*	*M*	*SD*
	28 vs. 34		27 vs. 28		27 vs. 28		26 vs. 24		25 vs. 22	
Self-care maintenance										
Intervention group	47.50	25.36	76.39	14.58	78.24	12.46	73.75	15.54	70.70	14.60
Control group	53.23	15.64	65.89	13.81	66.25	14.51	65.63	12.39	68.18	10.67
Self-care management										
Intervention group	60.98	18.34	81.94	13.42	75.00	12.10	75.00	19.01	76.88	13.19
Control group	64.84	22.71	70.42	19.40	69.12	24.95	74.22	19.08	59.38	11.08
Sleep quality (PSQI)										
Intervention group	7.57	4.33	8.74	5.53	8.37	4.76	7.27	4.53	6.52	4.59
Control group	8.82	5.09	10.18	5.41	10.82	4.89	9.46	4.77	7.36	4.50
Depression (PHQ-9)										
Intervention group	6.75	5.57	4.81	4.54	4.52	4.77	5.62	5.81	5.08	4.98
Control group	9.97	7.45	7.82	8.31	8.18	6.57	9.67	6.09	6.32	6.93

Note. PSQI = Pittsburg Sleep Quality Index; PHQ-9 = nine-item Patient Health Questionnaire.

Self-Care Management

After discharge, the intervention group reached a cutoff score of 70 for each time point. Similar to the finding for self-care maintenance, the ITT but not PP analysis showed a significant difference in self-management changes over time between the intervention group and the control group ($F = 2.65, p = .035$). Post hoc comparisons identified a significant interaction between group and time at the 12th month (Table 3).

Sleep Quality

Forty-two (68%) of participants reported poor quality of sleep, with a PSQI score greater than 5. Twenty-four of these participants were in the control group, and 18 were in the intervention group. The linear mixed model analysis of the PSQI using ITT and PP approaches indicated no significant differences in changes over time between the groups (Table 3).

Depression

Symptoms of clinical depression, indicated by a PHQ-9 score greater than 10, were reported by 35% ($n = 22$) of the participants. However, the analysis of PHQ-9 scores did not show significant differences in change over time between the groups using either the ITT or PP approach (Table 3).

Heart-Failure-Related Readmissions

Seven participants in the intervention group were readmitted for HF during the year compared with 12 participants in the control group (Table 4 and Figure 2). Among these, two in the intervention group and five in the control group were readmitted more than once during the 1-year period. The average time to first readmission was 4.6 months for the intervention group and 3.3 months for the control group. The censored observations were the 43 participants who were never readmitted. The time to first readmission model (Cox proportional hazards model) showed that the intervention group had 53% fewer, albeit not significantly fewer, first readmissions than the control group (hazard ratio = 0.47, 95% CI [0.17, 1.26]) after adjusting for the NYHA functional classification and left ventricular ejection fraction. The time to the first three readmissions model (AG, AG with robust sandwich estimator, and PWP) showed that the intervention group also had fewer first three readmission events (AG = 0.39, 95% CI [0.16, 0.92]; PWP TT = 0.52, 95% CI [0.23, 1.17]; PWP GT = 0.49, 95% CI [0.22, 1.08]). None of the participants in the intervention group required more than two readmissions over the year compared with the five participants in the control group with three hospital readmissions each.

Discussion

Compared with the data provided by Reyes et al. (2016) on the demographics of Asian patients with HF, the participants in this study were younger and included more women. However, Yu et al. (2011) reported that 58% of the participants in their epidemiological study were men, with an average age of 62 years, which is similar to this study. The age of hospitalized patients with HF is decreasing (Yu et al., 2011).

To reduce the bias results caused by a single analysis, both ITT and PP approaches were used in this study for data analysis, with propensity scores estimated with the NYHA status and left ventricular ejection fraction used to adjust for confounding effects and to increase precision, compensating for the nonrandomized research design (D'Agostino, 1998). The

Table 3

Results of a Two-Factor (Intervention and Time) Linear Mixed Modeling Analysis of Outcome Data for Participants

Effect	Self-Care Maintenance				Self-Care Management				Sleep Quality				Depression			
	ITT		PP		ITT		PP		ITT		PP		ITT		PP	
	F	*p*	*F*	*p*	*F*	*p*	*F*	*p*	*F*	*p*	*F*	*p*	*F*	*p*	*F*	*p*
Intervention	4.61	.036	8.98	.004**	2.46	.122	4.93	.031	1.73	.192	2.79	.101	4.56	.036*	5.64	.021*
Time	29.43	< .001***	25.51	< .001***	11.78	< .001***	10.59	< .001***	2.11	.082	2.07	.088	2.78	.028*	1.98	.100
Intervention × Time	4.22	.003**	2.35	.057	2.65	.035*	2.56	.065	0.31	.872	0.31	.874	0.77	.549	0.90	.466
Propensity score	1.51	.223	3.50	.067	0.35	.558	1.44	.235	0.48	.492	0.06	.810	0.02	.876	0.12	.728
Post hoc comparisons (IG vs. CG)																
Baseline to 1 month	13.95	< .001***			0.75	.453										
Baseline to 3 months	11.71	< .001***			1.13	.261										
Baseline to 6 months	5.78	.017*			1.45	.149										
Baseline to 12 months	1.77	.184			3.07	.002**										

Note. Data reflect 100 imputations. IG = intervention group; CG = control group; ITT = intention-to-treat analysis (n = 62); PP = per-protocol analysis (n = 47).
*p < .05. **p < .01. ***p < .001.

results of PP analysis estimate the true effect of an intervention for participants who complete the full course of a study. However, this analysis approach is not appropriate for studies affected by high dropout rates, as real-world treatment effects may be overestimated (Ranganathan et al., 2016). Although ITT analysis is suitable for randomized clinical trials, it has been recommended for nonequivalence trials because it takes into account the degree of noncompliance. Therefore, a full analysis was conducted in this study using ITT using multiple imputations of the missing data (Porta et al., 2007). The discrepancies between these two analyses were the findings of self-care maintenance and self-care management. This result differs from previous studies by showing that the PP analysis provides promising outcomes (Porta et al., 2007). It is possible that more participants in the control group complied with self-care requirements and completed the full course of the study.

Table 4

Comparisons of the First Three Readmissions Between the Intervention Group and the Control Group (N = 62)

No. of Readmissions	Intervention Group (IG)		Control Group (CG)		Time to the First Readmission			Recurrent Events Model
					IG vs. CG			IG vs. CG
	n	Average Time to Readmission (Months)	*n*	Average Time to Readmission (Months)	Variable	*B*	Hazard Ratio (95% CI)	Hazard Ratio (95% CI)
1	7	4.6	12	3.3	Group	−0.76	0.47 [a] [0.17, 1.26]	0.39 [b] [0.16, 0.92]
2	3	8.3	5	4.2	Propensity score	−0.93	0.40 [a] [0.02–9.41]	0.52 [c] [0.23, 1.17]
3	0	n/a	5	8.4				0.49 [d] [0.22, 1.08]

[a] Cox model, adjusted for New York Heart Association functional class and left ventricular ejection fraction. [b] Anderson and Gill model. [c] Prentice, Williams, and Peterson total time model. [d] Prentice, Williams, and Peterson gap time model.

Figure 2

Kaplan-Meier Survival Curves for First Readmission

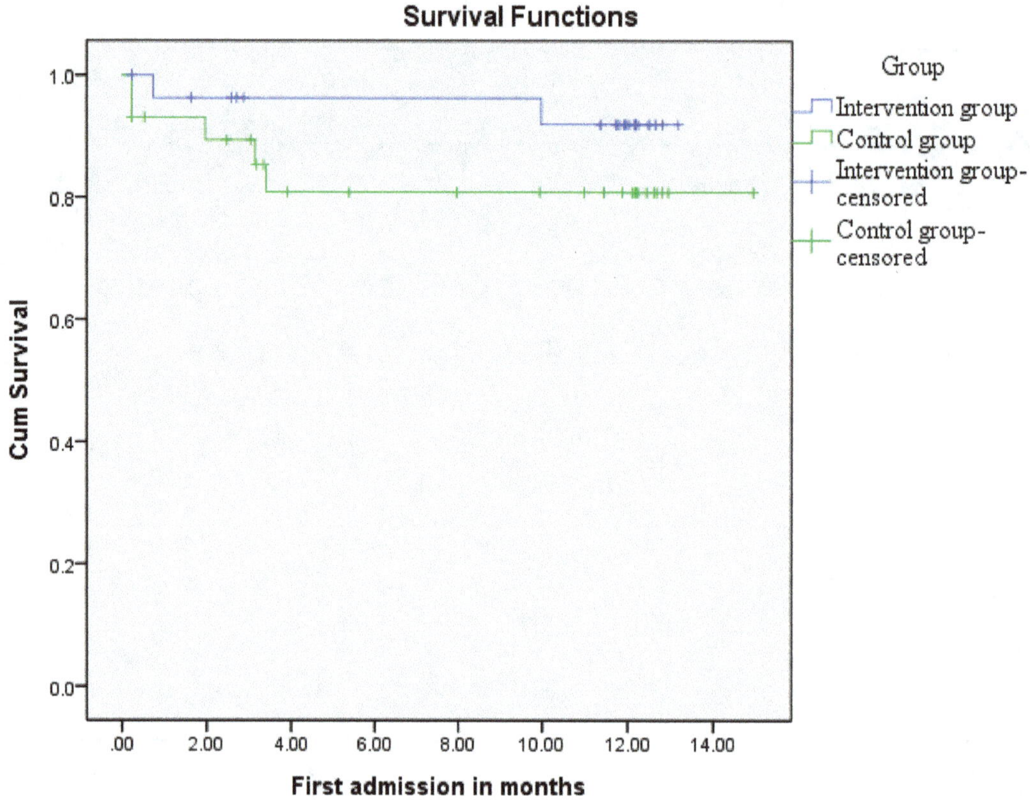

Self-Care Maintenance

At baseline, the mean self-care maintenance score indicates that the participants practiced inadequate self-care (score < 70) and that they likely did not engage in self-care behaviors before hospitalization. The intervention group reached and exceeded the cutoff score of 70 after discharge during the 12-month follow-up. The control group failed to reach the cutoff score, reporting an inadequate self-care status throughout the entire study. However, the PP analysis did not identify a significant difference in self-care maintenance between the two groups. According to the ITT analysis, although the education intervention improved self-care maintenance 6 months after discharge from the hospital, that improvement was not significantly sustained at 12 months. Initiating and sustaining self-care practices is a challenge if not continuously supported and encouraged. Therefore, empowerment throughout the HF trajectory with sufficient support from family and healthcare providers is necessary to initiate and sustain the self-care engagement of patients (Jaarsma et al., 2017).

Four self-care maintenance behaviors, including monitoring weight daily, avoiding illness, eating a low-sodium diet, and asking for low-sodium food when eating out, achieved sustained and significant improvements over the 1-year period of this study. Similarly, Shao et al. (2013) found that, 12 weeks after a self-management program, patients with HF showed significantly improved self-efficacy with regard to sodium and fluid control and consequently had fewer HF-related symptoms. In one large international study covering 15 countries, although poor adherence to most self-care behaviors was found regardless of country, Taiwanese participants had the highest percentage of adherence to HF behaviors in terms of restricting sodium intake (91%), performing regular exercise (68%), monitoring weight (74%), and getting a flu shot (53%; Jaarsma et al., 2013).

Self-Care Management

At baseline, self-care management for the participants in this study fell below the cutoff score of 70, indicating poor self-care management. However, the intervention group improved self-care management from 1 month after discharge, suggesting the sustained effect of this educational intervention on self-care management. The finding that the between-group difference was present only at Month 12 may indicate a delayed effect of this educational intervention on self-care management. In addition, over the yearlong follow-up period, individual medical management of each participant's HF may have changed with the addition of diuretics prescribed by physicians.

Sleep Quality and Depression

More than 73% of patients with HF report sleep disturbances (Lainsamputty & Chen, 2018), which is similar to the findings of this study. Clinical HF symptoms such as orthopnea and nocturia may interfere with sleep quality. However, sleep quality is a multifaceted issue, which may explain the lack of a direct effect of HF education on this outcome measure. Furthermore, one third of participants in this study reported signs of clinical depression, a finding that is higher than a study conducted in the United States. Bhatt et al. (2016), using a cutoff score of 10 or more on the PHQ-9, reported a depression prevalence of 26% among patients with HF. The rate of depression among patients with HF is more than twice that of the general population. There was no effect of the educational intervention on the prevalence of depression, suggesting that depression may be a mediator of self-care practices. Further investigation with larger sample sizes is needed.

Heart-Failure-Related Readmissions

Prevention of early readmission is an important goal of HF treatment (Ponikowski et al., 2016). Although not significant, participants receiving the educational intervention were less likely to be rehospitalized and had a longer time to readmission during the 1-year follow-up period. Telephone follow-ups and access to consultation services provide opportunities to ask and clarify questions such as how to address symptom reoccurrence or a worsening of current symptoms. In this study, participant skills in symptom management, attitudes toward self-care, and decision-making knowledge were reinforced during follow-up visits.

Limitations

The nonequivalent control group design may have introduced bias because of an imbalance in important prognostic factors between the intervention and control groups. In the future, a randomized clinical trial with a larger sample size should be conducted to validate the findings of this study. Retention strategies to maintain participants in studies are needed, as the dropout rate in this study was high, especially in the control group. The results regarding readmission had low statistical power to detect the difference and should be interpreted with caution.

Conclusions

Overall, the effect of this study intervention was not substantial in terms of improving self-care, sleep quality, depression, and readmission, indicating the need to design more efficacious and powerful interventions. However, the finding that participants with HF who received the focused educational program were more likely to report appropriate self-care practices and to have fewer readmission events over the course of a year highlights the importance of predischarge educational interventions. Adding nurse-led postdischarge follow-ups may help patients better manage symptom reoccurrence and further postpone HF readmissions.

Implications of the Findings

It is important that hospitalized patients receive education that promotes self-care knowledge and home-care-related skills before hospital discharge. Thus, nurses should be encouraged to provide patient-appropriate, predischarge educational programs. Strategies are needed to help nurses provide patient education in a quick and effective manner. For example, well-illustrated educational pamphlets, videos, or phone apps given to patients and families on the first day of hospitalization may help patients understand the critical issues before attending the educational session. Finally, postdischarge follow-ups and available consultation services should be offered to clarify questions.

Acknowledgment

The study was funded by the Ministry of Science and Technology, ROC (101-2314-B-037-059-MY2).

Author Contributions

Study conception and design: HMC, SJW, CSL, LMT
Data collection: HMC, SJW, CSL, LMT
Data analysis and interpretation: HMC, STW
Drafting of the article: HMC, STW, LMT
Critical revision of the article: HMC, SJF, LMT

References

Albert, N. M., Cohen, B., Liu, X., Best, C. H., Aspinwall, L., & Pratt, L. (2015). Hospital nurses' comfort in and frequency of delivering heart failure self-care education. *European Journal of Cardiovascular Nursing, 14*(5), 431–440. https:doi.org/10.1177/1474515 114540756

Amorim, L. D., & Cai, J. (2015). Modelling recurrent events: A tutorial for analysis in epidemiology. *International Journal of Epidemiology, 44*(1), 324–333. https://doi.org/10.1093/ije/dyu222

Benjamin, E. J., Blaha, M. J., Chiuve, S. E., Cushman, M., Das, S. R., Deo, R., de Ferranti, S. D., Floyd, J., Fornage, M., Gillespie, C., Isasi, C. R., Jiménez, M. C., Jordan, L. C., Judd, S. E., Lackland, D., Lichtman, J. H., Lisabeth, L., Liu, S., Longenecker, C. T., ... Muntner, P. (2017). Heart disease and stroke statistics—2017 update: A report from the American Heart Association. *Circulation, 135*(10), e146–e603. https://doi.org/10.1161/cir.0000000000000485

Bhatt, K. N., Kalogeropoulos, A. P., Dunbar, S. B., Butler, J., & Georgiopoulou, V. V. (2016). Depression in heart failure: Can PHQ-9 help? *International Journal of Cardiology, 221*, 246–250. https://doi.org/10.1016/j.ijcard.2016.07.057

Buysse, D. J., Reynolds, C. F. 3rd, Monk, T. H., Berman, S. R., & Kupfer, D. J. (1989). The Pittsburgh Sleep Quality Index: A new instrument for psychiatric practice and research. *Psychiatry Research, 28*(2), 193–213. https://doi.org/10.1016/0165-1781(89)90047-4

Carlson, B., Hoyt, H., Gillespie, K., Kunath, J., Lewis, D., & Bratzke, L. C. (2019). Predictors of heart failure readmission in a high-risk primarily Hispanic population in a rural setting. *The Journal of Cardiovascular Nursing, 34*(3), 267–274. https://doi.org/10.1097/jcn.0000000000000567

Chang, H.-Y., Wang, C. C., Wu, Y. W., Chu, P. H., Wu, C.-C., Hsu, C. H., Wen, M.-S., Voon, W.-C., Lin, W.-S., Huang, J.-L., Chen, S.-M., Yang, N.-I., Chang, H. C., Chang, K. C., Sung, S.-H., Shyu, K.-G., Lin, J.-L., Mar, G. Y., Chan, K. C., ... Yin, W. H. (2017). One-year outcomes of acute decompensated systolic heart failure in Taiwan: Lessons from TSOC-HFrEF Registry. *Acta Cardiologica Sinica, 33*(2), 127–138. https://doi.org/10.6515/ACS20170202A

Che, H. L., Yeh, M. Y., Jiang, R. S., & Wu, S. M. (2016). Taiwanese nurses' experiences of difficulties in providing patient education in hospital settings. *Nursing & Health Sciences, 18*(1), 113–119. https://doi.org/10.1111/nhs.12266

D'Agostino, R. B. Jr. (1998). Propensity score methods for bias reduction in the comparison of a treatment to a non-randomized control group. *Statistics in Medicine, 17*(19), 2265–2281.

Domingues, F. B., Clausell, N., Aliti, G. B., Dominguez, D. R., & Rabelo, E. R. (2011). Education and telephone monitoring by nurses of patients with heart failure: Randomized clinical trial. *Arquivos Brasileiros de Cardiologia, 96*(3), 233–239. https://doi.org/10.1590/s0066-782x2011005000014

Hsieh, F. Y., & Lavori, P. W. (2000). Sample-size calculations for the Cox proportional hazards regression model with nonbinary covariates. *Controlled Clinical Trials, 21*(16), 552–560. https://doi.org/10.1016/s0197-2456(00)00104-5

Huang, T. Y., Moser, D. K., & Hwang, S. L. (2018). Identification, associated factors, and prognosis of symptom clusters in Taiwanese patients with heart failure. *The Journal of Nursing Research, 26*(1), 60–67. https://doi.org/10.1097/jnr.0000000000000199

Jaarsma, T., Cameron, J., Riegel, B., & Stromberg, A. (2017). Factors related to self-care in heart failure patients according to the middle-range theory of self-care of chronic illness: A literature update. *Current Heart Failure Reports, 14*(2), 71–77. https://doi.org/10.1007/s11897-017-0324-1

Jaarsma, T., Strömberg, A., Ben Gal, T., Cameron, J., Driscoll, A., Duengen, H.-D., Inkrot, S., Huang, T. Y., Huyen, N. N., Kato, N., Köberich, S., Lupón, J., Moser, D. K., Pulignano, G., Rabelo, E. R., Suwanno, J., Thompson, D. R., Vellone, E., Alvaro, R., ... Riegel, B. (2013). Comparison of self-care behaviors of heart failure patients in 15 countries worldwide. *Patient Education and Counseling, 92*(1), 114–120. https://doi.org/10.1016/j.pec.2013.02.017

Köberich, S., Lohrmann, C., Mittag, O., & Dassen, T. (2015). Effects of a hospital-based education programme on self-care behaviour, care dependency and quality of life in patients with heart failure—A randomised controlled trial. *Journal of Clinical Nursing, 24*(11–12), 1643–1655. https://doi.org/10.1111/jocn.12766

Kroenke, K., Spitzer, R. L., & Williams, J. B. W. (2001). The PHQ-9 validity of a brief depression severity measure. *Journal of General Internal Medicine, 16*(9), 606–613. https://doi.org/10.1046/j.1525-1497.2001.016009606.x

Lainsamputty, F., & Chen, H. M. (2018). The correlation between fatigue and sleep quality among patients with heart failure. *NurseLine Journal, 3*(2), 100–114. https://doi.org/10.19184/nlj.v3i2.8580

Liao, H. Y., Chiu, C. C., Ko, Y. Y., & Chen, H. M. (2018). Factors associated with demoralisation syndrome in patients before and after cardiac surgery. *Journal of Clinical Nursing, 27*(3–4), e559–e568. https://doi.org/10.1111/jocn.14094

Liou, H.-L., Chen, H.-I., Hsu, S.-C., Lee, S.-C., Chang, C.-J., & Wu, M.-J. (2015). The effects of a self-care program on patients with heart failure. *Journal of the Chinese Medical Association, 78*(11), 648–656. https://doi.org/10.1016/j.jcma.2015.06.004

Mueller, K. E., Lavange, L. M., Ramey, S. L., & Ramey, C. T. (1992). Power calculations for general linear multivariate models including repeated measures applications. *Journal of the American Statistical Association, 87*(420), 1209–1226.

Nadrian, H., Shojafard, J., Mahmoodi, H., Rouhi, Z., & Rezaeipandari, H. (2018). Cognitive determinants of self-care behaviors among patients with heart failure: A path analysis. *Health Promotion Perspectives, 8*(4), 275–282. https://doi.org/10.15171/hpp.2018.39

Ponikowski, P., Voors, A. A., Anker, S. D., Bueno, H., Cleland, J. G., Coats, A. J., Falk, V., González-Juanatey, J. R., Harjola, V. P., Jankowska, E. A., Jessup, M., Linde, C., Nihoyannopoulos, P., Parissis, J. T., Pieske, B., Riley, J. P., Rosano, G. M., Ruilope, L. M., Ruschitzka, F., ... van der Meer, P. (2016). 2016 ESC guidelines for the diagnosis and treatment of acute and chronic heart failure: The task force for the diagnosis and treatment of acute and chronic heart failure of the European Society of Cardiology (ESC). Developed with the special contribution of the Heart Failure Association (HFA) of the ESC. *European Journal of Heart Failure, 18*(8), 891–975. https://doi.org/10.1002/ejhf.592

Porta, N., Bonet, C., & Cobo, E. (2007). Discordance between reported intention-to-treat and per protocol analyses. *Journal of Clinical Epidemiology, 60*(7), 663–669. https://doi.org/10.1016/j.jclinepi.2006.09.013

Ranganathan, P., Pramesh, C. S., & Aggarwal, R. (2016). Common pitfalls in statistical analysis: Intention-to-treat versus per-protocol analysis. *Perspectives in Clinical Research, 7*(3), 144–146. https://doi.org/10.4103/2229-3485.184823

Reyes, E. B., Ha, J.-W., Firdaus, I., Ghazi, A. M., Phrommintikul, A., Sim, D., Sim, D., Vu, Q. N., Siu, C. W., Yin, W. H., & Cowie, M. R. (2016). Heart failure across Asia: Same healthcare burden but differences in organization of care. *International Journal of Cardiology, 223*, 163–167. https://doi.org/10.1016/j.ijcard.2016.07.256

Riegel, B., Dickson, V. V., & Faulkner, K. M. (2016). The situation-specific theory of heart failure self-care: Revised and updated. *The Journal of Cardiovascular Nursing, 31*(3), 226–235. https://doi.org/10.1097/jcn.0000000000000244

Riegel, B., Lee, C. S., Dickson, V. V., & Carlson, B. (2009). An update on the self-care of heart failure index. *Journal of Cardiovascular Nursing, 24*(6), 485–497. https://doi.org/10.1097/JCN.0b013e3181b4baa0

Riegel, B., Lee, C. S., & Dickson, V. V. (2011). Self care in patients with chronic heart failure. *Nature Reviews Cardiology, 8*(11), 644–654. https://doi.org/10.1038/nrcardio.2011.95

Ryan, C. J., Bierle, R., & Vuckovic, K. M. (2019). The three Rs for preventing heart failure readmission: Review, reassess, and reeducate. *Critical Care Nurse, 39*(2), 85–93. https://doi.org/10.4037/ccn2019345

Shao, J.-H., Chang, A. M., Edwards, H., Shyu, Y.-I. L., & Chen, S.-H. (2013). A randomized controlled trial of self-management programme improves health-related outcomes of older people with heart failure. *Journal of Advanced Nursing, 69*(11), 2458–2469. https://doi.org/10.1111/jan.12121

Sun, R. J., & Cotton, D. (2010). *Analysis of survival data with recurrent events using SAS®*. Paper presented at the SAS Global Forum 2010, Seattle, USA. http://support.sas.com/resources/papers/proceedings10/255-2010.pdf

Teo, L. Y. L., Lim, C. P., Neo, C. L., Teo, L. W., Ng, S. L. E., Chan, L. L., Kaushik, M., & Sim, K. L. D. (2016). Ultrafiltration in patients with decompensated heart failure and diuretic resistance: An Asian centre's experience. *Singapore Medical Journal*, *57*(7), 378–383. https://doi.org/10.11622/smedj.2016014

Tsai, P. K., Wang, R. H., Lee, C. S., Tsai, L. M., & Chen, H. M. (2015). Determinants of self-care decision-making in hospitalised patients with heart failure. *Journal of Clinical Nursing*, *24* (7–8), 1101–1111. https://doi.org/10.1111/jocn.12722

Tsai, P.-S., Wang, S.-Y., Wang, M.-Y., Su, C.-T., Yang, T.-T., Huang, C.-J., & Fang, S.-C. (2005). Psychometric evaluation of the Chinese version of the Pittsburgh Sleep Quality Index (CPSQI) in primary insomnia and control subjects. *Quality of Life Research*, *14*(8), 1943–1952. https://doi.org/10.1007/s11136-005-4346-x

Yu, S. B., Cui, H. Y., Qin, M., Kong, B., Liu, T., Zhao, Q. Y., Huang, H., Yang, B., & Huang, C. X. (2011). Characteristics of in-hospital patients with chronic heart failure in Hubei province from 2000 to 2010. *Chinese Journal of Cardiovascular Diseases*, *39*(6), 549–552. (Original work published in Chinese)

23

End-of-Life Care Discussion for Residents With Dementia in Long-Term Care Facilities

Hsiu-Li HUANG[1]* • Li-Chueh WENG[2] • Wen-Yu HU[3] • Yea-Ing Lotus SHYU[4]
Wen-Pin YU[5] • Kang-Hua CHEN[6]

ABSTRACT

Background: Healthcare professionals play an important role in end-of-life care decisions. Although the factors affecting end-of-life care in long-term care facilities have been well studied in Western contexts, few studies have examined factors affecting end-of-life care discussions for residents with dementia among multidisciplinary professionals in Asian or Taiwanese contexts.

Purpose: The aim of this study was to explore the factors related to the end-of-life care discussions of registered nurses, social workers, and physicians with residents with dementia and their families.

Methods: This is a cross-sectional and correlational study. A stratified random sampling was conducted, and self-administered questionnaires were mailed to physicians, registered nurses, and social workers who work in long-term care facilities with accreditation ranks ≥ Grade A in Taiwan.

Results: Questionnaires were returned by 478 participants (response rate = 94.1%). Fewer than 10% of the participants reported often discussing end-of-life care with residents with dementia and their families. Physicians were significantly more likely to discuss life-sustaining treatment than nurses and social workers. The frequency of professionals discussing advance directives and life-sustaining treatment for residents with dementia was predicted by higher confidence in end-of-life care skills and greater perceived facility support.

Conclusions/Implications for Practice: Most professionals did not frequently discuss end-of-life care with residents with dementia and their caregivers. Discussions of end-of-life care in long-term care facilities should be promoted by enhancing the confidence of these professionals in providing end-of-life care and creating a supportive environment for end-of-life discussions and care.

Key Words:
long-term care facility, dementia, advance directives, end-of-life care, healthcare professionals.

Introduction

Dementia is not only a major determinant of nursing home placement (Lithgow, Jackson, & Browne, 2012) but also the most common cause of death in nursing homes (Gjerberg, Førde, & Bjørndal, 2011). Indeed, approximately 70% of dementia-related deaths in the United States (Hicks, Rabins, & Black, 2010) and 50%–92% of those in European countries occur in nursing homes (Houttekier et al., 2010). However, end-of-life (EOL) care in these settings has been shown to be poor (Vandervoort et al., 2013). Many nursing home residents with dementia (RWDs) are transferred to hospitals and receive intrusive medical intervention that has no demonstrated benefit to their quality of life or quality of death (Givens, Selby, Goldfeld, & Mitchell, 2012).

People with advanced dementia at the end of their lives typically experience acute conditions that require family members and healthcare professionals to make decisions about life-sustaining or palliative care, particularly in long-term care facilities. The quality of EOL care for these RWDs and the satisfaction of their family caregivers with EOL care have been shown to improve significantly with advance care planning (ACP; Givens, Jones, Shaffer, Kiely, & Mitchell, 2010; Liu, Guarino, & Lopez, 2012). These findings highlight the need to improve EOL care and discuss ACP in long-term care facilities (Givens et al., 2010). Nevertheless, most studies on this topic have been conducted in Western countries, and their outcomes have limited applicability in Asian contexts because of cultural differences and dissimilar medical systems. Taiwan is a newly developed Asian country in which the aging population and prevalence of dementia are increasing faster than those in most other developed countries (Wu et al., 2013). As in Western countries, a high proportion of nursing home residents in Taiwan (64.5%) experiences dementia (Chen et al., 2007). Therefore, providing EOL care to RWDs is an inevitable challenge for long-term care facility staff members in Taiwan and is a major component of their work.

[1]*PhD, RN, Associate professor, Department of Long-Term Care, National Taipei University of Nursing and Health Sciences* • [2]*PhD, RN, Associate Professor, School of Nursing, College of Medicine, Chang Gung University, and Associate Research Fellow, Department of General Surgery, Chang Gung Memorial Hospital* • [3]*PhD, RN, Professor, School of Nursing, National Taiwan University, and Director, Department of Nursing, National Taiwan University Hospital* • [4]*PhD, RN, Professor, School of Nursing, College of Medicine, Chang Gung University, and Research Fellow, Traumatological Division, Department of Orthopedics, Chang Gung Memorial Hospital, and Professor, Department of Gerontological Care and Management, Chang Gung University of Science and Technology* • [5]*MSN, RN, Deputy Director, Department of Nursing Management, Administration Center, Chang Gung Medical Foundation, and Assistant Professor, Department of Nursing, Chang Gung University of Science and Technology* • [6]*PhD, RN, Associate Professor, School of Nursing, College of Medicine, Chang Gung University, and Assistant Research Fellow, Department of Cardiovascular Surgery, Chang Gung Memorial Hospital.*

EOL care involves many complex treatment decisions. However, people with dementia are often unable to participate in their own EOL care decisions. To ensure that the autonomy of residents is respected, the use of advance directives (ADs) is encouraged. Taiwan's Legislative Yuan passed the Hospice Palliative Care Act in 2000, encouraging people to make ADs that reflect their preferences regarding whether to receive palliative or life-sustaining treatments (LSTs) at EOL (Chen, 2009). Discussions of EOL care and ADs in Taiwan have typically focused on patients with cancer, and patients with dementia have often been neglected in this respect (Huang, Weng, & Yeh, 2011). However, Taiwan's National Health Insurance program has covered the hospice fees of EOL patients with eight noncancer chronic diseases, including advanced dementia, since 2009 (Huang et al., 2011). This policy has not only raised awareness of dementia-related EOL care but also increased the availability of palliative care for RWDs. Discussion and communication are vital processes in these decisions, irrespective of the ultimate decision regarding ADs and palliative care (van der Steen et al., 2014). However, to date, information is lacking concerning how professionals discuss EOL care with RWDs and their families and what factors influence these discussion processes.

For appropriate EOL care decisions to be reached, RWDs and their caregivers must be informed about their right to make ADs and communicate their concerns regarding palliative care and LSTs. The key professionals in long-term care facilities who communicate with RWDs and their family surrogates regarding EOL care are physicians (Ampe, Sevenants, Smets, Declercq, & Van Audenhove, 2016; van Soest-Poortvliet et al., 2015), registered nurses (Rurup, Onwuteaka-Philipsen, Pasman, Ribbe, & van der Wal, 2006), social workers (Lacey, 2005), and management staff (Ampe et al., 2016).

Understanding the factors that influence the practice of EOL care by these professionals for RWDs may enable policy makers and managers of long-term care facilities to provide more focused support. Moreover, this understanding may help ensure that these influencing factors are addressed to improve the quality of EOL care for RWDs as well as the satisfaction of family surrogates with EOL care decision-making. Physicians, nurses, and families of RWDs in the Netherlands were reported to have different attitudes toward EOL care decisions for RWDs because of differences in religious beliefs and responsibilities (Rurup et al., 2006). Moreover, social workers in the United States reportedly perceive that discussing ADs with RWDs and their families is vital (Lacey, 2005). A qualitative study (Casey et al., 2011) and a mixed-method study (Marshall, Clark, Sheward, & Allan, 2011) further suggested that the EOL care delivery of long-term care professionals in Ireland (Casey et al., 2011) and New Zealand (Marshall et al., 2011) was influenced by their perceptions of their working environment and organizational culture. Nevertheless, these studies were conducted in Western countries and lacked comprehensive quantitative data on the factors affecting the EOL care discussions of these key professionals for RWDs in long-term care facilities. Moreover, these studies have not addressed the importance of cultural sensitivity in EOL care discussions and the role of multidisciplinary cooperation in EOL care quality. These knowledge gaps necessitate that studies on EOL care discussions be conducted in a diverse range of cultural settings and with different categories of long-term care facility professionals. Therefore, the authors of this study hope that their findings may establish a future reference for developing culturally sensitive interventions to promote EOL care discussions for RWDs.

Purposes

The purpose of this study was to explore the factors related to how healthcare professionals approach EOL care for RWDs in long-term care facilities. Specifically, we aimed to (a) investigate the EOL care discussions for RWDs among healthcare professionals in long-term care facilities; (b) compare the EOL care knowledge, attitudes, confidence, perceived facility support, and practices of physicians, registered nurses, and social workers with regard to their discussing EOL care for RWDs; and (c) explore the factors influencing EOL care discussions for RWDs, particularly discussions about ADs and LSTs.

Methods

Design

A cross-sectional and correlational study was used to describe the current status of EOL care discussions for RWDs among healthcare professionals in long-term care facilities and to explore the factors associated with these EOL care discussions in Taiwan. For the sample to be representative and accessible, stratified random sampling and postal surveys were applied in this study.

Setting and Participants

In Taiwan, people with dementia reside in four types of long-term care facilities, including dementia-specific facilities, free-standing nursing homes, hospital-based nursing homes, and general long-term care facilities. Participants in the this study included physicians, registered nurses, and social workers at accredited long-term care facilities in Taiwan that were rated at Grade A or higher and had capacities of more than 50 beds (i.e., a middle-scale facility or larger). Long-term care facilities in Taiwan are accredited using five grades (from highest to lowest): excellent, A, B, C, and D. Eligible facilities were selected from two government accreditation reports: Nursing Home Accreditations (Ministry of Health and Welfare, Taiwan, ROC, 2013) and Senior Welfare Institution Accreditations (Ministry of the Interior, Taiwan, ROC, 2012). Because EOL care in long-term care facilities is a recent concept, we assumed that middle-scale facilities graded A and higher have more workers and resources to implement this care. The sample size was estimated using G*Power 3 (Faul, Erdfelder, Buchner, & Lang, 2009). Setting the α level at .05, effect size at .2, and power at .90, we estimated the sample size to be at least 207. Assuming the manpower requirement of a middle-scale nursing home (50–100 beds) to be at least four to seven nurses (nurse/residents = 1:15), one part-time social worker, and one contract physician (Ministry of Health and Welfare, Taiwan, ROC, 2013), 36–63 facilities would need to be recruited. Furthermore, we estimated that the number of eligible facilities must be doubled if the rate of facility agreement and participant response was 50%.

Eligible facilities were stratified by random sampling and weighted by the number of facilities in different areas of Taiwan (north, central, south, and east). Of the 201 eligible facilities in Taiwan, 63 were selected at random. The chief administrators of these 63 facilities were contacted about participating in the survey, with 15 refusing, yielding a final sample of 48 facilities (agreement rate = 76%). When the chief administrators agreed to take part in this survey and reported the numbers of each type of professional in their facilities, these professionals became the target sample. Five hundred twenty-nine potential participants (410 nurses, 71 social workers, and 48 physicians) were referred by the study facilities in 2011. Of the 529 questionnaires mailed to these potential participants, 498 were returned, yielding a return rate of 94.1%. Valid questionnaires were defined as those questionnaires that were at least 90% complete (n = 478).

Data Collection and Instruments

Data were collected from November 2010 to July 2011 using a standardized questionnaire that was mailed to physicians, registered nurses, and social workers in long-term care facilities in Taiwan. On the basis of information from the consenting chief administrators of targeted facilities, questionnaires were mailed to administrators with cover letters, informed consent forms, and self-addressed, prepaid envelopes. The administrators then sent a questionnaire, an informed consent form, and a self-addressed prepaid envelope to each potential participant. All of the participants were volunteers and remained anonymous, with this explained to them in the cover letter. Anonymity was assured by using no identifying code on the questionnaire. All participants were asked to send back the informed consent form and the completed questionnaire by prepaid mail if they agreed to participate.

Frequency of end-of-life care discussions for residents with dementia

The frequency of the discussion of EOL care for RWDs was assessed using a six-item scale on ACP with RWDs and their family surrogates (Lacey, 2005). Items on this scale involved questions about explaining AD forms and do-not-resuscitate orders; discussing artificial nutrition, artificial hydration, and antibiotics; and helping people clarify their thoughts concerning LSTs. The six-item scale that was used in this study is divided into two subscales: a discussion of ADs (three items) and a discussion of LSTs (three items). Responses are rated on a 5-point Likert-type scale from 1 (never) to 5 (always), with the potential total score for each subscale ranging from 3 to 15 and higher scores indicating that professionals more often discuss ADs and LSTs with RWDs and their families. The internal consistency reliability (Cronbach's α) of the Frequency of EOL Care Discussions for RWDs Scale was determined to be .71 (Lacey, 2005). Because this scale is an English version and was being used in Taiwan for the first time, translation, back-translation, and content validity index (CVI) were performed to confirm accuracy and cultural sensitivity. The English version was translated into Chinese by the first author, and the Chinese version was then back-translated by an English speaker. The back-translated English version was again confirmed by the second author. The CVI and the pilot study were conducted to test validity and reliability. (The detailed procedures are described in the next paragraph.) In this study, the CVI of the scale was determined to be .97, with the two subscales earning Cronbach's α values of .86 and .88. For the total scale, the Cronbach's α value was .88, and the test–retest reliability was .83.

The next four scales were developed from four sources: (a) relevant studies (Lacey, 2005; Rurup et al., 2006); (b) four focus groups with four to six long-term care facility nurses and social workers in each group; (c) content validity testing by six experts, including one professor of palliative care, one associate professor, one lecturer of gerontological nursing, two master-degree nurses, and one master-degree social worker, all of whom worked in dementia care units; and (d) a pilot study that was performed to test internal consistency reliability (Cronbach's α or Kuder-Richardson Formula 20 [KR-20]) and 2-week test–retest reliability with 14 nurses and four social workers who worked in two long-term care facilities.

End-of-life care knowledge

Ten statements were constructed to test the EOL care knowledge of long-term care facility professionals. The scale involves five statements concerning LST, including cardiopulmonary resuscitation side effects, EOL hunger, dehydration, artificial nutrition, and antibiotics (Lacey, 2005; Rurup et al., 2006); one statement concerning pneumonia prevention; and four statements on the Hospice Palliative Care Act and National Health Insurance payment in Taiwan. For each statement, the participants were required to answer "true," "false," or "do not know." During processing by the statistical software, each "correct" answer was counted as 1; each "incorrect" or "do not know" answer was equated with having incorrect knowledge or a lack of knowledge regarding EOL care and counted as 0. Higher scores indicated a higher level of knowledge. The CVI of the EOL care knowledge scale was determined to be .96, and the internal consistency reliability (KR-20) for this study was .63.

Attitudes toward the end-of-life care decision-making rights of residents with dementia

The five-item Attitudes toward RWDs' EOL Care Decision-Making Rights Scale was developed to measure the attitudes of professionals toward the right of RWDs to know about ADs, respect for RWDs' decisions related to EOL care (e.g., regularly informing RWDs about how to fill out ADs when they are admitted to the facility), respect for RWDs' choice to refuse food, the reliability of RWDs' decisions to accept or refuse treatments, and the ability of residents with mild dementia to comprehend the meaning of ADs. Responses were rated on a 5-point Likert-type scale ranging from 1 (strongly disagree) to 5 (strongly agree). Total possible scores ranged from 5 to 25, with higher scores indicating greater respect for RWDs' decision-making rights and belief in the reliability of RWDs' EOL care decisions. The CVI of attitudes toward RWDs' EOL Care Decision-Making Rights Scale was determined to be .95, the Cronbach's α was .68, and the 2-week test–retest reliability was .66.

Confidence in end-of-life care and communication skills

The confidence of professionals in their ability to manage RWDs' problem behaviors and end-stage symptoms and in communicating with RWDs and their families about EOL care was assessed by applying the researcher-developed, 17-item Confidence in EOL Care and Communication Skills Scale. Responses were rated using a 4-point Likert-type scale ranging from 1 (no confidence) to 4 (highly confident). Total possible scores ranged from 17 to 68, with higher scores indicating greater confidence in management and communication regarding EOL care for RWDs. The CVI of the confidence in EOL care and communication skills scale was .92, the Cronbach's α was .97, and the 2-week test–retest reliability was .77.

Perceived facility support for end-of-life concerns

The perceptions of the participants regarding the support of their facilities on EOL issues were assessed using a researcher-developed 10-item Perceived Facility EOL Support Scale. This scale assesses professionals' perceptions of administrators' support for providing palliative care to RWDs and specifically addressed issues such as whether the facility has an explicit policy to forgo LST; if the facility educates or prepares its workers to provide palliative care; if the facility has a policy of routinely informing RWDs about ADs, a palliative care team, a special room for dying RWDs, and an available or cooperative referral hospice; if the facility has the ability to provide continuity of care to residents who are referred from a hospice unit and to build consensus among workers on palliative care for RWDs; and if the facility provides adequate palliative care to RWDs. Responses were rated using a 5-point Likert-type scale ranging from 1 (strongly disagree) to 5 (strongly agree). Total possible scores ranged from 10 to 50, with higher scores indicating greater perceived support from the facility. The CVI of perceived facility support for EOL concerns scale was .92, the Cronbach's α was .91, and the 2-week test–retest reliability was .76.

Demographics and related variables

Data were collected on the participants regarding their age, gender, level of education, work experience (years), and participation in continuing education on dementia and EOL care during the previous 2 years. If participants had taken part in continuing education, they were asked to report the number of education hours. The facilities where participants worked were categorized by type: dementia-specific facility, freestanding nursing home, hospital-based nursing home, and general long-term care facility.

Ethical Considerations

Before data collection, this study was approved (99–1005B) by the institutional review board of Chang Gung Memorial Hospital.

Data Analysis

All of the study variables were analyzed using predictive analytics software (IBM SPSS Statistics 22.0). Frequencies, percentages, means, standard deviations, and ranges were included as descriptive statistics to identify the demographic characteristics of participants, discussions about EOL care, and other relevant main variables. Frequency distributions of discussions about EOL care were measured using chi-square tests, mean-difference-related main variables with one-way analysis of variance, and Scheffe's post hoc analysis to determine any possible differences among the various professional groups. Factors that were identified as significantly associated with the practices of discussing EOL care for RWDs were analyzed using two multiple regression models, and all of the variables were entered into each regression model by forced entry. Model 1 was used to predict the factors that were associated with discussing ADs, and Model 2 was used to predict the factors that were associated with discussing LSTs. Moreover, p values of $< .05$ were considered statistically significant.

Results

Participant Characteristics

Of the 478 participants, 81.0% were registered nurses, 14.2% were social workers, and 4.8% were physicians. Their mean age was 35.5 ± 9.5 years. Approximately 93% of the survey participants in the sample were female. Most of the male participants were physicians. More than half of the participants had a bachelor's degree or higher (51.3%). However, in the nurse group, only 40.3% had a bachelor's degree or higher. Over half (62.6%) of the participants reported having never been exposed to curricula on dementia care in school, and exactly half (50.0%) had never taken curriculum-based lessons on EOL care in school. Most of the participants reported participating in continuing education on dementia care (77.2%) and EOL care (69.9%) during the previous

2 years. The mean number of hours of continuing education on dementia and EOL care was 10.0 ± 21.7 and 7.0 ± 16.4, respectively. The data on the characteristics of the participants and facilities are summarized in Table 1.

Most participants did not frequently discuss EOL care with RWDs or their families, with fewer than 10% reporting often or always providing documents about ADs, explaining how to fill in related documents, and discussing the benefits and risks of artificial nutrition and antibiotics. Less than 15% of the participants reported that often or always discussing items would facilitate decision-making regarding do-not-resuscitate orders (11.5%) and clarify problems related to life-extending treatments (11.5%). Although the three professional groups did not differ significantly regarding the three items of discussions about ADs with RWDs' families, the physician and nurse participants differed significantly from social workers in the three items of discussions about LSTs (benefits and risks of artificial nutrition, χ^2 = 71.21, $p < .001$; benefits and risks of antibiotics, χ^2 = 83.20, $p < .001$; and clarify problems related to life-extending treatments, χ^2 = 23.28, $p < .001$; see Table 2).

Knowledge of, Attitudes Toward, Perceived Facility Support for, and Confidence in End-of-Life Care of Residents With Dementia

The mean scores for perceived knowledge related to EOL care for RWDs differed significantly among registered nurses, social workers, and physicians (F = 2.96, p = .013); physicians' scores were significantly higher than those of social workers in a post hoc test. However, these professionals did not differ significantly in their attitudes toward RWDs' decision-making rights (F = 2.26, p = .106) and perceived support from their facilities (F = 0.03, p = .973). The mean confidence score of social workers was significantly lower than that of registered nurses and physicians (F = 5.85, p = .003), and physicians and nurses' scores were significantly higher than those of social workers in a post hoc test. Regarding discussing EOL care for RWDs, the three professional groups did not differ significantly in their frequency of discussing ADs (F = 0.40, p = .674), but they did differ significantly in their frequency of discussing LSTs (F = 29.48, $p < .001$). Physicians' scores were significantly higher than those of the nurses, and nurses' scores were also significantly higher than those of the social workers in a post hoc test (Table 3).

Factors Related to the Practice of Discussing End-of-Life Care for Residents With Dementia

The associations among all of the variables for discussing ADs and LSTs for RWDs were examined using two multiple regression models. The first model indicated that significant predictors of the frequency of professionals' discussions about ADs for RWDs included more hours of EOL-care-related continuing education (t = 4.25, 95% CI [0.02, 0.05], $p < .001$), more positive attitudes toward RWDs' decision-making rights (t = 2.68, 95% CI [0.03, 0.22], p = .008), more confidence in their EOL care and communication skills (t = 4.67, 95% CI [0.03, 0.08], $p < .001$), and higher perceived support from their facilities (t = 5.09, 95% CI [0.07, 0.16], $p < .001$).

The second model showed that nurses (t = −2.78, 95% CI [−2.47, −0.42], p = .006) and social workers (t = −5.51, 95% CI [−4.48, −2.12], $p < .001$) were significantly less likely to discuss LSTs for RWDs than physicians. In addition, the significant predictors of the frequency of discussing LSTs for RWDs were more hours of EOL care continuing education (t = 2.54, 95% CI [0.01, 0.03], p = .012), more confidence in EOL care and communication skills (t = 6.42, 95% CI [0.05, 0.09], $p <$ .001), and greater perceived support from their facilities (t = 2.87, 95% CI [0.02, 0.10], p = .004; Table 4).

Discussion

On the basis of a review of the literature, this study is the first to comprehensively examine the self-reported knowledge, attitudes, confidence, and frequency of EOL care discussion among registered nurses, social workers, and physicians working in a random, stratified sample of long-term care facilities.

The findings reveal that a large proportion of Taiwanese long-term care professionals never or rarely discuss EOL care for RWDs, which are similar to the results reported regarding managers of Norwegian nursing homes (Gjerberg et al., 2011). The low proportion of healthcare professionals discussing EOL care with RWDs may be attributed to various reasons. One reason may be the passage by Taiwan's Legislative Congress of the Hospice Palliative Care Act in 2000. However, the Hospice Palliative Care Act has neither a regulation component requiring that ADs be introduced to nursing home residents nor an incentive strategy to promote ADs or ACP (Lo, Wang, Liu, & Wang, 2010). Another reason may be that, in general, EOL care is discussed at the patient's EOL or at the diagnosis of a severe illness. However, the disease trajectory of dementia differs from that of cancer. Prognostications in relation to dementia are difficult. Thus, dementia is not usually considered as a life-limiting disease (Huang et al., 2011). A third reason may be that EOL care is still a taboo subject for Taiwanese people because they believe it will result in bad luck and unpleasant thoughts or that it means forgoing all treatment (Lo et al., 2010). Therefore, if professionals perceive that they have insufficient communication skills or confidence to discuss EOL care with RWDs or their families, they will be inclined to avoid talking about this issue.

This study found that more EOL-care-related continuing education and greater perceived confidence in EOL care planning were associated with an increased probability of participants discussing ADs and LSTs with RWDs and their

TABLE 1.

Participants' Demographic Characteristics by Profession (N = 478)

Variable	Total (*N* = 478) *n*	%	Nurse (*n* = 387) *n*	%	Social Worker (*n* =68) *n*	%	Physician (*n* = 23) *n*	%
Gender								
Male	33	6.9	2	0.5	9	13.2	22	95.7
Female	444	92.9	384	99.2	59	86.8	1	4.3
Missing	1	0.2	1	0.3				
Education								
Junior college or below	232	48.5	230	59.4	2	2.9	0	0
Bachelor's degree or above	245	51.3	156	40.3	66	97.1	23	100
Missing	1	0.2	1	0.3				
School education for dementia care								
No	299	62.6	234	60.5	52	76.4	13	56.5
Yes	168	35.1	144	37.2	15	22.1	9	39.1
Missing	11	2.3	9	2.3	1	1.5	1	4.4
School education for EOL care								
No	239	50.0	181	46.8	46	67.6	12	52.2
Yes	225	47.1	193	49.9	21	30.9	11	47.8
Missing	14	2.9	13	3.3	1	1.5		
Continuing education in dementia care								
No	101	21.1	79	20.4	13	19.1	9	39.1
Yes	369	77.2	301	77.8	54	79.4	14	60.9
Missing	8	1.7	7	1.8	1	1.5		
Continuing education in EOL care								
No	138	28.9	102	26.4	26	38.2	10	43.5
Yes	334	69.9	280	72.4	41	60.3	13	56.5
Missing	6	1.3	5	1.2	1	1.5		
Type of institution								
Dementia-specific facility	23	4.8	15	3.9	7	10.3	1	4.3
Freestanding nursing home	113	23.6	99	25.6	10	14.7	4	17.4
Hospital-based nursing home	208	43.5	170	43.9	23	33.8	15	65.2
General long-term care facility	130	27.2	99	25.6	28	41.2	3	13.0
Missing	4	0.8	4	1.0				
Geographic area of institution								
North	204	42.7	160	41.3	37	54.4	7	30.4
Central	68	14.2	60	15.5	6	8.8	2	8.7
South	175	36.6	140	36.2	23	33.8	12	52.2
East	31	6.5	27	7.0	2	2.9	2	8.7
	M	*SD*	*M*	*SD*	*M*	*SD*	*M*	*SD*
Age (years)	35.5	9.5	35.5	9.4	32.3	7.0	44.9	11.5
Range	21–72		21–64		23–54		31–72	
Work experience (months)	132.7	103.3	139.3	103.2	71.9	67.5	190.1	119.7
Range	2–505		2–468		6–360		44–505	
Continuing education in dementia care (hours)	10.0	21.7	10.1	23.2	11.1	16.4	6.0	7.9
Range	0–300		0–300		0–100		0–30	
Continuing education in EOL care (hours)	7.0	16.4	6.2	13.0	12.0	29.0	4.8	7.6
Range	0–124		0–120		0–124		0–30	

Note. EOL = end of life.

TABLE 2.
Profile of Discussions About EOL Care for RWDs by Profession (N = 478)

	Total (*N* = 478)		Nurse (*n* = 387)		Social Worker (*n* = 68)		Physician (*n* = 23)			
Frequency	*n*	%	*n*	%	*n*	%	*n*	%	χ^2	*p*
Discussion of advance directives										
Provide documents about advance EOL care planning										
Never	187	39.1	151	39.0	27	39.7	9	39.1	1.25	.870
Rarely/occasionally	253	52.9	207	53.5	35	51.5	11	47.8		
Often/always	35	7.3	27	7.0	5	7.4	3	13.0		
Missing	3	0.6	2	0.5	1	1.5				
Explain how to complete documents about advance EOL care planning										
Never	195	40.8	155	40.1	30	44.1	10	43.5	5.03	.285
Rarely/occasionally	245	51.3	205	53.0	31	45.6	9	39.1		
Often/always	36	7.5	26	6.7	6	8.8	4	17.4		
Missing	2	0.4		0.2	1	1.5				
Help make decisions for do-not-resuscitate order										
Never	150	31.4	119	30.7	25	36.8	6	26.1	6.13	.190
Rarely/occasionally	270	56.5	223	57.6	36	52.9	11	47.8		
Often/always	55	11.5	43	11.1	6	8.8	6	26.1		
Missing	3	0.6	2	0.5	1	1.5				
Discussion of life-sustaining treatments										
Discuss the benefits and risks of artificial nutrition or infusion										
Never	161	33.7	108	27.9	50	73.5	3	13.0	71.21	<.001
Rarely/occasionally	276	57.7	247	63.8	15	22.1	14	60.9		
Often/always	35	7.3	28	7.2	1	1.5	6	26.1		
Missing	6	1.3	4	1.0	2	2.9				
Discuss the benefits and risks of antibiotic use										
Never	142	29.7	92	23.8	48	70.6	2	8.7	83.20	<.001
Rarely/occasionally	284	59.4	254	65.6	17	25.0	13	56.5		
Often/always	45	9.4	36	9.3	1	1.5	8	34.8		
Missing	7	1.5	5	1.3	2	2.9				
Clarify problems related to life-extending treatments										
Never	104	21.8	76	19.6	25	36.8	3	13.0	23.28	<.001
Rarely/occasionally	312	65.3	264	68.2	36	52.9	12	52.2		
Often/always	55	11.5	42	10.9	5	7.4	8	34.8		
Missing	7	1.5	5	1.3	2	2.9				

Note. EOL = end of life; RWD = residents with dementia.

families. However, our results show that nearly one third of Taiwanese professionals working in long-term care have never had EOL-care-related continuing education. This finding corroborates earlier findings showing that lack of EOL care education was common among healthcare professionals in Western Europe (Lynch et al., 2010; Marshall et al., 2011). We observed that professionals who perceived higher levels of support from their facilities conducted more EOL care discussions for RWDs. This result is consistent with previous reports that the provision of effective EOL care is greatly impacted by organizational culture (Casey et al., 2011), work environment (Marshall et al., 2011), and ACP policies (Ampe et al., 2016; van Soest-Poortvliet et al., 2015). These findings suggest that nursing home managers should put EOL care into a continuing education routine and develop a supportive culture and strategies that guide professionals in initiating quality discussions on EOL care.

Furthermore, the findings of this study show that professionals with more positive attitudes toward RWDs' decision-making rights more frequently discuss ADs with RWDs and their families. This finding is noteworthy given the debate over the validity of ADs in the population with dementia (Hegde & Ellajosyula, 2016). Cognitive decline is often assumed to be accompanied by decreasing awareness. Indeed, persons with dementia are usually identified as lacking awareness, assigned the status of a "nonperson," and judged as being incapable of making or contributing to decisions about their own lives (Hegde & Ellajosyula, 2016). People who perceive that RWDs lack insight tend to show a lack of respect toward them, overrule them, and

TABLE 3.
Main Study Variables by Profession

Variable	Total		①Nurse		②Social Worker		③Physician				
	Mean	*SD*	Mean	*SD*	Mean	*SD*	Mean	*SD*	*F*	Post Hoc	*p*
Knowledge of EOL care	6.73	1.94	6.75	1.96	6.31	1.70	7.70	2.02	2.96*	③ > ②	.013
Attitudes toward RWDs' decision-making rights	17.36	2.87	17.25	2.91	17.52	2.84	18.55	1.71	2.26		.106
Perceived facility support	32.55	6.18	32.53	6.23	32.63	5.72	32.81	6.93	0.03		.973
Confidence in EOL care and communication skills	44.94	13.24	45.38	13.04	40.58	13.06	50.50	14.27	5.85	③ > ②, ① > ②	.003
Discussing EOL care											
Discussing ADs for RWDs	6.25	2.71	6.23	2.71	6.21	2.77	6.74	3.19	0.40		.674
Discussing life-sustaining treatments for RWDs	6.61	2.61	6.80	2.50	4.76	2.11	8.87	2.76	29.48	③ > ① > ②	< .001

Note. EOL = end of life; RWDs = residents with dementia; ADs = advance directives.
**p* < .05.

TABLE 4.
Factors Associated With Frequency of Discussing EOL Care for RWDs

Factor	Discussing Advance Directive				Discussing Life-Sustaining Treatment			
	B	*SE*	*t*	95% CI	*B*	*SE*	*t*	95% CI
Education (vs. bachelor's degree or above)								
Junior college or below = 1	−0.04	0.30	−0.10	[−0.62, 0.54]	0.16	0.27	0.63	[−0.37, 0.69]
Profession (vs. physician)								
Nurse	0.22	0.57	0.39	[−0.90, 1.35]	−1.45	0.52	−2.78**	[−2.47, −0.42]
Social worker	0.50	0.66	0.76	[−0.79, 1.79]	−3.30	0.60	−5.51***	[−4.48, −2.12]
Working experience (months)	0.01	0.01	0.99	[−0.01, 0.04]	0.0	0.01	1.25	[−0.01, 0.01]
Type of institution (vs. general LTC facility)								
Dementia-specific facility	−0.82	0.70	−1.18	[−2.20, 0.55]	−0.83	0.64	−1.30	[−2.09, 0.42]
Freestanding nursing home	0.40	0.36	1.21	[−0.28, 1.16]	0.42	0.33	1.26	[−0.24, 1.07]
Hospital-based nursing home	0.62	0.33	1.90	[−0.02, 1.26]	−0.18	0.30	−0.59	[−0.76, 0.41]
Continuing education (hours)								
On dementia care	0.0	0.01	1.61	[−0.01, 0.03]	0.01	0.01	1.05	[−0.01, 0.02]
On EOL care	0.03	0.01	4.25***	[0.02, 0.05]	0.02	0.01	2.54*	[0.01, 0.03]
Knowledge of EOL care	0.10	0.07	1.40	[0.04, 0.25]	0.12	0.07	1.73	[−0.02, 0.25]
Attitudes toward RWDs' decision-making rights	0.12	0.05	2.68**	[0.03, 0.22]	0.08	0.04	1.92	[−0.01, 0.16]
Confidence in EOL care and communication skills	0.05	0.01	4.67***	[0.03, 0.08]	0.07	0.01	6.42***	[0.05, 0.09]
Perceived facility support	0.12	0.02	5.09**	[0.07, 0.16]	0.06	0.02	2.87*	[0.02, 0.10]
Constant	−3.89	1.25	−3.10**	[−6.35, −1.43]	0.73	1.13	0.66	[−1.47, 2.97]
F and R^2	13.24	.36***			17.13	.42***		
Adjusted R^2		.33				.40		

Note. SE = standard error; CI = confidence interval; LTC = long-term care; EOL = end of life; RWDs = residents with dementia.
**p* < .05. ***p* < .01. ****p* < .001.

ignore their intentions and autonomy. A recent study showed that professionals who assume that people with dementia are incapable of making reliable decisions for themselves are not informed of RWDs' rights to ADs (De Vleminck et al., 2014). However, a diagnosis of dementia or a low score on the Mini-Mental State Examination is not a criterion for determining incapacity (Dening, Jones, & Sampson, 2011). Professionals who communicate effectively with RWDs are inclined to believe that RWDs can make valid ADs and express their wishes even at the advanced stages of dementia (Hegde & Ellajosyula, 2016; Rurup et al., 2006).

In this study, the registered nurse and social worker participants discussed LSTs with RWDs and their families significantly less often than the participants who were physicians. Although these professionals have different roles and responsibilities in long-term care facilities, physicians still have the greatest influence in the hierarchy of treatment decision-making (Rurup et al., 2006). Nevertheless, considering the current situation in long-term care facilities in Taiwan, nurses and social workers at these facilities constitute the primary professional workforce. They have the closest and most trusting relationships with RWDs and their families, and because physicians are not always in long-term care facilities, they are expected to assume more responsibility and to expand their professional roles in the EOL care process. Although nurses and social workers have less direct influence during EOL care decision-making, they are well positioned to play a valuable, indirect role in its initiation, functioning as RWDs' advocates, providing guidance and information, and supporting residents' families.

Although our findings indicate that the physician participants discussed LSTs more often than either the nurse or social worker participants, the LST discussion frequencies of the physician participants were still low. Approximately 70% of the physicians reported never or rarely discussing LSTs with RWDs and their families. This may be because physicians believe that RWDs or their families were reluctant to discuss EOL issues (Cheng et al., 2015) or because Taiwan lacks a consensus on or widely accepted medical or legal guidelines related to treating patients with advanced dementia at the EOL stage.

The three professional groups that were surveyed in this article did not differ significantly in their attitudes toward the decision-making rights of RWDs and their perceptions of facility support for discussing ADs with RWDs. However, the social worker participants had significantly lower perceived knowledge and confidence in EOL dementia care and discussed LSTs less frequently than their physician and registered nurse peers. Lower confidence in providing EOL care and less frequent discussion of LSTs are attributable to social workers not providing direct nursing care and having insufficient medical care training. Because they face increased demands for EOL care in long-term care facilities, facility administrators likely expand the roles of social workers to include not only discussing ADs with RWDs and their families but also maintaining ongoing discussions about the goals of medical care (Lacey, 2005). EOL care must be multidisciplinary, and promoting the knowledge and confidence of social workers regarding EOL care contributes to equitable cross-disciplinary dialogue.

Limitations

A strength of this study was its use of a randomized, stratified, nationwide sample of long-term care facilities. However, the generalizability of the results is limited to professionals in Grade A or higher long-term care facilities. The findings are also limited by only 23 physicians (4.8%) having responded to the questionnaires, with most of these (65.2%) working at hospital-based nursing homes. In addition, data were not collected on other potentially vital factors that are associated with EOL care practices such as facility staffing characteristics and facility policies regarding ADs. We suggest controlling for these factors in future studies. Furthermore, the instruments used to measure the knowledge of, attitudes toward, perceived facility support for, and confidence in EOL care were developed for this study, and this is the first time that they have been used. The validity and reliability of these measures should be retested. Finally, caution must be taken in interpreting these findings because self-reported information may not reflect the actual practice of discussing EOL care.

Conclusions

This study profiled discussions about ADs and LSTs in long-term care facilities in Taiwan. Healthcare professionals at these facilities did not frequently discuss ADs and LSTs with RWDs and their family caregivers. Greater perceived confidence in EOL care and communication skills, as well as facility support, were associated with more frequent discussions of ADs and LSTs with RWDs and their families. Professionals with more positive attitudes toward the decision-making rights of RWDs more frequently discussed ADs with RWDs and their families.

This study further determined that the frequency of professionals' discussions about ADs and LSTs was significantly and positively related to higher perceived confidence in EOL care and higher perceived support from the facility. We recommend that training for long-term care facility professionals should focus on promoting their confidence in EOL care and ability to communicate about EOL care with RWDs and their family caregivers. In addition, facility managers should establish explicit EOL care policies to guide professional staff in routinely discussing EOL care for RWDs. Managers should also work with staff members to mobilize the internal resources of their facility by promoting staff knowledge and multidisciplinary communication, organizing palliative care teams, and collaborating with external resources such as cooperative referral hospice units and palliative care providers to make professionals more comfortable and confident to engage in EOL care discussions. Moreover, we determined that the frequency of discussing ADs for RWDs was significantly predicted by the degree of positivity held by professionals toward RWDs' decision-making rights. This result suggests that the attitudes of professionals toward the awareness and decision-making rights of RWDs must be addressed to improve the ability of professionals to communicate with RWDs.

Acknowledgments

This work was supported by grants from the National Science Council (NSC 99-2314-B-182-044) and Chang Gung Memorial Hospital Research Programs (CMRPD1B0331) in Taiwan. We wish to thank the healthcare professionals in all of the practices who donated their time to complete the questionnaire survey and the administrative staffs for their cooperation.

References

Ampe, S., Sevenants, A., Smets, T., Declercq, A., & Van Audenhove, C. (2016). Advance care planning for nursing home residents with dementia: Policy vs. practice. *Journal of Advanced Nursing, 72*(3), 569–581. https://doi.org10.1111/jan.12854

Casey, D., Murphy, K., Ni Leime, A., Larkin, P., Payne, S., Froggatt, K. A., & O'Shea, E. (2011). Dying well: Factors that influence the provision of good end-of-life care for older people in acute and long-stay care settings in Ireland. *Journal of Clinical Nursing, 20*(13–14), 1824–1833. https://doi.org/10.1111/j.1365-2702.2010.03628.x

Chen, R. C. (2009). The spirit of humanism in terminal care: Taiwan experience. *The Open Area Studies Journal, 2*, 7–11.

Chen, T. F., Chiu, M. J., Tang, L. Y., Chiu, Y. H., Chang, S. F., Su, C. L., … Chen, R. C. (2007). Institution type-dependent high prevalence of dementia in long-term care units. *Neuroepidemiology, 28*(3), 142–149. https://doi.org/10.1159/000102142

Cheng, S. Y., Suh, S. Y., Morita, T., Oyama, Y., Chiu, T. Y., Koh, S. J., … Tsuneto, S. (2015). A cross-cultural study on behaviors when death is approaching in East Asian countries: What are the physician-perceived common beliefs and practices? *Medicine, 94*(39), e1573. doi:0000000000001573

Dening, K. H., Jones, L., & Sampson, E. L. (2011). Advance care planning for people with dementia: A review. *International Psychogeriatrics, 23*(10), 1535–1551. https://doi.org/10.1017/S1041610211001608

De Vleminck, A., Pardon, K., Beernaert, K., Deschepper, R., Houttekier, D., Van Audenhove, C., … Vander Stichele, R. (2014). Barriers to advance care planning in cancer, heart failure and dementia patients: A focus group study on general practitioners' views and experiences. *PLoS One, 9*(1), e84905. https://doi.org/10.1371/journal.pone.0084905

Faul, F., Erdfelder, E., Buchner, A., & Lang, A. G. (2009). Statistical power analyses using G*Power 3.1: Tests for correlation and regression analyses. *Behavior Research Methods, 41*(4), 1149–1160.

Givens, J. L., Jones, R. N., Shaffer, M. L., Kiely, D. K., & Mitchell, S. L. (2010). Survival and comfort after treatment of pneumonia in advanced dementia. *Archives of Internal Medicine, 170*(13), 1102–1107. https://doi.org/10.1001/archinternmed.2010.181

Givens, J. L., Selby, K., Goldfeld, K. S., & Mitchell, S. L. (2012). Hospital transfers of nursing home residents with advanced dementia. *Journal of the American Geriatrics Society, 60*(5), 905–909.

Gjerberg, E., Førde, R., & Bjørndal, A. (2011). Staff and family relationships in end-of-life nursing home care. *Nursing Ethics, 18*(1), 42–53. https://doi.org/10.1177/0969733010386160

Hegde, S., & Ellajosyula, R. (2016). Capacity issues and decision-making in dementia. *Annals of Indian Academy of Neurology, 19*(1, Suppl.), S34–S39. https://doi.org/10.4103/0972-2327.192890

Hicks, K. L., Rabins, P. V., & Black, B. S. (2010). Predictors of mortality in nursing home residents with advanced dementia. *American Journal of Alzheimer's Disease and Other Dementias, 25*(5), 439–445. https://doi.org/10.1177/1533317510370955

Houttekier, D., Cohen, J., Bilsen, J., Addington-Hall, J., Onwuteaka-Philipsen, B. D., & Deliens, L. (2010). Place of death of older persons with dementia. A study in five European countries. *Journal of the American Geriatrics Society, 58*(4), 751–756. https://doi.org/10.1111/j.1532-5415.2010.02771.x

Huang, H. L., Weng, L. C., & Yeh, C. M. (2011). Palliative care for persons with dementia. *Journal of Nursing, 58*(1), 91–96.

Lacey, D. (2005). Predictors of social service staff involvement in selected palliative care tasks in nursing homes: An exploratory model. *American Journal of Hospice & Palliative Care, 22*(4), 269–276. https://doi.org/10.1177/104990910502200407

Lithgow, S., Jackson, G. A., & Browne, D. (2012). Estimating the prevalence of dementia: Cognitive screening in Glasgow nursing homes. *International Journal of Geriatric Psychiatry, 27*(8), 785–791. https://doi.org/10.1002/gps.2784

Liu, L. M., Guarino, A. J., & Lopez, R. P. (2012). Family satisfaction with care provided by nurse practitioners to nursing home residents with dementia at the end of life. *Clinical Nursing Research, 21*(3), 350–367. https://doi.org/10.1177/1054773811431883

Lo, Y., Wang, J. J., Liu, L. F., & Wang, C. N. (2010). Prevalence and related factors of do-not-resuscitate directives among nursing home residents in Taiwan. *Journal of the American Medical Directors Association, 11*(6), 436–442. https://doi.org10.1016/j.jamda.2009.10.006

Lynch, T., Clark, D., Centeno, C., Rocafort, J., de Lima, L., Filbet, M., … Wright M. (2010). Barriers to the development of palliative care in Western Europe. *Palliative Medicine, 24*(8), 812–819. https://doi.org/10.1177/0269216310368578

Marshall, B., Clark, J., Sheward, K., & Allan, S. (2011). Staff perceptions of end-of-life care in aged residential care: A New Zealand perspective. *Journal of Palliative Medicine, 14*(6), 688–695. https://doi.org/10.1089/jpm.2010.0471

Ministry of Health and Welfare, Taiwan, ROC. (2013). *The name list of general nursing home accreditation (2010–2013)*. Retrieved from http://www.mohw.gov.tw/MOHW_Upload/doc/100-1020042702002.pdf

Ministry of the Interior, Taiwan, ROC. (2012). *The results of senior welfare institution accreditations 2010*. Retrieved from http://webarchive.ncl.edu.tw/archive/disk19/26/23/80/56/92/201001083095/20120515/web/sowf.moi/04/19/19.htm

Rurup, M. L., Onwuteaka-Philipsen, B. D., Pasman, H. R., Ribbe, M. W., & van der Wal, G. (2006). Attitudes of physicians, nurses and relatives towards end-of-life decisions concerning nursing home patients with dementia. *Patient Education and Counseling, 61*(3), 372–380. https://doi.org/10.1016/j.pec.2005.04.016

van der Steen, J. T., Radbruch, L., Hertogh, C. M., de Boer, M. E., Hughes, J. C., Larkin, P., ... European Association for Palliative Care. (2014). White paper defining optimal palliative care in older people with dementia: A delphi study and recommendations from the European Association for Palliative Care. *Palliative Medicine, 28*(3), 197–209. https://doi.org/10.1177/0269216313493685

Vandervoort, A., van den Block, L., van der Steen, J. T., Volicer, L., Vander Stichele, R., Houttekier, D., & Deliens, L. (2013). Nursing home residents dying with dementia in Flanders, Belgium: A nationwide postmortem study on clinical characteristics and quality of dying. *Journal of the American Medical Directors Association, 14*(7), 485–492. https://doi.org/10.1016/j.jamda.2013.01.016

van Soest-Poortvliet, M. C., van der Steen, J. T., Gutschow, G., Deliens, L., Onwuteaka-Philipsen, B. D., de Vet, H. C., & Hertogh, C. M. (2015). Advance care planning in nursing home patients with dementia: A qualitative interview study among family and professional caregivers. *Journal of the American Medical Directors Association, 16*(11), 979–989. https://doi.org/10.1016/j.jamda.2015.06.015

Wu, Y. T., Lee, H. Y., Norton, S., Chen, C., Chen, H., He, C., ... Brayne, C. (2013). Prevalence studies of dementia in mainland China, Hong Kong and Taiwan: A systematic review and meta-analysis. *PLoS One, 8*(6), e66252. https://doi.org/10.1371/journal.pone.0066252

Cognitive Dysfunction and Its Predictors in Adult Patients With Cancer Receiving Chemotherapy

Dhuha Youssef WAZQAR

ABSTRACT

Background: Chemotherapy-related cognitive dysfunction, one of the most frequently reported symptoms in patients with cancer, has a negative impact on the daily lives of patients. No research has examined cognitive dysfunction and its potential predictors in adult patients with cancer receiving chemotherapy in Saudi Arabia.

Purpose: The purpose of this study was to examine the sociodemographic, clinical, and psychological factors associated with cognitive dysfunction in adult patients with cancer receiving chemotherapy.

Methods: A cross-sectional correlational study was carried out with a convenience sample of 100 adult patients with cancer receiving chemotherapy at a university teaching hospital in Saudi Arabia. The Montreal Cognitive Assessment, the Hospital Anxiety and Depression Scale, and sociodemographic and clinical surveys were completed by participants. Descriptive statistics and linear regression were used to analyze the data.

Results: The data showed that the participants experienced moderate-to-severe cognitive dysfunction. Participants performed poorly in the divided attention and memory cognitive domains. Age, educational level, and depression factors were found to be significant predictors of cognitive dysfunction.

Conclusions/Implications for Practice: Cognitive dysfunction is commonly seen in patients with cancer receiving chemotherapy. Chemotherapy, age, and psychological factors increase susceptibility to cognitive dysfunction in adult patients with cancer. Oncology nurses should be aware that patients with cancer may be extremely vulnerable to cognitive dysfunction. Furthermore, age and psychological factors must be considered when developing symptom management and supportive care intervention programs to reduce the incidence of negative cognitive outcomes in this population.

Key Words:
patients with cancer, chemotherapy, cognitive dysfunction, oncology nurses.

Introduction

The number of cancer cases worldwide, estimated at 14.1 million in 2012, is on the rise and projected to reach 23.6 million new diagnoses each year by 2030 (World Health Organization, 2018). In Saudi Arabia (SA), 15,653 cancer cases were reported to the Saudi Cancer Registry (SCR) in 2013 (SCR, 2016). Overall, cancer has been more prevalent among Saudi women (8,294, 53%) than Saudi men (7,359, 47%), with a female–male ratio of 120:100 (SCR, 2016). The top three malignancies among Saudi women are breast, thyroid, and colorectal cancers, whereas colorectal cancer, non-Hodgkin's lymphoma, and leukemia are the top three malignancies among Saudi men (SCR, 2016). Improved access to cancer screening, early detection, and effective cancer treatments have increased the cancer survival rate in recent years, with the 5-year age-standardized relative survival reaching as high as 65% in SA (Swaminathan, Lucas, & Sankaranarayanan, 2011). The increasing numbers of patients with cancer and survivors in SA indicate the need for comprehensive assessment and management of the physical and psychological side effects of cancer treatment modalities to ameliorate the impact of these treatments on daily functioning, quality of life, work activities, and community integration both during and after treatment. Research indicates that healthcare providers should identify and manage chemotherapy-related physical symptoms and side effects and provide psychoeducational interventions to reduce the anxiety and depressive symptoms of patients undergoing cancer treatment to improve quality of life (Dai, Yang, Chen, & Tang, 2017; Wu, Chen, Huang, Chang, & Hsu, 2018).

PhD, RN, Assistant Professor, Oncology Nursing and Cancer Care, Faculty of Nursing, Department of Medical Surgical Nursing, King Abdulaziz University, Jeddah, Kingdom of Saudi Arabia.

Cancer and its treatment modalities such as chemotherapy, radiation therapy, and hormone therapy may cause mental and physical changes, including neurological impairment, that have a negative impact on the capacity of patients to perform daily life activities (Ahles, Root, & Ryan, 2012; Asher & Myers, 2015). Most related studies indicate that 15%–35% of cancer survivors experience cognitive decline months to years after finishing their treatment and about 75% of patients with cancer experience cognitive dysfunction during treatment (Ahles et al., 2012; Janelsins et al., 2011). Chemotherapy is the backbone of treatment for different types of cancer, and although it significantly increases survival, this treatment modality causes various side effects both during and after treatment. Evidence shows, across different healthcare facilities and country settings, that chemotherapy is the most common cancer treatment modality associated with cognitive dysfunction and/or cognitive decline in patients with cancer, although the effects are not universal (Moon, Kim, & Kim, 2011; Oh, 2017; Pendergrass, Targum, & Harrison, 2018). Although potential psychological and physiological mechanisms (e.g., fatigue, depression, microvascular injury, central nervous system toxicity, DNA damage, and inflammation) have been identified (Ahles, 2012), the structural and functional brain changes that underlie the cognitive dysfunctions associated with chemotherapy are not well understood.

Cognitive dysfunction, a major concern among patients with cancer, is usually referred to as "chemo brain" in the lay community (Asher & Myers, 2015). Chemo brain is a common term used in cancer research to refer to the mental cloudiness that patients with cancer report experiencing during and after chemotherapy (Asher & Myers, 2015). Common cognitive changes associated with chemotherapy typically encompass impairments in visuospatial skills, concentration, executive function (e.g., judgment), attention, and memory that may lead to increased stress levels and decreased job performance when higher cognitive abilities are required (Asher & Myers, 2015; Moon et al., 2011). Numerous studies have examined cognitive dysfunction among patients with cancer during and after chemotherapy. One cross-sectional and controlled longitudinal study on patients with breast cancer found a cognitive decline in the areas of verbal fluency in participants receiving chemotherapy as compared with healthy controls at 3-month follow-up assessments (Ahles et al., 2010). Moreover, a longitudinal and prospective study conducted by Bender and his colleagues (2006) found cognitive declines in verbal working and visual memory in patients with breast cancer after chemotherapy treatment. In addition, prior research suggests that cognitive declines in patients with cancer receiving chemotherapy may have a later onset and persist for 20 years after treatment (Koppelmans et al., 2012). Ahles (2012) found that chemotherapy may cause acute cognitive dysfunction as well as delayed effects as the survivor ages, with a variety of factors affecting the slope of change. As most previous studies have examined cognitive decline in patients with breast and colon cancers only, the reasons for cognitive dysfunction in patients with other cancers receiving chemotherapy are largely unknown.

In addition to chemotherapy, other factors such as age, gender, educational level, treatment duration, number of chemotherapy cycles, fatigue, anemia, quality of life, emotional stress, depression, and anxiety have been proposed as related to cognitive dysfunction in patients with cancer. However, the evidence related to these factors is inconsistent (Oh, 2017; Ramalho, 2015; Veancombe et al., 2009). In a cross-sectional study on adult patients with cancer, Oh (2017) found that cognitive impairment was more obvious in patients who were women, were older, had received cumulative cycles of chemotherapy, and had severe depression and fatigue. Of these factors, age and number of chemotherapy cycles were identified as the strongest predictors, indicating that cognitive function declines with increasing age and numbers of chemotherapy cycles (Oh, 2017). Another cross-sectional study conducted by Von Ah and Tallman (2015) found a significant relationship between anxiety and cognitive dysfunction in a sample of patients with breast cancer receiving chemotherapy ($r = .51, p < .01$). In addition, a study that examined cognitive dysfunction in patients with cancer found that attention decreased in participants who were and were not anxious, visual/executive functions decreased significantly in anxious participants, and memory decreased in participants who were not anxious (Ramalho, 2015). Furthermore, two additional studies assessed the effect of anxiety and depression on memory test performance in different populations (Bender et al., 2008; Yochim, Mueller, & Segal, 2013). On the basis of these findings, anxiety and depression affect certain aspects of memory functioning. Bender et al. (2008) showed a significant positive relationship between depression and cognitive dysfunction after chemotherapy in patients with cancer ($p = .03$). However, some researchers have found that symptomology falling short of the Diagnostic and Statistical Manual of Mental Disorder standards for anxiety and depression, although not related to cognitive dysfunction, may be associated with the perceived cognitive problems frequently described by patients with cancer (Hermelink et al., 2010).

Anemia after chemotherapy treatment has also been associated with cognitive decline, and patients with cancer who become anemic experienced significant decreases in attention and visual memory test performance (Castel et al., 2017). However, only two studies investigated the influence of anemia on cognitive function during and after receiving chemotherapy and found no significant relationship (Oh, 2017; Veancombe et al., 2009). Vearncombe et al. (2009) found that, although previous studies identified the significance of clinical and psychological variables in patients with cancer, the supporting evidence was contradictory. However, examination of all the related factors has not been extensive, and further investigation is required.

The extent to which chemotherapy and other factors increase the risk of cognitive decline in adult patients with cancer remains unclear, as few studies outside Western nations have investigated cognitive dysfunction and its associated factors, particularly in patients with breast and colon cancers receiving chemotherapy. Moreover, results vary among studies in terms of the magnitude of cognitive dysfunction, as expressed in the effect sizes. Therefore, a study of adult patients with different types of cancer in a developing country such as SA should help extend the current scholarly understanding and deepen the knowledge of oncology nurses about this phenomenon and promote improvements in the quality of nursing care delivered to adult patients with cancer. This study may also be a beneficial guide for developing symptom management and supportive care interventions for cognitive dysfunction related to chemotherapy in adult patients with cancer. The purpose of this study was to examine the sociodemographic, clinical (chemotherapy cycles/anemia), and psychological (anxiety and depression) factors associated with cognitive dysfunction in adult patients with cancer receiving chemotherapy in SA.

Methods

Design and Sample

This cross-sectional correlational study was designed to identify factors influencing the cognitive functioning in a convenience sample of adult patients with cancer receiving chemotherapy in King Abdulaziz University Hospital (KAUH) in Jeddah City, SA. Green (1991) proposed that the minimum sample size for regression analyses should be 50 with eight additional observations per term. Thus, this study required a sample size of 98 participants for a multiple regression analysis with six independent variables. An initial sample of 112 eligible patients was invited to participate, with 12 later excluded (eight declined to participate and four participants submitted questionnaires with missing data on the main study variables and the Hospital Anxiety and Depression Scale [HADS]). Thus, data from 100 participants were used in the analysis (response rate: 89%). Eligibility criteria included older than 18 years old, diagnosed with cancer at KAUH, had no evidence of a concurrent disease, and currently receiving chemotherapy. Otherwise, eligible patients were excluded if they were older than 65 years old, were on medications that might affect current cognitive function (i.e., anxiolytics, antidepressants, or narcotic analgesics), had a history of psychiatric or neurological disorders, had a history of alcohol or drug abuse, or had evidence of metastatic cancer or relapse. The medical files of all the participants were checked to confirm eligibility and to provide target demographic and clinical data.

Measures

Sociodemographic and clinical characteristics

The sociodemographic data that were collected included age, gender, nationality, marital status, and level of education. Furthermore, data on cancer type and stage, chemotherapy agents used, hemoglobin level, and number of chemotherapy cycles were collected.

Montreal Cognitive Assessment

The one-page Montreal Cognitive Assessment (MoCA) was used to assess the eight cognitive domains of attention (6 points), visuospatial/executive functions (5 points), short-term memory (5 points), naming (3 points), language (3 points), orientation (6 points), and abstraction (2 points). One point was added to the total score for participants with ≤ 12 years of formal education. The MoCA has been translated into several languages and is freely available on the Internet. It covers tasks such as naming, clock drawing, serial subtraction, sentence repetition, and delayed recall task, with a total possible score of 30 points and a score of less than 26 considered abnormal, as defined by the MoCA's authors (Nasreddine et al., 2005). According to the validation study, the specificity and sensitivity of the MoCA for detecting cognitive decline were 90% and 87%, respectively, compared with 18% and 100%, respectively, for the Mini-Mental Status Examination. The internal consistency of MoCA was also found to be good (Cronbach's alpha for the standardized items = .83; Nasreddine et al., 2005). The Cronbach's alpha value for the overall MoCA scale was .79 in this study.

Hospital Anxiety and Depression Scale

The HADS is utilized to assess the risk of depression and anxiety and incorporates 14 items, of which seven measure anxiety (HADS-A) and seven measure depression (HADS-D). There are four possible answers (0–3) for each item, and scores range from 0 to 21 for each subscale. The recommended cutoff point for a diagnosis of anxiety or depression is 8. The HADS questionnaire has been validated using both exploratory and confirmatory factor analyses and item response theory. The reported Cronbach's alpha ranges from .68 to .93 for HADS-A and from .67 to .90 for HADS-D (Zigmond & Snaith, 1983). In this study, the Cronbach's alpha for the overall HADS was .82.

Data Collection Procedures

Trained research nurse assistants consecutively invited qualified patients during regular visits to different oncology units in KAUH between January and May 2018. Participants signed written consent forms before enrollment, which included the purpose of research, the usefulness of the study, detailed instructions about completing the questionnaire, and a confidentiality statement. Participants were informed that they were free to withdraw from the study at any time without penalty and that there would be no financial or other gain from their participation. The questionnaires for assessing cognitive function and anxiety and depression risks, including sociodemographic and clinical items, were administered to all of the participants. Assessments of cognitive function by a trained research assistant occurred in each participant's room using standard instructions. The cognitive function assessment and self-report questionnaire took approximately 25–30 minutes to complete. The study was approved by KAUH's Research Ethics Board (Protocol reference no. 509-17).

Statistical Analysis

Data were analyzed using IBM SPSS Statistics Version 24 (IBM, Inc., Armonk, NY, USA). Descriptive statistics were used to characterize the sociodemographic and clinical variables of the participants. The data were screened for linearity, outliers, normality, and collinearity. Multiple linear regression analysis using the enter method was conducted to identify possible predictors of cognitive dysfunction. The MoCA (cognitive domains) was considered as a dependent variable, whereas age, education, chemotherapy cycles, hemoglobin level, anxiety, and depression were treated as independent variables. The level of significance was set at .05 for all analyses. Cronbach's alpha values were also calculated to estimate the internal consistency of the MoCA and HADS.

Results

Sociodemographic and Clinical Characteristics of the Participants

Most participants were female (78%), mean participant age was 44.0 (*SD* = 11.7, range: 18–60) years, most of the participants (63%) were non-Saudi nationals, and 75% were married. Less than one third (29%) had not completed high school, 33% had completed high school, and 38% had a college degree. Cancer stage distribution was as follows: Stage I, 17%; Stage II, 40%; and Stage III, 43%. The average number of chemotherapy cycles was 7.0 (*SD* = 4.9, range: 1–32) cycles, and the mean hemoglobin level was 10.8 (*SD* = 1.7) g/dl. Participants were receiving one or a combination of chemotherapy agents (5-fluorouracil), paclitaxel (Genexol), oxaliplatin (Eloxatin), topotecan (Hycamtin), doxorubicin (Adriamycin), cyclophosphamide (Cytoxan, Endoxan), methotrexate (Trexall), hydroxyurea (Hydrea), and vincristine (Oncovin). Participants with a diagnosis of breast cancer accounted for approximately one third of the sample (34%), and the remainder were diagnosed with gastrointestinal cancer (24%), hematological cancers (23%), and other cancers (19%), respectively (Table 1).

TABLE 1.
Sociodemographic and Clinical Characteristics of the Participants (N = 100)

Variable	*M*	Range	*SD*
Age (years)	44.0	18–60	11.7
Chemotherapy cycle (cycles)	7.0	1–32	4.9
Hemoglobin level (g/dl)	10.8	7.4–16.0	1.7
	n	%	
Gender			
Male	22	22	
Female	78	78	
Nationality			
Saudi	37	37	
Non-Saudi	63	63	
Marital status			
Single	14	14	
Married	75	75	
Divorced	9	9	
Widowed	2	2	
Education			
Primary	20	20	
Intermediate	9	9	
High school	33	33	
At least college	38	38	
Cancer stage			
I	17	17	
II	40	40	
III	43	43	
Type of cancer			
Breast cancer	34	34	
Colorectal cancer	17	17	
Lymphomas	14	14	
Gastric cancer	7	7	
Leukemia	9	9	
Bone cancer	6	6	
Skin cancer	5	5	
Lung cancer	5	5	
Prostate cancer	3	3	

Table 2 shows the results of the effect of chemotherapy on the eight domains of the MoCA and HADS scores. The mean MoCA score was 22 (*SD* = 4.73), with scores ranging from 10 to 29. It should be noted that 56% of participants experienced moderate-to-severe cognitive dysfunction and 24% experienced mild cognitive dysfunction. Participants showed lower scores for the cognitive domains of divided attention and short-term memory. The mean HADS-A score was 5.94 (*SD* = 3.28), with scores ranging from 0 to 13, and 21% of participants identified as experiencing moderate-to-severe anxiety. The mean HADS-D score was 7.25 (*SD* = 4.07), with scores ranging from 0 to 19 and 10% of participants experiencing moderate-to-severe depression.

Regression Analyses

Table 3 shows the predictors of cognitive dysfunction based on multiple regression analyses. In the regression model, age ($\beta = -.098$), level of education ($\beta = .588$), and depression ($\beta = -.160$) were the significant predictors of cognitive dysfunction. Of all of the predictors, level of education was the strongest, whereas depression, age, and education together accounted for 42% of the variance in both MoCA and cognitive test scores. The R^2 (AR^2) of the regression model, including the three significant predictors, was .415 (.396),

TABLE 2.
Descriptive Statistics for Anxiety, Depression, and Cognitive Function Assessment Scores (N = 100)

Variable	*n*	%	Mean	*SD*	Possible Range	Actual Range
MoCA			22.00	4.73	0–30	10–29
≤ 23	56	56				
24–26	24	24				
≥ 27	20	20				
Visuospatial/Executive function			3.52	1.52	0–5	1–5
Naming			2.71	0.49	0–3	1–3
Attention			3.44	1.34	0–6	0–6
Language			1.73	1.01	0–3	0–3
Abstraction			1.78	0.50	0–2	0–2
Memory			2.36	1.64	0–5	0–5
Orientation			5.53	0.86	0–6	2–6
HADS			13.19	6.13	0–42	1–31
HADS-A			5.94	3.28	0–13	0–13
0–7 (normal)	55	55				
8–10 (mid)	24	24				
11–21 (moderate–severe)	21	21				
HADS-D			7.25	4.07	0–21	0–19
0–7 (normal)	65	65				
8–10 (mid)	25	25				
11–21 (moderate–severe)	10	10				

Note. MoCA = Montreal Cognitive Assessment; HADS-A = Hospital Anxiety and Depression Scale-Anxiety; HADS-D = Hospital Anxiety and Depression Scale-Depression.

$F = 22.660$, $p < .001$. As predicted, depression, lower education, and older age were core factors explaining worse cognitive testing.

Discussion

The purpose of this study was to explore the impact of sociodemographic, clinical, and psychological factors on the cognitive dysfunction that adult patients with cancer commonly report during chemotherapy. Findings from this study indicated that 56% of the participants had moderate-to-severe cognitive dysfunction, which is consistent with previous studies that found a significantly higher incidence and a severe cognitive decline in patients with cancer who undergo or receive chemotherapy (Lange et al., 2014; Vitali et al., 2017). Moreover, of the various cognitive function domains, only attention (ability to process multiple information or activities simultaneously) and short-term memory were marked by significant decrements in this study. Similarly, prior studies on patients with stomach, breast, and colorectal cancers receiving different chemotherapy agents have identified negative impacts on the attention and memory domains in subgroup analyses (Cruzado et al., 2014; Oh, 2017). Attention is the basis for cognitive function, and decreasing attention negatively affects aspects of daily living such as community integration and work activities (Pendergrass et al., 2018). Physiological evidence supports the theory that chemotherapy affects the integrity of white matter in the brain and reflects cognitive dysfunction (Monje & Dietrich, 2012). Reduced white matter and hippocampal functionality may cause cognitive deficit symptoms in terms of processing speed, memory, and attention (Monje & Dietrich, 2012). However, other studies did not support a relationship between cognitive dysfunction and chemotherapy in patients with cancer but rather reported high rates of depression, anxiety, and

TABLE 3.
Significant Predictors of Cognitive Dysfunction in the Participants

Variable	Cognitive Function Score *B*	*SE*	β	*t*	*p*
Age	−0.039	.032	−.098	−1.235	.022
Education	2.467	.332	.588	7.421	.000
HADS-D	−0.231	.113	−.160	−2.049	.043

Note. R^2 (AR^2) = .415 (.396), $F(p)$ = 22.660 (< .001). AR^2 = adjusted R^2; HADS-D = Hospital Anxiety and Depression Scale-Depression.

fatigue (Abu-Helalah, Al-Hanaqta, Alshraideh, Abdulbaqi, & Hijazeen, 2014; Moon et al., 2011) that may negatively influence cognitive function. Further research is required to examine the relationships between cognitive dysfunction and psychological factors.

Age, education, and depression were associated with cognitive function in univariate analysis and were identified as significant predictors in multiple regression models, with these three factors explaining 42% of cognitive deterioration. Similarly, a recent study conducted by Oh (2017) on patients with cancer receiving chemotherapy found that age, gender, and depression had significant, discrete effects on cognitive decline and that these variables together explained 49.6% of the cognitive decline. However, these findings are in contrast to Moon et al. (2011), who suggested that although age and educational level were related to cognitive function in a univariate analysis, they were not significant predictors in multiple regression models. Future research may consider whether age and educational level moderate the effects of depression on cognitive function. Given that 49% of the participants in this study were adults older than 50 years old, the observed cognitive dysfunction may relate to the effects of aging. With increasing research into the cognitive changes in adult patients with cancer receiving chemotherapy, the influence of chemotherapy on the prevalence of dementia in older adult patients has become a significant focus of concern (Lange et al., 2014). Therefore, this issue must be considered when developing intervention programs to enhance cognitive function in this population.

Previous research has examined the correlations between cognitive dysfunction and depression and anxiety. This study found that depression contributed to cognitive dysfunction ($\beta = .21$), which is consistent with the findings of three previous studies conducted on patients with cancer (Bender et al., 2006; Moon et al., 2011; Oh, 2017), although the effect in this study was small and weaker than the effect of either age or educational level. The nonsignificant relationship between anxiety and cognitive decline that was found in this study suggests that cognitive dysfunction in patients with cancer is more closely associated with sociodemographic and clinical variables than with psychological variables. Kaiser, Bledowski, and Dietrich (2014) suggest that cognitive decline in some patients with cancer may be more indicative of emotional suffering than actual cognitive deficits. In this study, 35% of the participants showed signs of depression and 45% showed signs of anxiety, suggesting that screening for mental health conditions such as anxiety and depression may be important because these conditions are common in patients with cancer and because their underlying mechanisms are difficult to identify (Oh, 2017).

It has been reported that low hemoglobin level (anemia) and number of chemotherapy cycles are contributors of cognitive dysfunction in patients with cancer (Castel et al., 2017; Oh, 2017). Vearncombe et al. (2009) stated that hemoglobin was found to be independent of self-report measures and may provide a useful clinical indicator for risk of cognitive dysfunction. Furthermore, Oh (2017) noted that greater cognitive decline occurred in patients with cancer receiving chemotherapy in high doses over long periods. However, this study found no significant effect for either chemotherapy cycles or anemia.

Limitations

This study is affected by several limitations. The convenience sample of 100 adult patients with cancer in one geographic location (Jeddah, SA) reduces the generalizability of the findings. However, this study provides insights for decision makers and oncology nurses regarding the importance of developing symptom management and supportive care intervention programs targeting chemotherapy-related cognitive dysfunction for patients with cancer to improve quality of life in this vulnerable population. A second limitation of this study was the use of a cross-sectional design only at one point in time and without a control group. The impact of psychological factors on cognitive function during and after chemotherapy must be examined longitudinally. A third limitation was the lack of current studies in the field of oncology nursing on this topic in SA to allow for a direct comparison of findings. Thus, the direct comparison of results with existing studies was limited. A replication of this study on a large sample of older and middle-aged adult and pediatric patients with cancer being treated in public and private cancer care settings at different geographic locations in SA will be required to compare and contrast specific findings. Finally, study findings were obtained from adult patients with various cancers undergoing treatment with various chemotherapy agents. Thus, it remains unclear whether the observed cognitive dysfunction may be associated with certain cancers or chemotherapy agents or even other treatment modalities.

Conclusions

Cognitive dysfunction is commonly seen in adult patients with cancer. More of the participants receiving chemotherapy exhibited a moderate-to-severe decline in cognitive function, with some affected by significant levels of anxiety and depression. Notably, most of the participants in this study were affected by reduced attention and memory loss, which may significantly affect many aspects of life. The results of this study support previous research on cognitive dysfunction in patients with cancer receiving chemotherapy. Age, educational level, and depression were shown to be significant predictive factors for cognitive dysfunction in patients with cancer, explaining 42% of the variance. Further research in this area is necessary. In clinical settings, patients with cancer should be screened for cognitive dysfunction and oncology nurses should consider the effect of mood changes on cognitive function. A multidisciplinary approach involving assessment, education, monitoring, and rehabilitation will be necessary to improve the cognitive functioning of this population in SA.

Acknowledgments

The author would like to thank Barehen Nahouli, Enas Noorwall, Dena Baker, Razan Bugis, and Myan Abukhashba for their help in collecting data from the study participants. Special thanks go out to Ms. Kholood Mansouri, a statistical analyst who helped the author conduct the statistical analysis and interpretation.

References

Abu-Helalah, M., Al-Hanaqta, M., Alshraideh, H., Abdulbaqi, N., & Hijazeen, J. (2014). Quality of life and psychological well-being of breast cancer survivors in Jordan. *Asian Pacific Journal of Cancer Prevention, 15*(14), 5927–5936. https://doi.org/10.7314/APJCP.2014.15.14.5927

Ahles, T. A. (2012). Brain vulnerability to chemotherapy toxicities. *Psycho-Oncology, 21*(11), 1141–1148. https://doi.org/10.1002/pon.3196

Ahles, T. A., Root, J. C., & Ryan, E. L. (2012). Cancer- and cancer treatment-associated cognitive change: An update on the state of the science. *Journal of Clinical Oncology, 30*(30), 3675–3686. https://doi.org/10.1200/JCO.2012.43.0116

Ahles, T. A., Saykin, A. J., McDonald, B. C., Li, Y., Furstenberg, C. T., Hanscom, B. S., ... Kaufman, P. A. (2010). Longitudinal assessment of cognitive changes associated with adjuvant treatment for breast cancer: Impact of age and cognitive reserve. *Journal of Clinical Oncology, 28*(29), 4434–4440. https://doi.org/10.1200/JCO.2009.27.0827

Asher, A., & Myers, J. S. (2015). The effect of cancer treatment on cognitive function. *Clinical Advances in Hematology and Oncology, 13*(7), 441–450.

Bender, C. M., Pacella, M. L., Sereika, S. M., Brufsky, A. M., Vogel, V. G., Rastogi, P., ... Ryan, C. M. (2008). What do perceived cognitive problems reflect? *The Journal of Supportive Oncology, 6*(5), 238–242.

Bender, C. M., Sereika, S. M., Berga, S. L., Vogel, V. G., Brufsky, A. M., Paraska, K. K., & Ryan, C. M. (2006). Cognitive impairment associated with adjuvant therapy in breast cancer. *Psycho-Oncology, 15*(5), 422–430. https://doi.org/10.1002/pon.964

Castel, H., Denouel, A., Lange, M., Tonon, M. C., Dubois, M., & Joly, F. (2017). Biomarkers associated with cognitive impairment in treated cancer patients: Potential predisposition and risk factors. *Frontiers in Pharmacology, 8*, 138. https://doi.org/10.3389/fphar.2017.00138

Cruzado, J. A., Lopez-Santiago, S., Martínez-Marín, V., Jose-Moreno, G., Custodio, A. B., & Feliu, J. (2014). Longitudinal study of cognitive dysfunctions induced by adjuvant chemotherapy in colon cancer patients. *Support Care in Cancer, 22*(7), 1815–1823. https://doi.org/10.1007/s00520-014-2147-x

Dai, Y. L., Yang, C. T., Chen, K. H., & Tang, S. T. (2017). Changes in and determinants of quality of life in patients with advanced non-small-cell lung cancer undergoing initial chemotherapy. *The Journal of Nursing Research, 25*(3), 203–215. https://doi.org/10.1097/jnr.0000000000000148

Green, S. B. (1991). How many subjects does it take to do a regression analysis. *Multivariate Behavioral Research, 26*(3), 499–510. https://doi.org/10.1207/s15327906mbr2603_7

Hermelink, K., Küchenhoff, H., Untch, M., Bauerfeind, I., Lux, M. P., Bühner, M., ... Münzel, K. (2010). Two different sides of 'chemobrain': Determinants and nondeterminants of self-perceived cognitive dysfunction in a prospective, randomized, multicenter study. *Psycho-Oncology, 19*(12), 1321–1328. https://doi.org/10.1002/pon.1695

Janelsins, M. C., Kohli, S., Mohile, S. G., Usuki, K., Ahles, T. A., & Morrow, G. R. (2011). An update on cancer- and chemotherapy-related cognitive dysfunction: Current status. *Seminars in Oncology, 38*(3), 431–438. https://doi.org/10.1053/j.seminoncol.2011.03.014

Kaiser, J., Bledowski, C., & Dietrich, J. (2014). Neural correlates of chemotherapy-related cognitive impairment. *Cortex, 54*, 33–50. https://doi.org/10.1016/j.cortex.2014.01.010

Koppelmans, V., Breteler, M. M., Boogerd, W., Seynaeve, C., Gundy, C., & Schagen, S. B. (2012). Neuropsychological performance in survivors of breast cancer more than 20 years after adjuvant chemotherapy. *Journal of Clinical Oncology, 30*(10), 1080–1086. https://doi.org/10.1200/JCO.2011.37.0189

Lange, M., Rigal, O., Clarisse, B., Giffard, B., Sevin, E., Barillet, M., ... Joly, F. (2014). Cognitive dysfunctions in elderly cancer patients: A new challenge for oncologists. *Cancer Treatment Reviews, 40*(6), 810–817. https://doi.org/10.1016/j.ctrv.2014.03.003

Monje, M., & Dietrich, J. (2012). Cognitive side effects of cancer therapy demonstrate a functional role for adult neurogenesis. *Behavioral Brain Research, 227*(2), 376–379. https://doi.org/10.1016/j.bbr.2011.05.012

Moon, S., Kim, S. H., & Kim, M. J. (2011). Perceived cognitive function and related factors in Korean women with breast cancer. *Asian Nursing Research, 5*(2), 141–150. https://doi.org/10.1016/S1976-1317(11)60022-4

Nasreddine, Z. S., Phillips, N. A., Bédirian, V., Charbonneau, S., Whitehead, V., Collin, I., ... Chertkow, H. (2005). The Montreal Cognitive Assessment, MoCA: A brief screening tool for mild cognitive impairment. *Journal of the American Geriatrics Society, 53*(4), 695–699. https://doi.org/10.1111/j.1532-5415.2005.53221.x

Oh, P. J. (2017). Predictors of cognitive decline in people with cancer undergoing chemotherapy. *European Journal of Oncology Nursing, 27*, 53–59. https://doi.org/10.1016/j.ejon.2016.12.007

Pendergrass, J. C., Targum, S. D., & Harrison, J. E. (2018). Cognitive impairment associated with cancer: A brief review. *Innovation in Clinical Neuroscience, 15*(1-2), 36–44.

Ramalho, M. P. M. (2015). *Cognitive decline among breast cancer patients.* (Unpublished doctoral dissertation). Retrieved from https://pdfs.semanticscholar.org/06ee/147b53eedd9e1388da19b3099cc22d892113.pdf

Saudi Cancer Registry. (2016). *Cancer incidence report Saudi Arabia.* Retrieved from https://nhic.gov.sa/eServices/Documents/2013.pdf

Swaminathan, R., Lucas, E., & Sankaranarayanan, R. (2011). Cancer survival in Africa, Asia, the Caribbean and Central America: Database and attributes. *IARC Scientific Publications*, 162, 23–31.

Vearncombe, K. J., Rolfe, M., Wright, M., Pachana, N. A., Andrew, B., & Beadle, G. (2009). Predictors of cognitive decline after chemotherapy in breast cancer patients. *Journal of the International Neuropsychological Society*, *15*(6), 951–962. https://doi.org/10.1017/S1355617709990567

Vitali, M., Ripamonti, C. I., Roila, F., Proto, C., Signorelli, D., Imbimbo, M., ... Lo Russo, G. (2017). Cognitive impairment and chemotherapy: A brief overview. *Critical Reviews in Oncology/Hematology*, *118*, 7–14. https://doi.org/10.1016/j.critrevonc.2017.08.001

Von Ah, D., & Tallman, E. F. (2015). Perceived cognitive function in breast cancer survivors: Evaluating relationships with objective cognitive performance and other symptoms using the functional assessment of cancer therapy-cognitive function instrument. *Journal of Pain and Symptom Management*, *49*(4), 697–706. https://doi.org/10.1016/j.jpainsymman.2014.08.012

World Health Organization. (2018). *Worldwide cancer statistics*. Retrieved from http://www.cancerresearchuk.org/health-professional/cancer-statistics/worldwide-cancer

Wu, P. H., Chen, S. W., Huang, W. T., Chang, S. C., & Hsu, M. C. (2018). Effects of a psychoeducational intervention in patients with breast cancer undergoing chemotherapy. *The Journal of Nursing Research*, *26*(4), 266–279. https://doi.org/10.1097/jnr.0000000000000252

Yochim, B. P., Mueller, A. E., & Segal, D. L. (2013). Late life anxiety is associated with decreased memory and executive functioning in community dwelling older adults. *Journal of Anxiety Disorders*, *27*(6), 567–575. https://doi.org/10.1016/j.janxdis.2012.10.010

Zigmond, A. S., & Snaith, R. P. (1983). The Hospital Anxiety and Depression Scale. *Acta Psychiatrica Scandinavica*, *67*(6), 361–370.

25

Psychometric Evaluation of the Chinese Respiratory Distress Observation Scale on Critically Ill Patients With Cardiopulmonary Diseases

Ya-Hsiang CHAN[1] • Hua-Shan WU[2]* • Chih-Ching YEN[3] • Margaret L. CAMPBELL[4]

ABSTRACT

Background: Respiratory distress is a common and distressing experience that strikes most critically ill patients with cardiopulmonary diseases. Now, most dyspnea assessment tools rely on patient's self-report. Only one instrument, the Respiratory Distress Observation Scale (RDOS), is valid for assessing respiratory distress when the patient cannot provide a dyspnea self-report.

Purpose: The aims of this study were to develop the Chinese version of RDOS through two-way translation and examine its reliability and validity.

Methods: The first step was the translation and back-translation to establish the Chinese RDOS and examine the semantic equivalence between the back-translation version and the original one. The second step was the psychometric testing of the Chinese RDOS including internal reliability, interrater reliability, concurrent validity, convergent validity, and content and construct validity.

Results: The Chinese RDOS was reported with an internal consistency (Cronbach's α value) of .73, an interobserver reliability of .97, and a content validity index of .97. In the conscious critically ill patients, significant correlations were found between the Chinese RDOS and Spielberger State Anxiety Inventory scores or Dyspnea Vertical Visual Analog Scale scores ($r = .69$ and $r = .76$, respectively; $p < .001$). In the unconscious critically ill patients, there was a significantly positive correlation between the Chinese RDOS scores and fraction of inspiration O_2 ($r = .26$, $p < .05$) and a significantly negative correlation between the Chinese RDOS scores and saturation peripheral oxygen (SpO_2; $r = -.42$, $p = .001$). In addition, it also could effectively identify the dyspnea differences between the first and last days in the intensive care units ($p < .001$).

Conclusions: The Chinese RDOS showed good reliability and validity in conscious critically ill patients. The assessment with the Chinese RDOS could be completed within a short period no matter whether the assessor has nursing background in respiratory care or not. It could help the professionals systematically manage and track the change of respiratory distress in patients.

KEY WORDS:
critically ill patients, cardiopulmonary diseases, respiratory distress, reliability, validity.

Introduction

Sunshine, air, and water are the major elements of human survival. Breathing no air makes patients experience near-death. Dyspnea is the difficult, tiring, and straitened experience in breathing, and its property and intensity can be clearly felt subjectively by patients (Parshall et al., 2012). Campbell (2011) pointed out that a patient's subjective statement was the important basis for assessing dyspnea, including "I breathe with difficulty," "I breathe very little air," "I feel chest pressure and discomfort," or even suffocation. Dyspnea results from anoxemia, hypercapnia, or inspiratory effort and signifies the risk of breathing failure or even death (Campbell, 2012). Therefore, to effectively control dyspnea and prevent the complication after it, it is especially important for clinical staff to accurately assess dyspnea.

The current assessment tool, such as a numerical rating scale or a visual analog scale, is used to assess the intensity of the patient's dyspnea. However, only conscious patients are able to make a clear self-report for the property and intensity of dyspnea (AbouEzzeddine et al., 2016; Parshall et al., 2012; Pianosi, Zhang, Hernandez, & Huebner, 2016). Some patients, such as patients with cognitive impairment, unconsciousness, intubation, the use of sedative drugs, terminal illness, brain damage, and limb weakness, are not able to make the self-report and depend on their proxy to provide information. However, the information provided by the proxy may not be as trustworthy as the patients' behavioral clues (Campbell, 2012, 2015). The critically ill patients with cardiopulmonary diseases in intensive care units are also unable to express their feeling of dyspnea because of long- or short-term cognitive impairment. Currently, most clinical personnel simply judge and decide whether further treatment is needed for the patients with cognitive impairment in accordance with the patient's breathing rate per minute or

[1]*MSN, RN, Department of Nursing, China Medical University Hospital, Taiwan, ROC* • [2]*PhD, RN, Associate Professor, Department of Nursing, Asia University, and Research Consultant, Department of Medical Research, China Medical University Hospital, China Medical University, Taiwan, ROC* • [3]*PhD, Associate Professor, Department of Respiratory Care, China Medical University, and Attending Physician, Department of Medicine, China Medical University Hospital, Taiwan, ROC* • [4]*PhD, RN, FPCN, Associate Professor, College of Nursing, Wayne State University, Michigan, USA.*

blood oxygen saturation. However, undertreatment or overtreatment might be practiced if simply one or two figures are used to make the judgment, resulting in more severe diseases, extension of hospitalization, or even less chance of survival (Campbell & Templin, 2015).

In clinical practice, dyspnea is hardly regularly and systematically monitored, especially among patients unable to do self-report (Persichini et al., 2015). So far, the assessment tools used in Taiwan for dyspnea are all for conscious patients able to express themselves, but not for those who are not. Overseas, Dr. Campbell developed the Respiratory Distress Observation Scale (RDOS) in 2008, which showed good reliability and validity among patients who were not able to report their dyspnea by themselves owing to such diseases as terminal cancer under palliative care, chronic obstructive pulmonary disease, cardiac failure, pneumonia, and so on (Campbell, 2008a; Campbell, Templin, & Walch, 2010). The RDOS consists of eight dyspnea-related indicators with less than 5 minutes in each assessment. Using RDOS, the assessor can learn the patient's degree of respiratory distress and the effect after treatment, which helps prevent mistakes caused by subjective judgment and avoid the inappropriate medical treatment or care that contributes to undertreatment or overtreatment resulting in death. The RDOS was developed in English and has been translated into Dutch and French. A Chinese version is needed.

Different cultures, races, societies, and medical environments may affect the feasibility of an assessment tool. Therefore, this study aimed at (a) developing the Chinese RDOS using two-way translation, namely, translation and back-translation, and (b) examining the reliability and validity of the Chinese RDOS, including internal consistency, interobserver reliability, and content, concurrent, convergent, and construct validity. Hopefully, the establishment of the Chinese RDOS could help domestic nursing personnel objectively and systematically assess respiratory distress in those patients who were unable to do self-report, and the data collected through the Chinese RDOS could be used to explore the factors that affected the respiratory distress and to plan effective interventions accordingly to improve the breathing problems in patients with severe cardiopulmonary diseases.

Methods

Participants

This study used purposive sampling to recruit participants from the respiratory intensive care units (RICUs) in a medical center in central Taiwan. To meet the inclusion criteria, the participants had to (a) be diagnosed with cardiopulmonary diseases, (b) stay in the RICUs for at least 1 day, (c) be from 20 to 90 years old, and (d) agree to participate in the study and be able to communicate in Mandarin or Taiwanese under consciousness or have a family member, who agreed to patients' participation in the study and did the communication on the participants' behalf. Participants were excluded if they (a) completely depended on a ventilator (the rates patients breathed were the same with those when a ventilator had been set) and (b) were diagnosed with central nervous system diseases because the original RDOS was determined to be invalid in quadriplegia and motor neuron disease. All the data were collected between July and November 2014.

Design

The principal investigator had received the letter of consent from the original creator of RDOS, who had kindly allowed us to develop the Chinese version of RDOS based on the two steps below.

The first step

This study proceeded with the translation, back-translation, and pilot test in accordance with Brislin's translation model.

In the beginning, the original RDOS was translated into Chinese by the principal investigator and a nursing instructor who obtained a Doctor of Philosophy specializing in critical care in the United States and obtained translation consistency; next, the Chinese RDOS was back-translated to English by a Doctor of Basic Medical Science who had long stayed in the United States and an attending chest physician who studied respiratory physiology in the United States and obtained back-translation consistency. Dr. Campbell, the creator of the original RDOS, examined the consistency of the original RDOS and the back-translated version, with a score of 4 representing complete consistency, 3 representing consistency, 2 representing partial consistency in need of modification, and 1 representing complete inconsistency in need of retranslation. A score of 3 and above indicated that the question items, after translation and back-translation, achieved high consistency with the original question items. The first consistency comparison resulted in two questions (Item 5: accessory muscle use, Item 8: look of fear) scoring 2, one question (Item 6: grunting at end-expiration) scoring 1, and the remaining questions and the instructions for use scoring 4. Therefore, on the basis of the expert's advice, the three question items were modified, translated, back-translated, and compared by Dr. Campbell for consistency again. The second consistency comparison showed that all the question items and the instructions for use scored 3 or above, which suggested semantic equivalence between the back-translated version and the original version. Finally, during the pilot test, six nursing personnel, including three specializing in chest or respiratory care and the other three specializing in other medical care, filled out the Chinese RDOS. It was discovered that all the nursing personnel, with or without the experience in chest or respiratory care, could comprehend the Chinese RDOS and complete the test within 2–3 minutes.

The second step

The reliability and validity of the Chinese RDOS were established by psychometric analysis as follows:

1. Internal consistency reliability: The research assistant assessed the participants' respiratory distress using the Chinese RDOS. The collected data were analyzed using Cronbach's α to examine the correlation among the question items in the Chinese RDOS for confirming the consistency and homogeneity of the question items.
2. Interrater reliability: In this study, we used a table of random numbers to choose 30 participants for interrater reliability analysis. While the research assistant was assessing respiratory distress conditions of a participant with the Chinese RDOS, a nurse who works in this RICU was doing the same assessment simultaneously to examine the stability of different assessors.
3. Content validity: Five experts, including an instructor specializing in chest and intensive nursing care, a head nurse in a chest ward, an instructor specializing in respiratory therapy, and two attending physicians specializing in chest and critical care medicine, were invited to examine the feasibility and semantic clarity of the question items in the Chinese RDOS. A score of 4 indicated that the question was highly feasible and understandable and modification was unnecessary, a score of 3 indicated that the question was feasible and understandable and modification was only partially needed when necessary, a score of 2 indicated that the question was unfeasible and confusing and ought to be either deleted or extensively modified, and a score of 1 indicated that the question item was highly unfeasible and confusing and had to be deleted. In the end, the content validity index (CVI) was calculated according to the scores given by the experts. Individual responses were summed and then divided by the number of examiners.
4. Concurrent validity: State anxiety is the feeling of nervousness, worry, and unrest that an individual experiences under specific circumstances (Chung & Long, 1984). Herigstad, Hayen, Reinecke, and Pattinson (2016) pointed out that patients would experience a higher degree of state anxiety if they experienced a higher degree of respiratory distress. For the conscious critically ill patients, we used the Chinese version of Spielberger State Anxiety Inventory (SSAI) developed by Chung and Long (1984) as the criterion of the Chinese RDOS. In addition to the Chinese RDOS scores, we also collected the Chinese SSAI scores to examine whether these scores were significantly correlated. For the unconscious critically ill patients, we collected their fraction of inspiration O_2 (FiO_2) to examine whether the Chinese RDOS scores were significantly correlated to the FiO_2 values.
5. Construct validity:
   (1) Convergent validity: In addition to the collection of all the participants' RDOS scores, for the conscious critically ill patients, their Dyspnea Vertical Visual Analog Scale (DVVAS) scores were also collected. For the unconscious critically ill patients, their values of peripheral oxygen saturation (SpO_2) were collected to examine whether the Chinese RDOS and the DVVAS scores or SpO_2 values were correlated; the same construct was measured.
   (2) Contrasted group testing: Among all the recruited participants, the participants who were discharged from the ICU at last were assessed using the Chinese RDOS on the day before the discharge. These Chinese RDOS scores were compared with the scores when the participants stayed in the ICU for at least 1 day to examine whether the Chinese RDOS could effectively distinguish different degrees of respiratory distress at different severity levels of illness.

Measures

The Chinese version of Respiratory Distress Observation Scale

We employed the RDOS developed by Campbell et al. (2010), consisting of eight indicators as follows: heart rate, respiratory rate, accessory respiratory muscle, paradoxical breathing, dysphoria, respiratory rattling, alar flaring, frightened facial expression, and so on. Zero to 2 points are assigned to each variable, and the points are summed. Scores range from 0 to 16, with 0 representing "none" and 16 representing "severe breathing difficulties." The higher the scores, the more severe dyspnea. The original RDOS has acceptable internal reliability (α = .64–.85), perfect interrater reliability with registered nurse (r = 1.0), convergent validity with patient self-report (r = .74, p < .01), discriminant validity with pain (F = 119.84, p < .01), and convergent validity with oxygenation (r = −.369, p < .01; Campbell, 2008b, 2010). The research assistant was asked to assess the participants who had been admitted to the ICU for at least 1 day with the Chinese RDOS and to score appropriately according to the results of his or her observations.

The Chinese version of Spielberger State Anxiety Inventory

The State-Trait Anxiety Inventory, translated by Chung and Long (1984), was used in this study. This State Anxiety Inventory mainly measured the subjects' feeling under specific circumstances, such as nervousness, overcaution, worry, anxiety, and so on, and stressed that the subjects had to answer the questions based on the "present feeling" (Chung & Long, 1984). The Chinese SSAI is mainly for teenagers and adults, consisting of 20 question items; 4-point Likert scale is used to measure the anxiety level of the subjects. Scores range from 1 to 4 as follows: 1 = *none*, 2 = *a little*, 3 = *quite*, and 4 = *very much*. Points are summed, ranging from 20, representing the least severe anxiety, to 80, the most severe anxiety (Chung & Long, 1984). The Cronbach's αof the Chinese SSAI was found to be .90, and the test–retest reliability was .74 at an interval of 7 days (Chung & Long, 1984). In this study, the conscious participants with the ability to write and read filled out the questionnaire by themselves. If they were unable to write and read, the research assistant would read the question items to them, listen to their response, and check at the most appropriate score according to their response.

Dyspnea vertical visual analog scale

The DVVAS represents the patient's self-report dyspnea. The scale is a vertical 100-mm measuring gauge with the highest point representing the most severe dyspnea and the lowest representing no dyspnea. The subjects point at the vertical gauge according to the level of dyspnea. The reliability and validity of DVVAS have been confirmed for individuals with dyspnea. The intraclass correlation coefficient was .96 for breathing distress in 58 patients with chronic obstructive pulmonary disease (Hu & Meek, 2005). With regard to concurrent validity, the DVVAS was significantly correlated with the numeric rating scale (r = .8) and the Peak Expiratory Flow Rate (r = .85; Gift, 1989; Gift & Narsavage, 1998). Construct validity was established by using DVVAS to differentiate the degree of difficulty breathing at times of severe versus low obstruction for patients with asthma and chronic obstructive pulmonary disease (Gift, 1989). In the study, the research assistant marked at the gauge according to the participant's report. The length from no dyspnea to the mark meant the level of dyspnea. The longer it was, the more severe dyspnea was.

Pulse oximetry (peripheral oxygen saturation)

Pulse oximeter is a noninvasive skin-penetrating infrared sensor apparatus. It is an instrument mainly used to measure the proportion of oxygen saturated hemoglobin, which represents a patient's oxygenation ability (Tusman, Bohm, & Suarez-Sipmann, 2017). In this study, the research assistant used a finger-sensored pulse oximeter (Rossmax model SB100, size = 63.5 × 34 × 35 mm; Rossmax Innotek Corp., Taipei, Taiwan) to measure a participant's degree of blood oxygen saturation. The total weight of pulse oximeter was 37 g (excluding battery), with the precision of ± 2%. After measuring for 1 minute, the participant's SpO_2 and heart rate on the meter were recorded.

Basic information about the participants

(1) Demographic characteristics were age, gender, and marriage. (2) Information about disease and treatment were disease diagnosis, days in the ICU, Glasgow Coma Scale scores, and treatment outcome (decease, transfer to the general ward, transfer to a subacute respiratory care center, etc.). (3) Information about respiratory treatment were modes of respiratory therapy, SpO_2 value and FiO_2 values.

Ethical Considerations

This study had been approved by the institutional review board of a medical center in central Taiwan (Approval no. CMUH102-REC3-121). Before collecting data, the principal researcher explained to the eligible participants and their family members the purpose, content, procedure, privacy protection, rights to reject or end participation, right for medical care, and obligations. Data would not be collected until the written informed consent was obtained. The interval of the data collection would be no more than 10 minutes.

Data Analysis

The collected data in this study were analyzed using SPSS 18.0 for Windows. The basic information and the distribution of variables were analyzed using descriptive statistics. For reliability assessment, internal consistency was measured with Cronbach's α; test–retest reliability and interrater reliability were measured with Pearson correlation. For validity assessment, content validity was quantified using CVI; concurrent and convergent validities were measured using Pearson correlation to examine the correlation between the Chinese RDOS scores and the Chinese SSAI scores, DVVAS values, and FiO_2 values, respectively; and contrasted group testing was completed using a paired t test to compare the differences of the Chinese RDOS scores at different levels of illness severity.

Results

Basic Information About the Participants

In the 114 eligible participants, four refused participation and two were deceased. One hundred eight participants' data were collected and analyzed. Participants' characteristics are summarized in Table 1. Among the participants, 69.4% were male, with a mean age of 66.4 (SD = 15.9) years ranging from 21 to 89 years; educational degree was mainly elementary school and junior high school, followed by senior high school; diagnoses of the participants in the ICU were acute respiratory failure (46.2%, n = 50), followed by pneumonia (32.4%, n = 35); the most used respiratory therapy mode was pressure-control ventilation (82.4%, n = 89); the average oxygen concentration was 59.8%; the average Glasgow Coma Scale score was 8.0 (SD = 3.7), representing severe coma; the average stay in the ICU was 10.5 (SD = 5.5) days, most of whom were transferred to the general ward (38.0%) or subacute respiratory care center (34.3%) for treatment; and discharge due to terminal illness or decease were 18.5% (n = 20).

Reliability of the Chinese Version of Respiratory Distress Observation Scale

The internal consistency (Cronbach's α) of the Chinese version of RDOS was found to be .73 (Table 2). The correlation of the Chinese RDOS scores measured by the research assistant (mean = 2.23, SD = 1.98) and a nurse who works in the RICU (mean = 2.13, SD = 1.89) at the same time was .97 ($p < .001$), representing a highly

TABLE 1.

Demographic Characteristics (N = 108)

Characteristic	*n*	%
Gender		
Male	75	69.4
Female	33	30.6
Age (years; *M* and *SD*)	66.4	15.9
Education		
Illiterate	15	13.9
Literate	4	3.7
Elementary school	24	22.2
Junior high school	26	24.1
Senior high school	21	19.4
College	18	16.7
Disease diagnosis		
Acute respiratory failure	50	46.2
Pneumonia	35	32.4
Congestive heart failure	11	10.2
Lung cancer	6	5.6
Pneumothorax	3	2.8
Asthma	2	1.9
Lung abscess	1	0.9
Days in ICU (*M* and *SD*)	10.5	5.5
Glasgow Coma Scale (scores; *M* and *SD*)	8.0	3.7
Modes of respiratory therapy		
O2 cannula/Venturi mask/nonrebreathing mask	14	13.0
Pressure-control ventilation	89	82.4
Pressure support	2	1.9
Bi-PAP	3	2.8
FiO_2 (%; *M* and *SD*)	59.8	28.3
SpO_2 (value; *M* and *SD*)	97.0	3.3
Treatment outcome		
Transfer to the general ward	41	38.0
Transfer to subacute RCC	37	34.3
Transfer to respiratory care ward	7	6.5
Against advice discharge	5	4.6
Decease	15	13.9
Maybe discharged	3	2.8

Note. Participants' age ranged from 21 to 89 years, days in ICU ranged from 4 to 29, Glasgow Coma Scale scores ranged from 3 to 15, FiO_2 ranged from 21% to 100%, and SpO_2 ranged from 76% to 100%. ICU = intensive care unit; Bi-PAP = bilevel positive airway pressure; FiO_2 = fraction of inspiration O_2; SpO_2 = saturation peripheral oxygen; RCC = respiratory care center.

positive correlation and therefore good interrater reliability (Table 3).

Validity of the Chinese Version of Respiratory Distress Observation Scale

1. Content validity: Five experts, including a clinical respiratory therapist, a teacher specializing in chest nursing, two attending physicians specializing in chest and critical care medicine, and a head nurse in a chest ward, were invited to examine the feasibility and semantic clarity of the question items in the scale, scoring from 1 to 4. The CVI was calculated according to the scores given by the experts. The CVI of feasibility was 1.0, and that of semantic clarity was 0.97.

2. Concurrent validity: For the conscious critically ill patients ($N = 47$), the correlation coefficient was .69 ($p < .001$), representing that there was a moderate positive correlation between the Chinese RDOS and the Chinese SSAI scores. However, for the unconscious critically ill patients ($N = 61$), the correlation coefficient was .26 ($p < .05$; Table 4), representing that there was a low positive correlation between the Chinese RDOS scores and FiO_2.

3. Convergent validity: To the conscious critically ill patients ($N = 47$), the correlation coefficient was .76 ($p < .001$), representing that there was a high positive correlation

TABLE 2.

The Internal Consistency Analysis of the Chinese RDOS (N = 108)

Item	Cronbach's α (Cronbach's α Based on Standardized Items)	Cronbach's α if Item Was Deleted
RDOS	.73 (.75)	
Heart rate per minute		.73
Respiratory rate per minute		.67
Restlessness: purposeless movement		.72
Paradoxical respiratory movement		.72
Use of respiratory accessory muscle		.65
Gurgling sound at the end of expiration		.74
Flaring of nares		.74
Facial expression of frightening		.72

Note. RDOS = Respiratory Distress Observation Scale.

TABLE 3.

The Concurrent and Convergent Validity Analysis of the Chinese RDOS for Conscious Patients (N = 47)

Item	Total RDOS Score	Chinese SSAI Score	Chinese DVVAS Score
Total RDOS scores	1.00	.69**	.76**
Chinese SSAI scores	.69**	1.00	
Chinese DVVAS scores	.76**		1.00

Note. RDOS = Respiratory Distress Observation Scale; DVVAS = Dyspnea Vertical Visual Analog Scale; SSAI = Spielberger State Anxiety Inventory.
**$p < .01$.

TABLE 4.

The Concurrent and Convergent Validity Analysis of the Chinese RDOS for Unconscious Patients (N = 61)

Item	Total RDOS Score	FiO_2	SpO_2 Value
Total RDOS scores	1.00	.26*	−.42**
FiO_2	.26*	1.00	
SpO_2 value	−.42**		1.00

Note. RDOS = Respiratory Distress Observation Scale; FiO_2 = fraction of inspiration O_2; SpO_2 = saturation peripheral oxygen.
$*p < .05$. $**p < .01$.

between the Chinese RDOS scores and the DVVAS scores (Table 3). To the unconscious critically ill patients (*N* = 61), the correlation coefficient was −.42 ($p = .001$; Table 4), representing that there was a moderate negative correlation between the Chinese RDOS scores and the SpO_2 value and that there was the same "respiratory distress" construct among the Chinese RDOS, DVVAS, and SpO_2, showing good convergent validity.

4. Contrasted group validity: To the 88 patients who were transferred to the general wards, subacute respiratory care units, and chronic respiratory care wards and discharged from the hospital, the use of a paired *t* test found a significant difference ($t = 8.81$, $p < .001$) between the RDOS scores when they stayed in the ICU for at least 1 day and on the last day before discharge (Table 5).

Discussion

In accordance with the aim of this study, we translated the RDOS developed by Dr. Campbell into Chinese and applied it to the cardiopulmonary patients in critical care to assess the reliability and validity of the scale. The internal consistency reliability of the Chinese RDOS using Cronbach's α is .73, which corresponds to that of the original RDOS ranging from .64 to .85. According to Lu (2011), internal consistency reliability is the correlation or consistency among the similar questions in a questionnaire. Cronbach's α between .7 and .9 means high internal consistency, and Cronbach's α < .35 means low internal consistency; Cronbach's α of .6 or higher is generally acceptable. Accordingly, the Chinese RDOS shows good internal consistency reliability similar to the original RDOS.

As for the interobserver reliability, in Dr. Campbell's study in 2010 on RDOS, different assessors were invited to obtain the RDOS scores of five patients with terminal disease at the same time and the scores represented perfect ($r = 1.0$) interobserver reliability. This study increased the number of subjects to 30, and two assessors were invited. Similar interobserver reliability was obtained ($r = .97$), indicating that the Chinese RDOS, with two assessors assessing the same subject at the same time, showed high stability and would not be affected owing to different assessors.

The original RDOS did not proceed to obtain expert and comprehensive concurrent validity. This study invited five experts to examine the feasibility and semantic clarity of the questionnaire, and the obtained CVI values were 1.0 and 0.97, respectively, indicating that each question item was feasible and semantically well organized and that the assessor, with or without the background in chest or respiratory care, could use the Chinese RDOS. In addition, for the critically ill patients who were cognitive and conscious, there was a highly positive correlation between the Chinese RDOS and the Chinese SSAI scores. In other words, when the subject was found to have a higher level of respiratory distress, he or she had a higher level of state anxiety, which indicated that the Chinese RDOS showed good concurrent validity for the conscious patients. However, for the critically ill patients who were unconscious, there was a significantly low correlation ($r = .26$) between the Chinese RDOS and FiO_2. It is the same as the study of Campbell (2010), which also reported a significantly low correlation between the RDOS scores and FiO_2 ($r = .315$) in the 89 patients with terminal illnesses (23% were unconscious, and 65% have cognitive impairment). Maybe, it is because the use of FiO_2 exhibited a proof effect for critically ill patients and the correlation between the Chinese/original RDOS scores and FiO_2 was not very high. Mahler et al. (2009) indicated that dyspnea rating was significantly related to the disease severity. Perhaps, disease severity index is more suitable as a concurrent criterion.

As for convergent validity, Campbell (2008a) reported a significantly negative correlation between the RDOS scores and SpO_2 ($r = -.24$) and a significantly positive correlation

TABLE 5.

Contrasted Group Validity (N = 88)

	The First Day Staying in the ICU (A)		The Last Day Before Discharging From the ICU (B)		(A)-(B)			
Item	Mean	*SD*	Mean	*SD*	Mean	*SD*	*t*	95% CI
RDOS scores	3.60	2.83	0.93	1.20	2.67	2.84	8.81***	[2.07, 3.27]

Note. ICU = intensive care unit; RDOS = Respiratory Distress Observation Scale.
$***p < .001$.

between the RDOS scores and DVVAS (r = .389) in 70 pulmonary rehabilitation (conscious) patients who were experiencing hypoxemia. Afterward, Campbell (2010) also reported a significantly negative correlation between the RDOS scores and SpO_2 (r = −.369) in the patients with terminal illnesses (some of them were unconscious). Comparing this study with the study of Campbell (2008a, 2010), this study obtained better results as Dr. Campbell did regardless of consciousness or unconsciousness. Moreover, although only a moderate correlation (r = −.42) between the RDOS scores and SpO_2 for unconscious patients was obtained in this study, it was shown that the Chinese RDOS was more suitable for unconscious people who cannot self-report dyspnea in considering the case of low correlation (r = −.24) in conscious patients of Dr. Campbell's study. Likewise, because respiratory distress can be confirmed by measuring the oxygen saturation of hemoglobin in the blood, the SpO_2 obtained by noninvasive pulse oximetry was used to replace SaO_2 measured by invasive arterial blood gas analysis (Amalakanti & Pentakota, 2016). However, pulse oximetry was 84.6% sensitive to hypoxemia in patients with respiratory failure (Amalakanti & Pentakota, 2016). Maybe because of this, the correlation was not high between the RDOS scores and SpO_2.

As well as construct validity, Campbell (2010) also reported a significant decrease in RDOS over time corresponding with treatment time in 89 patients with terminal illnesses. This study used the comparison group to examine the construct validity of the Chinese RDOS. The Chinese RDOS could effectively differentiate the levels of respiratory distress on the first day in the ICU and the last day before discharge, showing that the level was significantly lower on the last day before discharge than on the first day in the ICU, which also illustrated the Chinese RDOS' sensitivity to change when treatment is applied.

This study has the following limitations. First, the subjects were critical cardiopulmonary patients in a single medical center in central Taiwan, so the findings in this study may not be applied to the critical cardiopulmonary patients in other areas. Second, it is suggested that disease severity (e.g., the Acute Physiology and Chronic Health Evaluation scores) and SaO_2 could be respectively used to evaluate the concurrent and convergent validities in unconscious patients. Third, in regard to criterion-related validity, this study work has provided concurrent validity of the Chinese RDOS, but not predictive validity. In the future, the correlation coefficient between the Acute Physiology and Chronic Health Evaluation scores before discharge (criterion) and the Chinese RDOS scores on the first day can be examined to obtain predictive validity.

Conclusions

This Chinese version of RDOS shows good reliability and validity for conscious patients who cannot provide a dyspnea self-report and is a handy and timesaving assessment tool for the assessor with or without chest or respiratory care background. This tool will help the professionals in the ICU to systematically manage and track the changes of dyspnea under clinical treatments in conscious critically ill patients unable to self-report dyspnea. As for the use of unconscious patients, the scores measured by the Chinese RDOS can be a reference. To make the professionals do an adequate management, the information measured by multiple tools or methods was required. In the future, the studies on respiratory distress in conscious patients unable to self-report in the ICU, such as the factors that affect the level of respiratory distress, the interventions that improve respiratory distress, the timing of intubation, and so on, can choose the Chinese RDOS as a tool for more objective and overall comparison and analysis.

Acknowledgment

The authors thank the Taiwan Nurses Association, which supported this study work (Grant number TWNA-1032016).

References

AbouEzzeddine, O. F., Lala, A., Khazanie, P. P., Shah, R., Ho, J. E., Chen, H. H., ... NHLBI Heart Failure Clinical Research Network. (2016). Evaluation of a provocative dyspnea severity score in acute heart failure. *American Heart Journal, 172*, 34–41. https://doi.org/10.1016/j.ahj.2015.10.009

Amalakanti, S., & Pentakota, M. R. (2016). Pulse oximetry overestimates oxygen saturation in COPD. *Respiratory Care, 61*(4), 423–427. https://doi.org/10.4187/respcare.04435

Campbell, M. L. (2008a). Psychometric testing of a respiratory distress observation scale. *Journal of Palliative Medicine, 11*(1), 44–50. https://doi.org/10.1089/jpm.2007.0090

Campbell, M. L. (2008b). Respiratory distress: A model of responses and behaviors to an asphyxial threat for patients who are unable to self-report. *Heart and Lung, 37*(1), 54–60. https://doi.org/10.1016/j.hrtlng.2007.05.007

Campbell, M. L. (2010). Assessing respiratory distress when the patient cannot report dyspnea. *The Nursing Clinics of North America, 45*(3), 363–373. https://doi.org/10.1016/j.cnur.2010.03.001

Campbell, M. L. (2011). Dyspnea. *American Association of Critical-Care Nurses, 22*(3), 257–264.

Campbell, M. L. (2012). Dyspnea prevalence, trajectories, and measurement in critical care and at life's end. *Current Opinion in Supportive & Palliative Care, 6*(2), 168–171. https://doi.org/10.1097/SPC.0b013e328352b67f

Campbell, M. L. (2015). Caring for dying patients in the intensive care unit: Managing pain, dyspnea, anxiety, delirium, and death rattle. *AACN Advanced Critical Care, 26*(2), 110–120; quiz 121-122. https://doi.org/10.1097/NCI.0000000000000077

Campbell, M. L., & Templin, T. N. (2015). Intensity cut-points for the respiratory distress observation scale. *Palliative Medicine, 29*(5), 436–442. https://doi.org/10.1177/0269216314564238

Campbell, M. L., Templin, T., & Walch, J. (2010). A respiratory distress observation scale for patients unable to self-report dyspnea. *Journal of Palliative Medicine, 13*(3), 285–289. https://doi.org/10.1089/jpm.2009.0229

Chung, S., & Long, C. (1984). A study of the revised State-Trait Anxiety Inventory. *Psychological Testing, 31*, 27–36.

Gift, A. G. (1989). Validation of a vertical visual analogue scale as a measure of clinical dyspnea. *Rehabilitation Nursing, 14*(6), 323–325. https://doi.org/10.1002/j.2048-7940.1989.tb01129.x

Gift, A. G., & Narsavage, G. (1998). Validity of the numeric rating scale as a measure of dyspnea. *American Journal of Critical Care, 7*(3), 200–204.

Herigstad, M. M., Hayen, A., Reinecke, A., & Pattinson, K. T. (2016). Development of a dyspnoea word cue set for studies of emotional processing in COPD. *Respiratory Physiology & Neurobiology, 223*, 37–42. https://doi.org/10.1016/j.resp.2015.12.006

Hu, J., & Meek, P. (2005). Health-related quality of life in individuals with chronic obstructive pulmonary disease. *Heart & Lung, 34*(6), 415–422. https://doi.org/10.1016/j.hrtlng.2005.03.008

Lu, C. J. (2011). Reliability and validity of research tools. In S. Lee (Ed.), *Nursing research: Principles and practice* (4th ed., pp. 327–340). Taipei City, Taiwan, ROC: Farseeing. (Original work published in Chinese)

Mahler, D. A., Ward, J., Waterman, L. A., McCusker, C., ZuWallack, R., & Baird, J. C. (2009). Patient-reported dyspnea in COPD reliability and association with stage of disease. *Chest, 136*(6), 1473–1479. https://doi.org/10.1378/chest.09-0934

Parshall, M. B., Schwartzstein, R. M., Adams, L., Banzett, R. B., Manning, H. L., Bourbeau, J., ... American Thoracic Society Committee on Dyspnea. (2012). An official American Thoracic Society statement: Update on the mechanisms, assessment, and management of dyspnea. *American Journal of Respiratory and Critical Care Medicine, 185*(4), 435–452. https://doi.org/10.1164/rccm.201111-2042ST

Persichini, R., Gay, F., Schmidt, M., Mayaux, J., Demoule, A., Morélot-Panzini, P. C., & Similowski, T. (2015). Diagnostic accuracy of respiratory distress observation scales as surrogates of dyspnea self-report in intensive care unit patients. *Anesthesiology, 123*(4), 830–837. https://doi.org/10.1097/ALN.0000000000000805

Pianosi, P. T., Zhang, Z., Hernandez, P., & Huebner, M. (2016). Measuring dyspnea and perceived exertion in healthy adults and with respiratory disease: New pictorial scales. *Sports Medicine Open, 2*, 17. https://doi.org/10.1186/s40798-015-0038-4

Tusman, G., Bohm, S. H., & Suarez-Sipmann, F. (2017). Advanced uses of pulse oximetry for monitoring mechanically ventilated patients. *Anesthesia and Analgesia, 124*(1), 62–71.

Readiness for Behavior Change in Patients Living With Ischemic Heart Disease

Nidal F. ESHAH

ABSTRACT

Background: Readiness for behavioral change may be evaluated by assessing the patient's stage of change, as described in the transtheoretical model. Identifying readiness to change in patients with ischemic heart disease may enhance the effectiveness of interventions that target risk reduction and lifestyle modification.

Purpose: This study was designed to assess the readiness of patients with ischemic heart disease to change health behaviors as well as to identify the factors that significantly predict this change.

Methods: A descriptive correlation design approach was adopted, and a convenience sample of 122 patients with ischemic heart disease was recruited from an outpatient cardiac clinic. Readiness for behavioral change was evaluated by assessing the stages of change of the participants, as described in the transtheoretical model. Data on readiness to change were collected using the "readiness for lifestyle change inventory."

Results: A total of 62.2% and 43.4% of the participants were in the precontemplation phase of change for "cease smoking" and "be physically active," respectively; about 33% of the patients were in the maintenance phase for "control weight"; 36.1% were in the maintenance phase for "reduce consumption of high-fat foods"; and 51.6% and 57.4% were in the maintenance phase for "eat fruits and vegetables" and "practice relaxation," respectively. Participants who were overweight or obese showed higher readiness to practice physical activity, and those with high cholesterol levels showed a higher readiness to reduce the amount of fat in their diet. Higher income was found to predict higher readiness to eat fruits and vegetables.

Conclusions: Patients are not adequately ready to change their health-related behaviors. Higher cardiovascular risk predicts higher readiness to change health behaviors.

Key Words:
behavior, change, heart, readiness, stage of change.

Introduction

Among cardiovascular diseases, ischemic heart disease (IHD) is the leading cause of death worldwide (Go et al., 2013). Previous studies have documented the associations among risk factors, unhealthy lifestyles, and suffering from IHD. A high prevalence of risk factors as well as unhealthy behaviors among patients experiencing cardiovascular diseases and IHD have also been observed (Masana, Ros, Sudano, Angoulvant, & Lifestyle Expert Working Group, 2017; Micha et al., 2017). Jordan faces a high prevalence of IHD, which is the leading cause of death in the country and responsible for 17% of all deaths there (World Health Organization, 2015). Adult Jordanians are widely challenged by cardiovascular risk factors, including obesity (34.5% of adult Jordanians), smoking (26.5%), hypertension (23.2%), and elevated blood glucose (17.7%; World Health Organization, 2015). Moreover, a previous Jordanian study documented a critical shortage of public knowledge about IHD and its risk factors, which has made IHD a largely unrecognized killer in Jordan (Eshah, 2014).

The successful management of IHD depends on successfully controlling the related risk factors (Go et al., 2013). Fortunately, most risk factors are modifiable, and patients may reduce the risk of experiencing IHD if they control these risk factors and pursue a healthy lifestyle (Go et al., 2013). Therefore, researchers started building intervention programs that targeted risk factors and lifestyle modifications (Wolever et al., 2011). Several previous studies dealt with risk behaviors and risk factors as possible predictors of the motivation to change behaviors (Larson et al., 2018; Morris, Ko, Hutcheson, & Quyyumi, 2018; Noureddine & Massouh, 2019).

As a part of these intervention programs, researchers looked for possible indicators of the successful achievement of their interventions as well as the significant predictors of risk reduction and lifestyle modification. Researchers subsequently became interested in assessing the concept of readiness to change as a possible indicator and predictor of lifestyle modification (Frame, Green, Herr, & Taylor, 2003; Prugger et al., 2015; Steptoe, Kerry, Rink, & Hilton, 2001; Wolever et al., 2011). Many studies highlight the importance of considering stages of change as described by the Transtheoretical Model (TTM) when designing and implementing cardiac rehabilitation and risk reduction programs (Mochari-Geenberger, Terry, & Mosca, 2010; Toth-Capelli, Brawer, Plumb, & Daskalakis, 2013).

PhD, RN, CNS, Associate Professor, Faculty of Nursing, Zarqa University, Jordan.

The TTM of health behavior change, described by James Prochaska and colleagues in 1977 (Prochaska & DiClemente, 2005), facilitates the monitoring of changes in daily-lifestyle-related health behaviors. This model was gradually refined into its current form over the following two decades. The model, based on several related psychotherapy theories, has generated significant interest in the literature in recent years (Prochaska & DiClemente, 2005).

The TTM includes several constructs, including stage of change, process of change, decisional balance, self-efficacy, and temptation (Norcross, Krebs, & Prochaska, 2011), which produce a tool to help understand changes in health-related behaviors in humans.

This study focuses on the stage of change construct. "Change of behavior" may be defined as the process of passing through different stages over time (Norcross et al., 2011). The TTM defines five stages of behavior change, including precontemplation, contemplation, preparation, action, and maintenance. Precontemplation is the stage at which a patient is not yet ready to change and does not think that she or he needs to change her or his behavior. Contemplation is the stage at which a patient begins to weigh up the pros and cons of changing a behavior. Preparation is the stage at which a patient develops the intention to start changing her or his behavior in the near future. Action is the stage at which a patient has changed her or his behavior for a period of less than 6 months. Finally, maintenance is the stage at which a patient has changed her or his behavior for a period of longer than 6 months (Norcross et al., 2011).

The model has been used for various issues, including stress management (McKee, Bannon, Kerins, & FitzGerald, 2007), depression prevention (Levesque et al., 2011), hypertension management (Drevenhorn, Bengtson, Allen, Säljö, & Kjellgren, 2007), adherence to lipid-lowering agents (Johnson et al., 2006), weight control (Ceccarini, Borrello, Pietrabissa, Manzoni, & Castelnuovo, 2015), and smoking cessation (Chouinard & Robichaud-Ekstrand, 2005).

Studies that assessed stages of change in cardiac patients highlighted some interesting findings about factors that relate to readiness for behavior change. Doherty, Steptoe, Rink, Kendrick, and Hilton (1998) found higher-risk patients more ready to change their behaviors than lower-risk peers. For example, they found patients with higher cholesterol levels more ready to reduce fat in their diet and those who were physically inactive and overweight more ready to increase physical activities (Doherty et al., 1998). In an interventional study that targeted control over modifiable cardiac risk factors, researchers reported significant improvements in the readiness of patients to reduce consumption of fats, increase physical activities, and cease smoking (Steptoe et al., 2001). Another study reported an improvement in patient readiness to reduce fat intake and increase fruit and vegetable intake (Frame et al., 2003). Another study that assessed readiness to change in patients with heart failure reported the surprising finding that, although all of the participants committed to avoid tobacco, engage in regular physical activity, and lose weight, an assessment of the stages of change conducted afterward revealed that only a small number had actually achieved the recommended level of behavioral change (Sneed & Paul, 2003).

In this study, TTM is used to link the data from the measurement tool to the five stages of change to produce a clear picture of the readiness of patients with IHD to change their health-related behaviors. "Readiness to change" has been defined as a psychologically impeded intent to adopt a new pattern of doing things (Andreasen, 1991). Identifying the stages of change in patients describes their current readiness to change their health behaviors, which in turn provides nurses with a clear picture and a reference point to prepare patients to modify their health-related behaviors. Therefore, nurses and other related healthcare providers should focus on increasing patient readiness to change by using special techniques such as motivational interventions, which have proven to be a successful tool for achieving behavior change in at-risk patients (Eaton et al., 2018). Because of the scarcity of cardiac rehabilitation centers in Jordan, nurses may practice health education about lifestyle modification either in their patients' rooms before discharge or in outpatient clinics. The therapeutic behaviors of motivational interview consist of open-ended questions, reflective listening, and supportive statements (Miller & Rollnick, 2012) that lead patients to self-exploration (Borsari & Carey, 2005).

In addition, considering the stages of change may help build better, more successful cardiac rehabilitation programs by allowing the preparation of content that is specific to each stage of behavior change. Therefore, this study aims to assess readiness to change of patients with IHD to identify the stage of change for each of the targeted modifiable risk factors and to identify the factors that significantly predict the readiness of patients to change their health-related behaviors.

This study asked the following research questions: (a) "How are the patient participants with IHD distributed over the five stages of change in terms of health-related behaviors (i.e., smoking cessation, physical activity, weight control, control over eating a high-fat diet, eating fruits and vegetables, and practicing relaxation)?" and (b) "What are the predictors of health behavior change in patients with IHD?"

Methods

Design and Sample

This study implemented a cross-sectional descriptive correlation design. The required sample size, which was calculated by setting a medium effect size = 0.15, power = 80%, and $\alpha = .05$, was 118 participants for testing 10 predictors (gender, age, educational level, employment status, monthly income, marital status, smoking status, physical activity, cholesterol level, and body mass index) using a logistic regression model. The 10 predictors were proposed based on the literature related to the risk factors of cardiovascular diseases. These factors were chosen and treated as possible predictors based on assumptions grounded in the "health belief model," which states that perceived susceptibility to a certain disease will affect a person's future behaviors related to that disease (Green & Murphy, 2014).

A convenience sample was recruited by inviting patients with IHD who attended an outpatient clinic at one of the biggest private healthcare centers in the Jordanian capital, Amman, for regular routine follow-up care. Eligibility criteria included a previous medical history confirming myocardial infarction or angina for more than 1 year and no mental or physical disability that may limit the ability to change behaviors.

Data Collection Procedures

Data were collected from March to September 2017. A research assistant met patients in the waiting room. The goal of the study was explained to all potentially eligible patients. To confirm patient diagnosis, the medical files of those patients who were willing to participate in the study were checked. Next, meetings with those patients who satisfied the study's inclusion criteria were arranged to collect demographical and clinical history and to provide the study questionnaire.

The questionnaires were completed either independently by the patient or, when a patient was illiterate or unable/unwilling to read the instrument, by the research assistant. In cases of the latter, the research assistant did not influence responses and simply recorded the patients' choices.

Measures

Data related to the readiness to change stage were collected using the "readiness for lifestyle change inventory." This scale was developed by Krisko-Hagel (2009) to assess the association between the readiness to change stage and commitment to a cardiac rehabilitation program. The scale, consisting of six multiple-choice questions, was designed to evaluate readiness for change in terms of the following six behaviors: smoking cessation, physical activity, weight control, control over eating a high-fat diet, eating fruits and vegetables, and practicing relaxation (Krisko-Hagel, 2009).

Patients were asked a question regarding each of these behaviors and asked to respond using the answer that best reflected their condition. The questions were worded in a positive format to reflect the desired healthy outcome (e.g., "Do you exercise regularly?"). Five possible answers were given for each question, with each answer reflecting a specific stage of behavior change as described in the TTM. Example of these possible answers are "Yes, and I have been for more than 6 months" (maintenance stage); "Yes, and I have been for less than 6 months" (action stage); "No, but I intend to start in the next month" (preparation stage); "No, but I intend to start in the next 6 months" (contemplation stage); and "No, and I do not intend to start in the next 6 months" (precontemplation). The two questions addressing behaviors related to smoking cessation and weight control had, respectively, one additional response, namely, "No, I have never smoked" and "No, I do not need to lose weight." Patients were requested to choose the answer that best reflected their actual status (Krisko-Hagel, 2009).

Although multiple-choice questions are used frequently in nursing research, debate about the best methods of assessing the validity and reliability of multiple-choice questions continues (Considine, Botti, & Thomas, 2005; Masters et al., 2001). According to Haladyna (2004), the multiple-choice question format provides high reliability because of the objective scoring system used. The face validity for "readiness for lifestyle change inventory" was initially evaluated and supported by the scale developer (Krisko-Hagel, 2009).

Ethical Considerations

Approval number 1-1/2015 was assigned to this study by the responsible institutional review boards. Each patient was told explicitly that participation in the study was voluntary, that the collected data would be used only for scientific purposes, and that results would be reported in groups for the whole sample without any personal identifiers. Patients who decided to participate signed an informed consent form before receiving the study questionnaire.

Data Analysis

Data were analyzed using SPSS Version 22 (IBM, Armonk, NY, USA). Descriptive statistics were used to describe the sample, present the demographic and clinical characteristics of the participants, identify the prevalence of risk factors among the participants, and summarize the status of participants with regard to stages of change. Means and standard deviations were calculated for the continuous variables, whereas frequencies and proportions were calculated for categorical variables. Data regarding the stages of change for the six healthy behaviors were categorized dichotomously ("ready for change" and "not ready for change"). The cutoff point distinguishing "ready for change" from "not ready for change" was identified based on the TTM, in which, for each health behavior, participants in the precontemplation, contemplation, and preparation phases are considered "not ready for (behavior) change" and those in the action and maintenance phases are considered "ready for (behavior) change." Next, a binary logistic regression model was used for each of the six healthy behaviors to predict readiness for behavioral change. The proposed predictors entered the regression model as one block (enter method).

Results

The study enrolled 122 participants with confirmed diagnoses of IHD. Of these, 25.4% experienced myocardial infarction and 74.6% experienced unstable angina. The age of the participants ranged from 35 to 83 years, with an average age of 54.3 years, and the average duration with IHD up to the point of data collection was 7.3 years. Most participants were men (60.7%), were married (86.1%), had a low educational background (56.6%), were retired (61.5%), and earned a low monthly income (72.1%; Table 1).

Screening for prevalence of cardiovascular-related risk factors revealed a high frequency of smoking behaviors (60.7%), being overweight or obese (63.9%), hyperlipidemia (60.6%), and physical inactivity (68.9%; Table 1).

Stages of Change and Health Behaviors

Two thirds (62.2%) and 43.4% of the participants who were active smokers (n = 74) were in the precontemplation phase for "cease smoking" and "be physically active," respectively (Table 1). Although 108 of the participants self-reported being aware of the need to control their weight, only one third (33.3%) of this subgroup self-reported as being in the maintenance phase for "control weight" (Table 2).

TABLE 1.

Participant Characteristics and Prevalence of Cardiovascular Risk Factors (N = 122)

Variable	*n*	%
Gender		
Male	74	60.7
Female	48	39.3
Marital status		
Single	17	13.9
Married	105	86.1
Educational level		
Secondary school or below	69	56.6
More than secondary school	53	43.4
Employment status		
Retired	75	61.5
Currently employed	47	38.5
Monthly income		
Low	88	72.1
Intermediate or high	34	27.9
Smoking cigarettes		
No	48	39.3
Yes	74	60.7
Smoking water pipe		
No	85	69.7
Yes	37	30.3
Weight or BMI		
Normal	44	36.1
Overweight or obese	78	63.9
Cholesterol level		
Not elevated	48	39.4
Elevated	74	60.6
Physical activity		
Active	38	31.1
Inactive	84	68.9
Family history of CVDs		
Negative	81	66.4
Positive	41	33.6

Note. BMI = body mass index; CVDs = cardiovascular diseases.

In addition, slightly over one third of the participants (36.1%) were in the maintenance phase for "reduce consumption of high-fat foods," whereas 51.6% and 57.4% reported being in the maintenance phase for "eating fruits and vegetables" and "practice relaxation," respectively (Table 2).

Predictors of Readiness for Behavior Change

Although the binary logistic regression model explained 27% of the variance in readiness for behavior change related to "cease smoking" (Nagelkerke R^2 = .27), it was not statistically significant in predicting whether participants were ready to change their smoking behaviors (χ^2 = 13.43, p = .49).

However, the binary logistic regression model significantly predicted readiness for behavior change in the category "practicing physical activity" (χ^2 = 55.32, p = .001), with body mass index serving as the most significant predictor (Table 3). This model explained 52% of the variance in readiness to change for "practicing physical activity" (Nagelkerke R^2 = .526), with participants in the "normal weight" category 0.71 times less likely to be ready to practice physical activity than their peers in the "overweight and obese" category (odds ratio = 0.71).

Although the binary logistic regression model explained 23% of the variance in readiness for behavior change related to "control weight" (Nagelkerke R^2 = .23), it was not statistically significant in predicting if participants were ready to change their weight control behaviors (χ^2 = 20.54, p = .11).

The binary logistic regression model significantly predicted behavior change readiness for "reduce consumption of high-fat foods" (χ^2 = 25.81, p = .02), with age and cholesterol level as the most significant predictors (Table 3). This model explained 25% of the variance in readiness to change for "reduce consumption of high-fat foods" (Nagelkerke R^2 = .25). A 1-year increase in age increased the probability of the participants being ready to control eating a high-fat diet by 1.07 (odds ratio = 1.07). Furthermore, participants in the "normal cholesterol level" category were 0.55 times less likely to be ready to control eating a high-fat diet than their "high cholesterol level" peers (odds ratio = 0.55).

The binary logistic regression model significantly predicted the readiness for behavior change for "eating fruits and vegetables" (χ^2 = 35.91, p = .001), with income and employment status as the most significant predictors (Table 3). This model explained 36% of the variance in readiness to change for "eating fruits and vegetables" (Nagelkerke R^2 = .36). Moreover, participants in the "intermediate and high income" category were 13.31 times more likely to be ready to eat fruits and vegetables than their "low-income" peers (odds ratio = 13.31). In addition, participants who were currently working were 4.06 times more likely to be ready to eat fruits and vegetables than their retired peers (odds ratio = 4.06).

The binary logistic regression model significantly predicted readiness for behavior change for "practice relaxation" (χ^2 = 33.51, p = .002), with smoking cigarettes, physical activity, educational level, and age as the most significant predictors (Table 3). This model explained 33% of

TABLE 2.

Stages of Change for the Six Health Behaviors (N = 122)

		Stage of Change									
		Precontemplation		Contemplation		Preparation		Action		Maintenance	
Behavior	*n*	*n*	%	*n*	%	*n*	%	*n*	%	*n*	%
Cease smoking	74[a]	46	62.2	7	9.5	8	10.8	5	6.8	8	10.8
Be physically active	122	53	43.4	19	15.6	16	13.1	15	12.3	19	15.6
Control weight	108[b]	38	35.2	3	2.8	16	14.8	15	13.9	36	33.3
Reduce consumption of high-fat foods	122	36	29.5	10	8.2	10	8.2	22	18.0	44	36.1
Eat fruits and vegetables	122	20	16.4	–	–	15	12.3	24	19.7	63	51.6
Practice relaxation	122	13	10.7	16	13.1	10	8.2	13	10.7	70	57.4

[a]Not intended to be answered by all patients, because some stated they never smoked cigarettes. [b]Not intended to be answered by all patients, because some stated they were at an ideal body weight.

the variance in readiness to change for "practice relaxation" (Nagelkerke R^2 = .33). Moreover, participants who were smokers were 0.15 times less likely to be ready to practice relaxation than their nonsmoker peers (odds ratio = 0.15), those who were physically inactive were 4.6 times more likely to be ready to practice relaxation than their physically active peers (odds ratio = 4.6), and those with better than a secondary school education were 2.96 times more likely to be ready to practice relaxation than their less educated peers (odds ratio = 2.96). Finally, every 1-year increase in age was associated with a 1.05-times increase in probability of being ready to practice relaxation (odds ratio = 1.05).

Discussion

This study included patients with an established diagnosis of IHD. About two thirds experienced unstable angina, whereas the remaining one third experienced myocardial infarction. Consistent with previous Jordanian studies (Eshah, 2013; Haddad, Saleh, & Eshah, 2017), the results of this study documented a high prevalence of cardiac-related risk factors. The high prevalence of these risk factors among the study sample may be responsible for the participants previously experiencing IHD and may increase the risks of their suffering from other episodes of IHD in the future.

Irrespective of the high prevalence of risk factors in the study sample, only a limited number of patients in this study showed a readiness to change their health-related behaviors. Similar to previous studies (Noureddine & Massouh, 2019; Prugger et al., 2015), about two thirds of the smokers in this study reported being in the preaction stage of behavior change, which indicates little or no intention to cease smoking. Moreover, about half of the sample had no intention of increasing their daily physical activity levels. Similar findings were reported by (Sneed & Paul, 2003), who stated that, although patients believe that they are doing well in controlling their risk

TABLE 3.

Significant Predictors for Change of Health Behaviors (N = 122)

Outcome Behavior and Predictor	*B*	Wald	*p*	Odds Ratio	95% CI for Odds Ratio
Be physically active					
Body mass index	−3.45	5.51	.01	0.71	[0.53, 0.94]
Reduce consumption of high fat foods					
Age	0.07	8.74	< .01	1.07	[1.02, 1.12]
Cholesterol level	−0.58	4.99	.02	0.55	[0.33, 0.93]
Eat fruits and vegetables					
Income	2.58	8.99	< .01	13.31	[2.45, 72.31]
Employment status	1.41	4.79	.02	4.06	[1.15, 14.26]
Practice relaxation					
Smoking cigarettes	−1.85	7.96	< .01	0.15	[0.04, 0.56]
Physical activity	1.52	5.48	.01	4.60	[1.28, 16.54]
Education	1.08	3.95	.04	2.96	[1.01, 8.66]
Age	0.05	3.93	.04	1.05	[1.00, 1.11]

Note. CI = confidence interval.

factors, a limited number of them actually performed activities to control these risk factors effectively. These findings may be attributed to a false belief among patients that they are controlling their own health status as well as a lack of appropriate and effective interventions that may improve awareness and correct self-perceptions regarding personal health status.

The stages of change as reflected by the TTM indicate that overall readiness to change healthy behaviors among the study sample fell below expectations. Specifically, the participants were more ready to change their behaviors related to practicing relaxation, eating fruits and vegetables, and reducing the amount of fat in their diets and were not ready for smoking cessation, physical activity, and weight control (Table 2). This finding is consistent with previous studies that reported higher levels of readiness among participants to change behaviors related to consuming more fruits and vegetables and reducing consumption of fats (Frame et al., 2003; Noureddine & Massouh, 2019).

Changing behaviors related to practicing relaxation, eating fruits and vegetables, and reducing fat intake may be achievable through simple intervention programs such as education interventions that increase patient knowledge and awareness about the importance of modifying these behaviors (Eshah, Bond, & Froelicher, 2010). However, behaviors such as smoking cessation, physical activity, and weight control may require interventions that are more advanced and specialized (McKee et al., 2007; Mochari-Greenberger, Terry, & Mosca, 2010; Steptoe et al., 2001). These latter interventions should combine activities such as education, counseling, and skill-building techniques. Moreover, changing these behaviors may require the availability of sufficient infrastructure and resources such as referrals to smoking cessation clinics and dieticians as well as the availability of walking yards and sports facilities (Eshah et al., 2010).

The low readiness among the participants to stop smoking, engage in physical activity, and practice weight control behaviors may relate to the lack of cardiac rehabilitation centers in Jordan and the general paucity of professional assistance available in-country to help patients quit smoking and achieve weight control (Eshah, 2011). Although Jordan has a relatively high level of healthcare for the region, attention to cardiac rehabilitation remains inadequate. This may relate to resource availability, the present focus on primary healthcare, and/or the lack of healthcare decision-maker attention on rehabilitation. Thus, healthcare providers and cardiac researchers must increasingly prioritize the importance of cardiac rehabilitation to convince decision makers regarding the important role of specialized cardiac rehabilitation centers in improving the quality of life of cardiac patients and in reducing cardiac-disease-related suffering and mortality.

Moreover, physical activity is not a daily routine in Jordan, and so cardiac patients are unlikely to respond to traditional instructions on increasing levels of daily physical activities (Eshah, 2011).

In terms of predicting readiness to change health-related behaviors, the results of this study echoed those of a previous study (Doherty et al., 1998) that found that suffering from higher risks predicted more advancement in the stage of change described by TTM and, consequently, greater readiness to change behaviors. In this study, greater readiness to practice physical activity was predicted by being overweight. In addition, readiness to control eating a high-fat diet was predicted by having a high cholesterol level. In this study, being at a higher risk may intensify the feeling of susceptibility to disease recurrence, which may in turn motivate behavior change.

Eating fruits and vegetables was predicted by a higher income and by being employed. Thus, this behavior may relate to economic status, as people with higher incomes and/or who are currently employed may have relatively more resources. This finding echoes that of Adams and White (2007), who stated that people with higher incomes are more ready to change their behavior than those with lower incomes. Jordan is a middle-income country, and most Jordanians earn a middle-to-low monthly income. Thus, people of lower economic status may perceive buying more fruits and vegetables as an extra burden on their budget and, consequently, are less ready to change their fruit and vegetable purchasing behaviors.

Being physically inactive and having a higher level of education predicted readiness to practice relaxation. People who are physically inactive may perceive themselves as "more fit" to practice relaxation and (falsely) believe that relaxation involves minimal physical exertion. Those who are highly educated may be more knowledgeable about relaxation techniques as well as the benefits of practicing relaxation. Surprisingly, in this study, tobacco smokers were less likely to practice relaxation. This finding is contradictory to a frequently used argument used by tobacco smokers that smoking leads to relaxation.

The generalizability of the study findings should be considered in light of several study limitations, including the relatively small size of the sample, the sampling technique used, the reliance on self-reported measurements, and the collection of the data from one site only. Future studies should collect data from larger samples and include patients from various healthcare settings. Furthermore, it will be helpful to compare the construct of readiness to change with the actual adoption of healthy lifestyles.

Finally, studying readiness for health-related behavioral change over an extended period using a longitudinal study design may provide researchers with valuable information to better understand behavior change processes.

Conclusions

Readiness to change health-related behaviors varies among patients with IHD. Two thirds of the participants in this study self-reported being ready to practice relaxation and to eat more fruits and vegetables. Furthermore, half of the participants self-reported being ready to reduce their fat intake and control their weight. However, only one third self-reported being ready to increase physical activity and to stop smoking.

Higher cardiovascular risk predicts higher readiness to change health behaviors. The participants who were overweight or obese showed a higher readiness to engage in regular physical activity, whereas those with high cholesterol levels showed a higher readiness to reduce the amount of fat in their diet. In addition, higher income predicts greater readiness to eat fruits and vegetables.

Implications for Nursing Practice

The findings of this study may assist nurses and other healthcare providers worldwide who are dealing with patients living with chronic heart diseases to modify current and develop new practices related to risk reduction and secondary intervention programs. Each of the points below may contribute positively to the improvement of these programs:

- The content and nature of interventions to modify lifestyle and control risk factors should be prepared and tailored individually based on the patient's stage of change.
- Nurses may utilize tools that are based on the TTM of behavioral change to evaluate patients' current stages of behavioral change.
- Clinical nurses should set realistic goals for moving patients forward gradually through the stages of change, starting from their current reference point.
- Interventions targeting specific behaviors may need to be changed or tailored based on patient needs. For instance, behaviors such as smoking, physical activity, and weight control may require different interventional strategies than those used for behaviors such as eating fruits and vegetables, reducing fat intake, and practicing relaxation.
- Nurses and other healthcare practitioners must tailor interventions to target lifestyle modification and focus on increasing the readiness to change of patients with IHD as a medium for behavior change.
- The five stages of change as described by TTM may be used to reflect the degree of patient readiness for behavior change.

Acknowledgment

This research was funded by the deanship of research in Zarqa University, Jordan.

References

Adams, J., & White, M. (2007). Are the stages of change socioeconomically distributed? A scoping review. *American Journal of Health Promotion, 21*(4), 237–247. https://doi.org/10.4278/0890-1171-21.4.237

Andreasen, A. R. (1991). Readiness to change: Theoretical, empirical and managerial issues. In G. Antonides, W. Arts, & W. F. van Raaij (Eds.), *The consumption of time and the timing of consumption* (pp. 138–148). Amsterdam, The Netherlands: North-Holland.

Borsari, B., & Carey, K. B. (2005). Two brief alcohol interventions for mandated college students. *Psychology of Addictive Behaviors, 19*(3), 2960. https://doi.org/10.1037/0893-164X.19.3.296

Ceccarini, M., Borrello, M., Pietrabissa, G., Manzoni, G. M., & Castelnuovo, G. (2015). Assessing motivation and readiness to change for weight management and control: An in-depth evaluation of three sets of instruments. *Frontiers in Psychology, 6*, 511. https://doi.org/10.3389/fpsyg.2015.00511

Chouinard, M. C., & Robichaud-Ekstrand, S. (2005). The effectiveness of a nursing inpatient smoking cessation program in individuals with cardiovascular disease. *Nursing Research, 54*(4), 243–254. https://doi.org/10.1097/00006199-200507000-00006

Considine, J., Botti, M., & Thomas, S. (2005). Design, format, validity and reliability of multiple choice questions for use in nursing research and education. *Collegian, 12*(1), 19–24. https://doi.org/10.1016/S1322-7696(08)60478-3

Doherty, S. C., Steptoe, A., Rink, E., Kendrick, T., & Hilton, S. (1998). Readiness to change health behaviours among patients at high risk of cardiovascular disease. *Journal of Cardiovascular Risk, 5*(3), 147–153. https://doi.org/10.1177/174182679800500302

Drevenhorn, E., Bengtson, A., Allen, J. K., Säljö, R., & Kjellgren, K. I. (2007). Counselling on lifestyle factors in hypertension care after training on the stages of change model. *European Journal of Cardiovascular Nursing, 6*(1), 46–53. https://doi.org/10.1016/j.ejcnurse.2006.03.007

Eaton, E. M., Magill, M., Capone, C., Cramer, M. A., Mastroleo, N. R., Reavy, R., ... Borsari, B. (2018). Mechanisms of behavior change within peer-implemented alcohol interventions. *Journal of Studies on Alcohol and Drugs, 79*(2), 208–216. https://doi.org/10.15288/jsad.2018.79.208

Eshah, N. F. (2011). Jordanian acute coronary syndrome patients' learning needs: Implications for cardiac rehabilitation and secondary prevention programs. *Nursing & Health Sciences, 13*(3), 238–245. https://doi.org/10.1111/j.1442-2018.2011.00608.x

Eshah, N. F. (2013). Knowledge of stroke and cerebrovascular risk factors among Jordanian adults. *Journal of Neuroscience Nursing, 45*(5), E13–E19. https://doi.org/10.1097/JNN.0b013e31829db99f

Eshah, N. F. (2014). Ischemic heart diseases: The unrecognized killer in the Jordanian community. *Journal of Behavioral Health, 3*(1), 58–64. https://doi.org/10.5455/jbh.20131226115903

Eshah, N. F., Bond, A. E., & Froelicher, E. S. (2010). The effects of a cardiovascular disease prevention program on knowledge and adoption of a heart healthy lifestyle in Jordanian working adults. *European Journal of Cardiovascular Nursing, 9*(4), 244–253. https://doi.org/10.1016/j.ejcnurse.2010.02.002

Frame, C. J., Green, C. G., Herr, D. G., & Taylor, M. L. (2003). A 2-year stage of change evaluation of dietary fat and fruit and vegetable intake behaviors of cardiac rehabilitation patients. *American Journal of Health Promotion, 17*(6), 361–368. https://doi.org/10.4278/0890-1171-17.6.361

Go, A. S., Mozaffarian, D., Roger, V. L., Benjamin, E. J., Berry, J. D., Borden, W. B., ... Turner, M.; On behalf of the American Heart

Association Statistics Committee and Stroke Statistics Subcommittee. (2013). Heart disease and stroke statistics—2013 update: A report from the American Heart Association. *Circulation, 127*(1), e6–e245. https://doi.org/10.1161/CIR.0b013e31828124ad

Green, E. C., & Murphy, E. (2014). *Health belief model. The Wiley Blackwell encyclopedia of health, illness, behavior, and society* (pp. 766–769). New York, NY: John Wiley & Sons. https://doi.org/10.1002/9781118410868.wbehibs410

Haddad, N. E., Saleh, M. N., & Eshah, N. F. (2017). Cardiac catheterisation and patients' anxiety levels. *British Journal of Cardiac Nursing, 12*(7), 353–358. https://doi.org/10.12968/bjca.2017.12.7.353

Haladyna, T. M. (2004). *Developing and validating multiple-choice test items* (3rd ed.). Abingdon, UK: Routledge.

Johnson, S. S., Driskell, M. M., Johnson, J. L., Dyment, S. J., Prochaska, J. O., Prochaska, J. M., & Bourne, L. (2006). Transtheoretical model intervention for adherence to lipid-lowering drugs. *Disease Management, 9*(2), 102–114. https://doi.org/10.1089/dis.2006.9.102

Krisko-Hagel, K. A. (2009). *Predictors for participation in a cardiac rehabilitation program feasibility study* (Doctoral dissertation). Retrieved from http://hdl.handle.net/11299/58442

Larson, N., Chen, Y., Wall, M., Winkler, M. R., Goldschmit, A. B., & Neumark-Sztainer, D. (2018). Personal, behavioral, and environmental predictors of healthy weight maintenance during the transition to adulthood. *Preventive Medicine, 113*, 80–90. https://doi.org/10.1016/j.ypmed.2018.04.027

Levesque, D. A., Van Marter, D. F., Schneider, R. J., Bauer, M. R., Goldberg, D. N., Prochaska, J. O., & Prochaska, J. M. (2011). Randomized trial of a computer-tailored intervention for patients with depression. *American Journal of Health Promotion, 26*(2), 77–89. https://doi.org/10.4278/ajhp.090123-QUAN-27

Masana, L., Ros, E., Sudano, I., & Angoulvant, D., , Lifestyle Expert Working Group. (2017). Is there a role for lifestyle changes in cardiovascular prevention? What, when and how. *Atherosclerosis Supplements, 26*, 2–15. https://doi.org/10.1016/S1567-5688(17)30020-X

Masters, J. C., Hulsmeyer, B. S., Pike, M. E., Leichty, K., Miller, M. T., & Verst, A. L. (2001). Assessment of multiple-choice questions in selected test banks accompanying text books used in nursing education. *Journal of Nursing Education, 40*(1), 25–32.

McKee, G., Bannon, J., Kerins, M., & FitzGerald, G. (2007). Changes in diet, exercise and stress behaviours using the stages of change model in cardiac rehabilitation patients. *European Journal of Cardiovascular Nursing, 6*(3), 233–240. https://doi.org/10.1016/J.EJCNURSE.2006.10.002

Micha, R., Peñalvo, J. L., Cudhea, F., Imamura, F., Rehm, C. D., & Mozaffarian, D. (2017). Association between dietary factors and mortality from heart disease, stroke, and type 2 diabetes in the United States. *JAMA, 317*(9), 912–924. https://doi.org/10.1001/jama.2017.0947

Miller, W. R., & Rollnick, S. (2012). *Motivational interviewing: Helping people change* (3rd ed.). New York, NY: Guilford Press.

Mochari-Greenberger, H., Terry, M. B., & Mosca, L. (2010). Does stage of change modify the effectiveness of an educational intervention to improve diet among family members of hospitalized cardiovascular disease patients. *Journal of the American Dietetic Association, 110*(7), 1027–1035. https://doi.org//10.1016/j.jada.2010.04.012

Morris, A. A., Ko, Y. A., Hutcheson, S. H., & Quyyumi, A. (2018). Race/ethnic and sex differences in the association of atherosclerotic cardiovascular disease risk and healthy lifestyle behaviors. *Journal of the American Heart Association, 7*(10), e008250. https://doi.org/10.1161/JAHA.117.008250

Norcross, J. C., Krebs, P. M., & Prochaska, J. O. (2011). Stages of change. *Journal of Clinical Psychology, 67*(2), 143–154. https://doi.org/10.1002/jclp.20758

Noureddine, S., & Massouh, A. (2019). Factors associated with continued smoking in Lebanese patients with acute coronary syndrome. *The Journal of Cardiovascular Nursing, 34*(1), 94–98. https://doi.org/10.1097/JCN.0000000000000514

Prochaska, J. O., & DiClemente, C. C. (2005). The transtheoretical approach. In J. C. Norcross & M. R. Goldfried (Eds.), *Handbook of psychotherapy integration* (2nd ed., pp. 147–171). New York, NY: Oxford.

Prugger, C., Wellmann, J., Heidrich, J., De Bacquer, D., De Backer, G., Périer, M. C., ... Kotseva, K. (2015). Readiness for smoking cessation in coronary heart disease patients across Europe: Results from the EUROASPIRE III survey. *European Journal of Preventive Cardiology, 22*(9), 1212–1219. https://doi.org/10.1177/2047487314564728

Sneed, N. V., & Paul, S. C. (2003). Readiness for behavioral changes in patients with heart failure. *American Journal of Critical Care, 12*(5), 444–453.

Steptoe, A., Kerry, S., Rink, E., & Hilton, S. (2001). The impact of behavioral counseling on stage of change in fat intake, physical activity, and cigarette smoking in adults at increased risk of coronary heart disease. *American Journal of Public Health, 91*(2), 265–269.

Toth-Capelli, K. M., Brawer, R., Plumb, J., & Daskalakis, C. (2013). Stage of change and other predictors of participant retention in a behavioral weight management program in primary care. *Health Promotion Practice, 14*(3), 441–450. https://doi.org/10.1177/1524839912460871

Wolever, R. Q., Webber, D. M., Meunier, J. P., Greeson, J. M., Lausier, E. R., & Gaudet, T. W. (2011). Modifiable disease risk, readiness to change, and psychosocial functioning improve with integrative medicine immersion model. *Alternative Therapies in Health and Medicine, 17*(4), 38–47.

World Health Organization. (2015). *Country statistics and global health estimates by WHO and UN partners*. Retrieved from https://www.who.int/gho/countries/npl.pdf

Permissions

All chapters in this book were first published by Wolters Kluwer; hereby published with permission under the Creative Commons Attribution License or equivalent. Every chapter published in this book has been scrutinized by our experts. Their significance has been extensively debated. The topics covered herein carry significant findings which will fuel the growth of the discipline. They may even be implemented as practical applications or may be referred to as a beginning point for another development.

The contributors of this book come from diverse backgrounds, making this book a truly international effort. This book will bring forth new frontiers with its revolutionizing research information and detailed analysis of the nascent developments around the world.

We would like to thank all the contributing authors for lending their expertise to make the book truly unique. They have played a crucial role in the development of this book. Without their invaluable contributions this book wouldn't have been possible. They have made vital efforts to compile up to date information on the varied aspects of this subject to make this book a valuable addition to the collection of many professionals and students.

This book was conceptualized with the vision of imparting up-to-date information and advanced data in this field. To ensure the same, a matchless editorial board was set up. Every individual on the board went through rigorous rounds of assessment to prove their worth. After which they invested a large part of their time researching and compiling the most relevant data for our readers.

The editorial board has been involved in producing this book since its inception. They have spent rigorous hours researching and exploring the diverse topics which have resulted in the successful publishing of this book. They have passed on their knowledge of decades through this book. To expedite this challenging task, the publisher supported the team at every step. A small team of assistant editors was also appointed to further simplify the editing procedure and attain best results for the readers.

Apart from the editorial board, the designing team has also invested a significant amount of their time in understanding the subject and creating the most relevant covers. They scrutinized every image to scout for the most suitable representation of the subject and create an appropriate cover for the book.

The publishing team has been an ardent support to the editorial, designing and production team. Their endless efforts to recruit the best for this project, has resulted in the accomplishment of this book. They are a veteran in the field of academics and their pool of knowledge is as vast as their experience in printing. Their expertise and guidance has proved useful at every step. Their uncompromising quality standards have made this book an exceptional effort. Their encouragement from time to time has been an inspiration for everyone.

The publisher and the editorial board hope that this book will prove to be a valuable piece of knowledge for researchers, students, practitioners and scholars across the globe.

List of Contributors

Ayfer KARAASLAN
Faculty of Health Sciences, Department of Nursing, Necmettin Erbakan University, Konya, Turkey

Manar ASLAN
Faculty of Health Sciences, Department of Nursing, Trakya University, Edirne, Turkey

Emel GÜR
Department of Nursing, Health Science Faculty, Çankırı Karatekin University, Turkey

Dilek EKICI
Department of Nursing, Health Science Faculty, Gazi University, Turkey

Yuan LI
West China School of Nursing, Sichuan University, Chengdu City, Sichuan Province, China

Jinbo FANG
Nursing Department, West China Hospital, Sichuan University, Chengdu City, Sichuan Province, China

Chunfen ZHOU
Mental Health Center of West China Hospital, Sichuan University, Chengdu City, Sichuan Province, China

Suyoung KIM
Public Health Center, Uijeongbu-si, Gyeonggi-do, Republic of Korea

Sanghee KIM
College of Nursing, Keimyung University, Daegu, Republic of Korea

Porkodi ARJUNAN
Faculty of Nursing, Sri Ramachandra Institute of Higher Education & Research (DU), Chennai, India

Ramakrishnan Venkatakrishnan TRICHUR
Department of Emergency Medicine, Sri Ramachandra Institute of Higher Education & Research (DU), Chennai, India

Li-Yin CHANG
Department of Nursing, China Medical University Hospital and Adjunct Assistant Professor, Department of Nursing, China Medical University

Hsiu-Hui YU
Department of Nursing, Taichung Veterans General Hospital

Yann-Fen C. CHAO
College of Nursing, Hungkuang University

Yi-Chien CHIANG
Department of Nursing, Chang Gung University of Science and Technology and Associate Research Fellow, Department of Pediatrics, Chang Gung Memorial Hospital at Linkou

Hsiang-Chun LEE
Department of Nursing, Chang Gung University of Science and Technology

Tsung-Lan CHU
Administration Center of Quality Management Department, Chang Gung Medical Foundation and Assistant Professor, Department of Nursing, Chang Gung University of Science and Technology

Chin-Yen HAN
Department of Nursing, Chang Gung University of Science and Technology and Associate Research Fellow, Department of Nursing, Chang Gung Memorial Hospital at Linkou

Ya-Chu HSIAO
Department of Nursing, Chang Gung University of Science and Technology and Research Fellow, Department of Nursing, Chang Gung Memorial Hospital at Linkou

Juh Hyun SHIN
College of Nursing, Ewha Womans University, Republic of Korea

Qiuling XING
Department of Nursing, Tianjin Medical University Metabolic Diseases Hospital, Tianjin, China

Mingxia ZHANG
Department of Endocrinology, Peking University People's Hospital, Beijing, China

Fang ZHAO
Department of Nursing, China-Japan Friendship Hospital, Beijing, China

Yingxia ZHOU
Department of Endocrinology, Rui Jin Hospital Shanghai Jiao Tong University School of Medicine, Shanghai, China

Yongzhen MO
Department of Nursing, Jiangsu Province Official Hospital, Nanjing, China

Li YUAN
Department of Endocrinology and Metabolism, West China Hospital, Sichuan University, Chengdu, China

Ulfiye CELIKKALP
Department of Public Health, School of Medicine, Trakya University, Edirne, Turkey

Sebnem BILGIC
Faculty of Health Sciences, Department of Nursing, Trakya University, Edirne, Turkey

Munire TEMEL
Department of Nursing, Health School Collage, Namık Kemal University, Tekirdag, Turkey

Gamze VAROL
Faculty of Medicine, Department of Public Health, Namık Kemal University, Tekirdağ, Turkey

Nursalam NURSALAM
Faculty of Nursing, Universitas Airlangga, Surabaya, Indonesia

Ching-Min CHEN
Research Center for Humanities and Social Sciences, Department of Nursing, College of Medicine, National Cheng Kung University, Taiwan

Ferry EFENDI
Faculty of Nursing, Department of Community and Mental Health, Universitas Airlangga, Surabaya, Indonesia

Eka Misbahatul Mar'ah HAS
Faculty of Nursing, Department of Community and Mental Health, Universitas Airlangga, Surabaya, Indonesia

Laily HIDAYATI
Faculty of Nursing, Department of Basic, Medical-Surgical and Critical Care, Universitas Airlangga, Surabaya, Indonesia

Setho HADISUYATMANA
Faculty of Nursing, Department of Community and Mental Health, Universitas Airlangga, Surabaya, Indonesia

Özüm ERKİN
Faculty of Health Sciences, Department of Nursing, İzmir Democracy University, Turkey

Özcan AYGÜN
Fethiye Faculty of Health Sciences, Department of Nursing, Mugla Sitki Kocman University, Turkey

Shengxiao NIE, Chao SUN, Lei WANG and Xia WANG
Department of Nursing, Beijing Hospital, National Center of Gerontology; Institute of Geriatric Medicine, Chinese Academy of Medical Sciences, People's Republic of China

Ayten ŞENTÜRK ERENEL, Şengül YAMAN SÖZBİR, Mehtap UZUN AKSOY, Sıdıka PELİT AKSU and Canan UÇAKCI ASALIOĞLU
Faculty of Health Sciences, Nursing Department, Gazi University, Ankara, Turkey

Esra ARSLAN GÜRCÜOĞLU
Faculty of Health Sciences, Nursing Department, Çankırı Karatekin University, Çankırı, Turkey

Filiz ÜNAL TOPRAK
Faculty of Health Sciences, Nursing Department, Abant Izzet Baysal University, Bolu, Turkey

Hadi RANJBAR
Mental Health Research Center, Iran University of Medical Sciences, Tehran, Iran

Soodabeh JOOLAEE
Center for Nursing Care Research, School of Nursing & Midwifery, Iran University of Medical Sciences and Iranian Academy of Medical Sciences, Tehran, Iran

Abouali VEDADHIR
Faculty of Social Sciences, Department of Anthropology, University of Tehran, Tehran, Iran

Abbass ABBASSZADEH
School of Nursing & Midwifery, Shahid Beheshti University of Medical Sciences, Tehran, Iran

Colleen BERNSTEIN
Department of Psychology, School of Human and Community Development, University of the Witwatersrand, Johannesburg, South Africa

Arzu Kader Harmanci Seren
Florence Nightingale Faculty of Nursing, Department of Nursing Administration, Istanbul University, Istanbul,Turkey

Rujnan Tuna and Feride Eskin Bacaksiz
Faculty of Health Sciences, Department of Nursing, Istanbul Medeniyet University, Istanbul, Turkey

Chia-Yun FU
Department of Nursing, Fooyin University, Kaohsiung, Taiwan

Chia-Chan KAO
Department of Nursing, I-Shou University, Kaohsiung, Taiwan

Ruey-Hsia WANG
College of Nursing, Kaohsiung Medical University, Kaohsiung, Taiwan and Department of Medical Research, Kaohsiung Medical University Hospital, Kaohsiung, Taiwan

Neda JAMALIMOGHADAM
Department of Nursing, Community Based Psychiatric Care Research Center, School of Nursing and Midwifery, Shiraz University of Medical Sciences, Shiraz, Iran

Shahrzad YEKTATALAB
Department of Mental Health and Psychiatric Nursing, School of Nursing and Midwifery, Shiraz University of Medical Sciences, Shiraz, Iran

Marzieh MOMENNASAB
Department of Nursing, School of Nursing and Midwifery, Shiraz University of Medical Sciences, Shiraz, Iran

Abbas EBADI
Faculty of Nursing, Behavioral Sciences Research Center, Life Style Institute, Baqiyatallah University of Medical Sciences, Tehran, Iran

Najaf ZARE
Department of Biostatistics, Shiraz School of Public Health, Shiraz University of Medical Sciences, Shiraz, Iran

Hsun-Kuei Ko, Chi-Chun Chin and Min-Tao Hsu
College of Nursing, Kaohsiung Medical University

HeeKyung CHANG
College of Nursing, Gyeongsang National University, Gyeongnam, ROK

Chorong GIL
Institute of Health Sciences, Gyeongsang National University, Gyeongnam, ROK

Hyejin KIM
Department of Nursing Science, Kyungsung University, Busan, ROK

Hanju BEA
Department of Nursing, Keimyung College University, Daegu, ROK

Tian ZHANG, Hongye HE, Qunhui LIU, Yongxia SONG and Jingfang HONG
School of Nursing, Anhui Medical University,Hefei, China

Xiaoqing LV
The First Affiliated Hospital of Anhui Medical University, Hefei, China

Hsing-Mei CHEN
Department of Nursing, College of Medicine, National Cheng Kung University, Taiwan

Shan-Tair WANG
Ditmanson Medical Foundation Chiayi Christian Hospital, Chiayi City, Taiwan; Institute of Gerontology, College of Medicine, National Cheng Kung University, Taiwan

Shyh-Jong WU
Department of Medical Laboratory Science and Biotechnology, Kaohsiung Medical University, Taiwan

Chee-Siong LEE
Division of Cardiology, Kaohsiung Medical University Hospital, Kaohsiung Medical University, Taiwan

Susan J. FETZER
Department of Nursing, University of New Hampshire, USA

Liang-Miin TSAI
Department of Internal Medicine, Tainan Municipal Hospital, Taiwan

Hsiu-Li HUANG
Department of Long-Term Care, National Taipei University of Nursing and Health Sciences

Li-Chueh WENG
School of Nursing, College of Medicine, Chang Gung University and Associate Research Fellow, Department of General Surgery, Chang Gung Memorial Hospital

Wen-Yu HU
School of Nursing, National Taiwan University and Director, Department of Nursing, National Taiwan University Hospital

Yea-Ing Lotus SHYU
School of Nursing, College of Medicine, Chang Gung University and Research Fellow, Traumatological Division, Department of Orthopedics, Chang Gung Memorial Hospital and Department of Gerontological Care and Management, Chang Gung University of Science and Technology

Wen-Pin YU
Department of Nursing Management, Administration Center, Chang Gung Medical Foundation and Department of Nursing, Chang Gung University of Science and Technology

Kang-Hua CHEN
School of Nursing, College of Medicine, Chang Gung University and Department of Cardiovascular Surgery, Chang Gung Memorial Hospital

Dhuha Youssef WAZQAR
Oncology Nursing and Cancer Care, Faculty of Nursing, Department of Medical Surgical Nursing, King Abdulaziz University, Jeddah, Kingdom of Saudi Arabia

Ya-Hsiang CHAN
Department of Nursing, China Medical University Hospital, Taiwan

Hua-Shan WU
Department of Nursing, Asia University and Research Consultant, Department of Medical Research, China Medical University Hospital, China Medical University, Taiwan

Chih-Ching YEN
Department of Respiratory Care, China Medical University and Attending Physician, Department of Medicine, China Medical University Hospital, Taiwan

Margaret L. CAMPBELL
College of Nursing, Wayne State University, Michigan, USA

Nidal F. ESHAH
Faculty of Nursing, Zarqa University, Jordan

Index

P

Q

R

S

T

W

www.ingramcontent.com/pod-product-compliance
Lightning Source LLC
LaVergne TN
LVHW081019210926
848485LV00004B/903